Transitions in Nursing
Preparing for Professional Practice
Third Edition

Transitions in Nursing
Preparing for Professional Practice
Third Edition

Edited by

Professor Esther Chang RN, CM, BAppSc(AdvNsg), DNE, MEdAdmin, PhD

Director of Research
School of Nursing and Midwifery
University of Western Sydney, NSW
Australia

Professor John Daly RN, BA, BHSc, MEd(Hons), GradCertEdMgmt, PhD, FRCNA

Dean and Professor of Nursing
Faculty of Nursing, Midwifery and Health
Head, WHO Collaborating Centre for Nursing
Midwifery and Health Development
University of Technology, Sydney, NSW
Australia

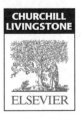

CHURCHILL LIVINGSTONE

ELSEVIER

Sydney   Edinburgh   London   New York   Philadelphia   St Louis   Toronto

Churchill Livingstone
is an imprint of Elsevier

Elsevier Australia. ACN 001 002 357
(a division of Reed International Books Australia Pty Ltd)
Tower 1, 475 Victoria Avenue, Chatswood, NSW 2067

ELSEVIER

National Library of Australia Cataloguing-in-Publication Data

---

Chang, Esther May Lan.

Transitions in nursing : preparing for professional practice / Esther Chang, John Daly.

3rd ed.

9780729540827 (pbk.)

Nursing.
Nursing—Practice.

Daly, John.

610.73

Publisher: Libby Houston
Developmental Editor: Elizabeth Coady
Publishing Services Manager: Helena Klijn
Project Coordinators: Lisa Shillan and Priya Dauntess
Cover design by Stella Vassiliou
Internal design by Trina McDonald
Edited by Liz Williams
Proofread by Stephanie Pickering
Index by Chris Boot
Typeset by Toppan Best-set Premedia Limited
Printed by China Translation and Printing Services

CONTENTS

SECTION 3: ORGANISATIONAL ENVIRONMENTS

PREFACE

Welcome to the third edition of *Transitions in Nursing: Preparing for professional practice.* As with the first and second editions, this book has been developed to assist undergraduate students, new registered nurses and other professionals interested in issues and challenges associated with the transition from higher education to practice. For the majority of new graduates this rite of passage is associated with a degree of stress, strain and culture shock. These are issues that have existed in nursing, internationally, for decades. The literature shows that this transition is a multidimensional and complex process. Intensive socialisation brings to the surface many challenges and opportunities for new registered nurses as they assimilate into their professional work roles. Research has shed much light on the issues associated with transition and has uncovered knowledge and strategies that can be useful in managing the process.

The book has been designed to provide comprehensive information on key issues associated with transition. Readers will find viewpoints that are challenging and sometimes disconcerting, but at the same time motivating and thought-provoking. The third edition is divided into three sections. Section 1 examines issues from student to graduate nurse. Section 2 looks at skills for dealing with the world of work. Section 3 discusses the organisational environment. This edition also includes two new chapters in the area of clinical leadership and continuing competence for practice.

Understanding the context in which we work is crucial to effective functioning in the workplace. Knowing how to provide care for patients and their families in the health system is not sufficient: we need to learn how to care for ourselves in order to care for our patients effectively. The exercises and learning activities that appear throughout the book offer readers a range of helpful suggestions in understanding the nursing context, managing stress and caring for themselves. In addition, each chapter includes recommended readings, case studies and reflective questions for further exploration.

Our intention was to involve clinicians and academics in producing a resource which is scholarly, accessible, reality-based and practical. More importantly, it is a resource for every student, practising nurse, educator and administrator in understanding the issues of transition for new registered nurses. By reading the book, reflecting on the issues and posing possible answers, readers should be able to gain a comprehensive view of the issues, challenges and opportunities ahead of them. The journey during this period can be rewarding with implications of a long-term career for new nurses, particularly when educators, administrators and clinicians collaboratively anticipate and manage the socialisation process.

We extend our sincere appreciation to the contributors to the work for their shared interest and concern with the issues and challenges of transition from student to registered nurse. This book would not be possible without them. We are thankful to Cheryl Murray for assistance in the initial stages of the manuscript, and to Debbie Taylor Robson at the University of Western Sydney. We would like to extend our special appreciation to Elizabeth Coady and the rest of the team at Elsevier for their encouragement and support. Elsevier Australia joins us in thanking the reviewers for their feedback on the manuscript. We would also like to thank our partners and families for their support. Finally we wish to dedicate this text to our past, present and future students.

Esther Chang and John Daly

CONTRIBUTORS

Christine Ashley RN, RM, FRCNA
Christine Ashley Consulting, NSW, Australia

Alan Barnard RN, BA, MA, PhD
Senior Lecturer, School of Nursing, Member, Institute of Health and Biomedical Innovation, Queensland University of Technology, Research Fellow, Redcliffe Hospital, QLD, Australia

Angela Brown BSc(Hons), MA
Head, School of Nursing, Midwifery and Indigenous Health, University of Wollongong, NSW, Australia

Esther Chang RN, CM, BAppSc(AdvNsg), DNE, MEdAdmin, PhD
Professor of Nursing and Director of Research, School of Nursing and Midwifery, University of Western Sydney, NSW, Australia

Jennifer Clauson RN, BN
New Graduate Nursing Program, Campbelltown and Camden Hospitals, NSW, Australia

Jane Conway RN, BNurs(Hons), Grad Cert HRM, DEd
Conjoint Associate Professor, School of Nursing and Midwifery, University of Newcastle, NSW, Australia

Elizabeth Crock PhD, RN, Cert in Infectious Diseases Nursing, BSc, Grad Dip Ed
Clinical Nurse Consultant HIV/AIDS, Royal District Nursing Service, VIC, Australia

Patrick Crookes PhD, BSc(Nurs), RN, RNT, CertEd
Dean, Faculty of Health and Behavioural Sciences, University of Wollongong, NSW, Australia

John Daly RN, BA, BHSc, MEd(Hons), GradCertEdMgmt, PhD, FRCNA
Dean and Professor of Nursing, Faculty of Nursing, Midwifery and Health, Head, WHO Collaborating Centre for Nursing, Midwifery and Health Development, University of Technology, Sydney, NSW, Australia

Patricia M Davidson RN, BA, Med, PhD
Professor and Director, Centre for Cardiovascular and Chronic Care, University of Technology, Sydney, NSW, Australia

Gary Day DHSM, MHM, BNurs, DipAppSc(Nursing Mgt), RN, RM, FCHSM
Director, Workforce Development and Learning, SA Health, Adjunct Associate Professor, the University of Adelaide, Adjunct Associate Professor, Griffith University, SA, Australia

Denise Dignam RN, DipSocSci(Dist), BA, PhD, MAICD
Professor, Faculty of Nursing, Midwifery and Health, University of Technology, Sydney, NSW, Australia

Kathleen Dixon PhD, MHA, BA, RN, RCNA
Associate Head of School, Senior Lecturer, School of Nursing and Midwifery, Hawkesbury Campus, University of Western Sydney, NSW, Australia

Christine Duffield RN, PhD
Professor of Nursing and Health Services Management, Associate Dean (Research), Director, Centre for Health Services Management and, Deputy Director, WHO Collaborating Centre for Nursing, Midwifery and Health Development, Faculty of Nursing, Midwifery and Health, University of Technology, Sydney, NSW, Australia

Maxine Duke PhD, Med, BApp(Sci), RN, FRCNA
Chair in Nursing Development, Head, School of Nursing and Midwifery, Deakin University, Melbourne, VIC, Australia

Bronwyn Everett RN, BAppSc(Nurs), MSc(Hons), PhD
Senior Lecturer, Faculty of Nursing Midwifery and Health, University of Technology, Sydney, NSW, Australia

Mary FitzGerald RN, DN, CertEd, MN, PhD, FRCNA
Professor of Nursing, School of Nursing and Midwifery, University of Tasmania and Southern Tasmanian Area Health Service, TAS, Australia

Helen Forbes RN, PhD, MedSt, BAppSc AdvNsgEd
Director of Teaching and Learning, School of Nursing and Midwifery, Faculty of Health, Deakin University, Melbourne, VIC, Australia

Kim Foster RN, DipAppSc, BN, MA, PhD, MRCNA, FACMHN
Associate Professor Mental Health Nursing, Sydney Nursing School, University of Sydney, NSW, Australia

Rhonda Griffiths AM, RN, RM, BEd(Nurs), MSc(Hons), DrPH, FRCNA
Dean of Nursing and Midwifery, University of Western Sydney, NSW, Australia

Deborah Hatcher RN, DipT(Phys Ed), BHSc(N), MHPEd, PhD
Senior Lecturer, Deputy Director of Undergraduate Studies, School of Nursing and Midwifery, University of Western Sydney, NSW, Australia

Debra Jackson RN, PhD
Professor of Nursing, Faculty of Nursing, Midwifery and Health, University of Technology, Sydney, NSW, Australia

Amanda Johnson PhD, MstHScEd, DipT(Ng), RN
Senior Lecturer (Aged Care Focus) and Director of Undergraduate Studies, School of Nursing and Midwifery, University of Western Sydney, NSW, Australia

Megan-Jane Johnstone RN, PhD, FRCNA, FCN
Chair in Nursing, Associate Head of School (Research), School of Nursing and Midwifery, Director, Centre for Quality and Patient Safety Research, Deakin University, Melbourne, VIC, Australia

Judy Lumby AM, RN, PhD, MHPEd, BA, Dip NurseEd
Director Joanna Briggs Foundation, Adjunct Professor The University of Adelaide, SA, Emeritus Professor UTS, Adjunct Professor The University of Sydney, Adjunct Professor UWS, NSW, Australia

Judy Mannix RN, BEd(Nsg), MN(Hons)
Senior Lecturer and Director of Postgraduate Studies, School of Nursing and Midwifery, University of Western Sydney, NSW, Australia

Margaret McMillan RN, PhD, OAM
Conjoint Professor, Faculty of Health, University of Newcastle, NSW, Australia

Kathleen Milton-Wildey RN, BA, DipEd, MA, PhD, FCN
Senior Lecturer, Faculty of Nursing, Midwifery and Health, University of Technology, Sydney, NSW, Australia

Annette Moore
Nurse Transition to Practice Coordinator, Practice Development Unit, Royal Hobart Hospital, TAS, Australia

Paul Morrison RMN, RGN, BA, PhD, PGCE, GradDip Counselling
Professor of Nursing and Health Studies, Dean, School of Nursing and Midwifery, Murdoch University, WA, Australia

Alison Natera RN, BN, Grad Cert Critical Care, Grad Dip in Teaching and Learning
Nurse Transition to Practice Coordinator, Royal Hobart Hospital, TAS, Australia

Stephen Neville RN, PhD, FCNA
Senior Lecturer, School of Health and Social Services, Massey University, New Zealand

Elaine Papps RN, BA, Med, PhD
Health and Research Consultant, Hawke's Bay, New Zealand

Claire Rickard RN, PhD, FRCNA
Professor, NHMRC Centre of Research Excellence in Nursing Interventions for Hospital Patients, Griffith University, QLD, Australia

Suzanne Rochester RN, RM, MA(Psych), MN(Hons)
Director Undergraduate Nursing Studies, Faculty of Nursing Midwifery and Health, University of Technology, Sydney, NSW, Australia

Jane Stein-Parbury RN, BSN, Med, PhD, FRCNA
Professor of Mental Health Nursing, University of Technology, Sydney, NSW, Australia

Lee Stewart DipT(Nsg), BHlthSc(Nsg), PGCertEd, MDisputeResolution, PhD, RN, RM
Head of School, School of Nursing, Midwifery and Nutrition, James Cook University, QLD, Australia

Lyn Stewart RN, RM, BHScN, Med, Cert1V (Teaching Conversational English)
Lecturer, School of Nursing and Midwifery, University of Western Sydney, NSW, Australia

Debra Thoms RN, RM, BA, MNA, Grad Cert Bioethics, Adv Dip Arts, FRCNA, FCN, FACHSM(Hon)
Chief Nursing and Midwifery Officer, Ministry of Health, NSW, Australia, Adjunct Professor, University of Technology, Sydney, NSW, Australia

Kim Usher RN, BA, DipNEd, DipHSc, MNSt, PhD, FACMHN, FRCNA
Professor of Nursing and Associate Dean for Graduate Research Studies, James Cook University, QLD, Australia

Rachael Vernon RN, BN, MPhil(Dist), MCNA(NZ)
Head of School Nursing, Eastern Institute of Technology, New Zealand

Carol Walker BHSC(Nsg), GradDip Health Service Management

Kenneth Walsh RPN, RGN, BNurs, PhD
Professor of Nursing Practice Development, School of Nursing, Midwifery and Indigenous Health, University of Wollongong, Director, Nursing Development and Research Unit, Illawarra Shoalhaven Local Health District, NSW Health, Wollongong, NSW, Fellow of the Joanna Briggs Institute, SA, Australia, Visiting Professor in the Department of Nursing and Applied Clinical Studies, Canterbury Christchurch University, Kent, England

Jill White AM, MEd, PhD
Chair, Australian Nursing and Midwifery Accreditation Council, Dean and Professor of Nursing, Sydney Nursing School, University of Sydney, NSW, Australia

Denise Wilson PhD, MA(Hons), BA, RN, FCNA(NZ)
Associate Professor Māori Health, AUT University, Auckland, New Zealand

REVIEWERS

Roy Brown RN, DPSN, PGCE(Adult), BA, DMS, MA
Senior Lecturer and Director-Bachelor of Nursing Programmes, School of Nursing, Midwifery and Indigenous Health, University of Wollongong, NSW, Australia

Karen Clark-Burg MBA(Executive), GBQ, BN, MRCNA, RN
Assistant Dean, Undergraduate Course Coordinator, School of Nursing and Midwifery, Fremantle Campus, University of Notre Dame, Australia

Leonie Cox RN, BA(Hons1), PhD, GCE-HE
Senior Lecturer, QUT School of Nursing and Midwifery, Queensland University of Technology, Brisbane, Australia

Sue Dean RN, BA, MA, Grad Dip Adult Ed, Grad Dip App Sc(Nurs), GCDEM
Lecturer, Faculty of Nursing, Midwifery and Health, University of Technology, Sydney, NSW, Australia

Elizabeth Denmead RN, ICURN, BSc, MHPEd
Educational Consultant, NSW, Australia

Helen Donovan RN, RMid, MEd, FRCNA
Lecturer, School of Nursing and Midwifery, Queensland University of Technology, Brisbane, Australia

Lyn Francis BN, MHM, LLB, LLM, Grad Cert TT
Academic, Acting BN Program Convenor, Faculty of Health, School of Nursing and Midwifery, University of Newcastle, Callaghan, NSW, Australia

Beryl McEwan MN, MRCNA
Lecturer in Nursing, School of Health, Charles Darwin University, NT, Australia

Marilyn Richardson-Tench PhD, MEdStud, BAppSc(AdvNsg), RN, RCNT
Senior Lecturer, School of Nursing and Midwifery, Victoria University, Melbourne, VIC, Australia

David Stanley NursD, MSc(HS), BA Ng, Dip HE(Nurs), Gerontic CERT, RN, RM, TF, MRCNA, ANTZ
Associate Professor in Nursing, University of Western Australia, School of Population Health, WA, Australia

Antonia van Loon RN, MN(Research), PhD
Senior Research Fellow, Silverchain RDNS SA Group, SA, Australia

CHAPTER 1

Managing the transition from student to graduate nurse

Esther Chang and John Daly

LEARNING OBJECTIVES

When you have completed this chapter you will be able to:

- describe the process of transition from student to graduate nurse
- appreciate a range of factors and issues that influence the transition from student to graduate nurse
- consider strategies to ease the tension associated with adjustment to the realities of nursing practice for new registered nurses
- recognise the importance of a positive, proactive approach to managing transition on an individual level
- identify and access resources which have been shown to facilitate adjustment to nursing practice for new registered nurses.

Keywords: transition, education, role stress, strategies, students, new graduate nurse

---

INTRODUCTION

Nursing attracts people from many walks of life, motivated largely by a concern and a desire to understand and help people who are confronted by a range of actual or potential health problems and challenges. Many of these experiences cause major disruption in people's lives – for example, illness, suffering, loss, grief and trauma. According to Englert,[1] 'such experiences are both the privilege and burden of nurses and of others who share the drama, the humour and the tragedy of other people's lives' (p 1). Englert, a leader in administration of nursing services, encouraged members of the nursing profession to 'reflect for a moment … to recall some of those high and low points of the beginning years as a registered nurse' (p 1). She went on:

> I believe that the situation of our nursing students and new graduates today is not so very different. Their motivations in entering nursing are much the same as were ours. They too share an idealism based on the desire to help their fellow human beings, an apprehension that they will be found wanting when the crisis occurs, a certain awkwardness in accepting advice, however kindly given, and an admiration for those whom they see as epitomising the best of nursing.[1]

The nursing profession in Australia and elsewhere continues to be concerned with the process of transition for graduates of undergraduate nursing courses on entry to the world of clinical practice.[2-6] This concern exists for several reasons. It has remained an issue of concern in nurse education in Australia because of ongoing changes in the clinical practice environment; research data which continue to show that it is a period which can be stressful[5]; and related questions about adequate preparation of new graduate nurses.

One key issue here is the relevance and quality of clinical education in undergraduate courses. Indeed, in recent times, access to an adequate number of quality clinical placements has become a serious challenge to educators in nursing, medicine and allied health. This has fostered a number of innovations, including the development of more sophisticated clinical simulation teaching and learning environments.[7] The impact of such innovations on clinical competence of graduates in the health professions will require ongoing research and evaluation.

These challenges are international, particularly in developed countries which are struggling with health sector reforms, cost containment challenges, the growing burden of chronic disease, ageing populations and human resources for health issues. In the USA, a provocative and scholarly report for the Carnegie Foundation for the Advancement of Teaching called recently for a reinvention of preregistration nursing education.[8] The authors' argument is based on a number of factors, one dimension being the relevance of current models of undergraduate nursing education in the present-day context of health system re-engineering. The Council of Australian Governments recently established Health Workforce Australia which has a role to play in creating solutions to clinical education challenges (www.hwa.gov.au). It has a concern with 'improving and expanding access to quality clinical training for health professionals in training across the public and private and non-government sectors. This will be achieved through funding programs which expand capacity, improve quality, reform delivery systems and offer diversity in learning opportunities' (p 2).[9]

In addition, recruitment and retention of new graduates are issues from time to time, both nationally and internationally. Demand for, and supply of, registered nurses is cyclical, and occasionally healthcare systems are confronted by a shortage of nurses. Such shortages can reach crisis proportions, a phenomenon that we are currently witnessing in Australia and overseas. In Australia and New Zealand supply will continue to be a problem because of our ageing workforce and ongoing undersupply of graduates in many areas.[10] It is important to note that this supply and demand imbalance is an international problem.

Other reasons for this concern with the experience of transition include changing attitudes in society towards nursing as a career, a decline in the number of people choosing to enter undergraduate nursing courses and the need to create sustainable nursing. It also appears that healthcare system reform has created an environment that has a negative impact on the quality of worklife for nurses and other health professionals, and on the quality of patient care. Nursing leaders are currently investigating these issues and searching for strategies to enhance the quality of undergraduate clinical education, the image of nursing as a career, transition for new graduates, quality of worklife and the recruitment and retention of qualified staff in the nursing workforce.

There is a large amount of literature on the process of transition from senior student to graduate nurse. It is clear from this literature that transition is multifaceted and complex, and that problems often described and discussed in relation to the process are not new.[11,12] In Australia nursing education has undergone rapid transformation since the late 1980s. The system of basic nurse education (BNE) is now university-based with 3-year degree programs leading to eligibility to register as a nurse. In addition, the national healthcare system has undergone radical change in the last decade in particular. Much of this system change has been driven by the shift to an economic model for designing and managing health services. This has led to changes in the nursing practice environment that have implications for new graduates entering employment.

To date, the Australian government has commissioned two national reviews[3,13] of undergraduate nurse education since the national shift of BNE from hospital schools of nursing to the higher-education sector. The second review (the Heath report) was published in 2002.[2] Two major matters of concern uncovered by the first national review committee were 'the adequacy of clinical education provided during pre-registration nursing courses and the best means of facilitating the transition from higher education to work' (p 4).[13] The first national review of BNE made a number of recommendations designed to enhance the quality of educational endeavours in both these areas and outcomes for course graduates and nursing services providers. These concerns remain and were also considered by the second national review[2] and the Australian Senate inquiry into nursing.[3] The National Nursing and Nursing Education Taskforce, which was established to implement the recommendations of the Heath report,[2] and which concluded its work in 2006, also considered the issue of transition.[4] In the Heath report,[2] transition was addressed through recommendation 14, standards for transition programs. It was recommended that:

> to ensure consistency and quality in the development and delivery of transition programs a national framework be developed for transition to provide guidelines and standards for institutions. State and territory nursing registration boards should accredit transition programs; employing institutions should be responsible for meeting the standards (p 22).[2]

Preregistration nursing courses today need to prepare graduates for a work environment that has undergone enormous change in the last decade. The practice environment is constantly changing and this has implications for the type of knowledge and skills that new graduates will require. University schools of nursing are constantly challenged to ensure that their courses are designed to give graduates the best possible preparation for entry to nursing practice as new registered nurses, and to optimise their ability to move through the transition process confidently and successfully. Experience has shown that this is best done in cooperation with nursing service leaders and providers. Preparation of new graduates in nursing is best viewed as a shared responsibility between the universities and nursing service sectors.[14]

University schools of nursing aim to prepare flexible, critical thinkers for the practice of professional nursing. They emphasise individual client- or patient-centred holistic care and lifelong learning as key values. All preregistration nursing courses are required to provide a clinical education component to ensure that course graduates meet the clinical competency expectations of beginning registered nurses. In many surveys, however, new graduates report that the clinical practice and clinical education components of their undergraduate course were too short and that the course was too theoretical.[12] Nursing service providers often report that new graduates 'are inadequately prepared for clinical practice in that they are deficient in certain skills' (p 17).[14] This reflects a clear mismatch in expectations of new graduate nurses between the education and service sectors.

Preregistration nursing courses do not aim to produce expert practitioners on graduation. Research has demonstrated that development of clinical expertise requires some years of constant immersion in clinical experience following entry to nursing practice as a registered nurse.[15] It would be ideal if newly registered nurses could meet all expectations required by the healthcare settings immediately following entry to the workforce. Experience has shown that few individuals are able to perform at this level, and for the majority of new graduates this is an unrealistic and difficult expectation.

Nursing has a long history of anti-intellectualism,[16] and at one time it was believed that nurses who are too academic tend to be hamstrung when it comes to clinical practice. Paradoxically, many authorities argue that contemporary nursing requires intelligent, flexible, critical thinkers and problem solvers who are able to demonstrate the ability to deliver safe, competent care in a range of environments. Many of the environments in which nurses work are highly complex and demand higher-order cognitive skills. The ability to 'do' is prized in clinical nursing – this is understandable to a large degree but there has to be acceptance of some middle ground in debates about these issues. Nursing requires adequate theoretical preparation and competence in clinical practice. Conway and McMillan[17] argue that the transition from student to graduate and practitioner requires the development of the ability to examine critically our own and others' practice and be accountable for our own actions. These abilities are often linked to the idea of being a lifelong learner and are seen as increasingly important to professional nursing practice in the 21st century.

It is important, therefore, that new graduates are provided with support, tolerance, patience and encouragement as they learn to assimilate values, beliefs and practices acquired in their undergraduate education with the practice values and beliefs that are dominant in the clinical work world. It is no surprise that in this context the transition process presents many challenges and potential rewards for the new graduate in nursing. The first 3–6 months as a new registered nurse have been identified as potentially the most challenging and stressful period in professional adjustment.[5,11,14,18–21] This period is 'crucial in determining new graduates' commitment to nursing as well as their acquisition of technical, clinical and patient management skills' (p 20).[14] Perhaps the key to successful negotiation of this phase is anticipation and psychological preparation. This requires you to be adequately informed of what is known about the process and what you can do to ease your transition into practice as a new registered nurse. In addition, nurses in service need to place greater emphasis on the clinical area as a place where learning is ongoing[22] and a lifelong process.

A survey of the table of contents in this book will show that component chapters are concerned with preparation for entry into the nursing workforce and the development of a successful, sustainable and rewarding career in nursing. Chapter topics can be classified according to a number of themes: managing self in clinical practice; caring for self; understanding the forces that shape the practice environment; learning to manage different approaches to nursing care delivery; collaborating and working with colleagues and patients/clients; and professional development strategies.

TRANSITION: A PROCESS

The transition from student to graduate nurse is characterised by a period of intense socialisation into the culture of the clinical work world. Socialisation, in this context, may be defined as 'a reciprocal process by which the neophyte nurses learn what others will demand of them in a specific role and, in turn, learn to exert control over their new environments' (p 1).[23] Myers and Arbor describe this process as one of 'give and take', a process through which new registered nurses 'learn to behave as nurses in the hospital setting'. It is through this process that the new nurse learns to behave 'according to the culturally prescribed rules and standards' of the clinical work world (pp 120–1).[23] Corwin[24] believes there is a 'turning point' between graduating from a nursing school and induction into employment for students. This turning point in a career produces role conflict between professional (idealised) role conceptions and bureaucratic (actualised) role conceptions in the working environment. Consequently, a sense of conflicting loyalties towards bureaucratic and professional systems of work organisation emerges.

The gap between what students are taught to expect and what is actually experienced in the early stages of work has been termed 'reality shock'.[25] Marlene Kramer, a nurse researcher, first recognised the problem in 1966. The difference between professional and bureaucratic role conceptions is a source of conflict for the nurse.[21,25,26] The strong dissimilarity in the expectations of these two systems often gives rise to nursing role conflicts.

Most studies of transition for new registered nurses have shown that there are challenges and difficulties associated with the process.[11,12,14,23,24,26,27–35] Common reactions to initial employment as a registered nurse include:

physical and emotional exhaustion; a sense of inadequacy; frustration; loss of ideals and, at the extreme, the abandonment of nursing as a career. In other cases, where they [new graduates] have received support and encouragement and advice from more experienced nurses and from their own peers and families, initiation into the world of nursing is reported to be less stressful (p 3).[12]

Common problems that surface during transition include the theory–practice gap[36] (where theory learnt in the classroom does not match the theory said to be required in clinical practice),[12] limited proficiency in managing and executing technical procedures, time management, drug administration, patient assessment and report-writing skills.[1] Other issues include:

- managing nursing care responsibilities for a number of patients simultaneously
- working in teams
- coping with a beginning level of skill as a new registered nurse relative to job demands and workload
- the acceptance of accountability
- independently taking action and making decisions
- coping with unexpected events
- supervising other nurses
- shift work
- learning how to collaborate with other nurses and health professionals, including liaison and discussion about the total care of patients
- developing competence in planning and organising.[11,27,31,37–42]

In some research studies, heavy patient loads were found to create excessive tiredness in many new graduate nurses because they were often allocated high-dependency patient loads. This was further affected by low staffing ratios, which resulted in additional stress for the graduates as they attempted to adjust to their new culture (p 56).[30] A common issue for new graduates in many studies was having inadequate staff and time to complete all client care.[11,31,37,38] What also appears to be operating for many new registered nurses is the fact that they are having to adjust not only to the registered nurse's role, but also to the health service organisation. Because of the pressures in hospitals, many new nurses felt they lacked a receptive climate in which to enact many of the aspects of what they perceived should comprise a professional nurse's role, such as having autonomy and more responsibility to assess and plan care. This need to care for others well has been found to be related to personal satisfaction, as has appreciation for one's efforts.[43]

Role ambiguity and role overload

Role ambiguity and role overload have also been identified as sources of stress during role transition and have been linked to organisational dynamics and subsequent job dissatisfaction and turnover. Many research studies, as far back as the 1970s, show a relationship between role ambiguity and voluntary turnover.[44–46] According to some authors, role ambiguity was more influential in an individual leaving the organisation than role conflict. In general, role ambiguity is defined as the lack of clear, consistent information about the behaviour expected in a role (p 23).[47]

There are two types of role ambiguity in relation to the uncertainty felt by the individual: the first type is known as objective ambiguity, which arises from lack of the information needed for role definition and role performance; the second type is subjective ambiguity, which is related to the social–psychological aspects of role performance. This occurs where individuals are concerned about how others perceive them in relation to attainment of their personal goals.[47] Studies with registered nurses have shown, in all relationships, that role conflict or role ambiguity was a basis of negative influence, causing decreased job satisfaction.[11,44,48,49]

Role ambiguity is often increased by the fact that each ward is a specialty unit in an organisation, and has different personnel and unique patient management. New graduates not only have to adjust to the nursing role, but also adapt to the transition within complicated social networks. Role ambiguity can be further compounded by role overload, when graduates lack skills in handling role demands, establishing priorities and allocating time wisely.[11,50,51]

Chang[11] conducted two longitudinal surveys on role stress. The first survey showed that role overload and ambiguity were negatively related to job satisfaction in the first few months of employment. However, in the second survey role overload was not significantly related to job satisfaction. In spite of the overload prevalent in the role of registered nurses, many of the graduates did not relate this to job satisfaction after 11–12 months of employment. It appears to be easier for graduates to deal with role overload after 1 year of employment. This may be a reflection of the graduates' coping abilities and experience gained in their role that can ultimately make a difference in dealing with problems in the work environment (p 140).[52]

Factors affecting role transition

According to a major Australian study undertaken by Madjar and colleagues in 1997[12]:

how well and how quickly newly graduated nurses are able to demonstrate mastery of their new role, acting in a safe, competent, sensitive, and confident manner, depends on a range of factors. In broad terms these may include:

- personal qualities of each beginning registered nurse, including age, maturity, previous work experiences, motivation, aspirations, and availability of personal supports;
- the quality and extent of the educational preparation, including the nature and duration of structured clinical experiences during the pre-registration course, and the quality and rigour of formative and summative assessments within the course;
- the quality and duration of orientation/transition programs for new graduates provided by employing institutions;
- the expectations, attitudes, reactions, and behaviour of more experienced clinical nurses, nurse managers and other staff toward new graduates, the role modelling of expected behaviour by more senior nurses, and the prevailing ethos of the institution;
- the exigencies of clinical situations, staffing levels, and other demands placed on the registered nurse (p 3).[12]

The complexity of the process of transition is illustrated by the many factors that can influence individual experience. For most new graduates this is a time of stress and strain, learning and assimilation. It is also a time of upheaval and adjustment affecting all aspects of life (p 79).[12] During this time decisions are made about a long-term commitment to nursing. It is reassuring to note, however, that the majority of participants in the study reported that the transition process was worthwhile and culminated in 'a sense of satisfaction and personal achievement' (p 79).[12]

NEW GRADUATES: SKILLS AND STRENGTHS

Against this background of challenges and difficulties it is important to acknowledge the skills and strengths that new graduates have on entry to the workforce.[11,53] In a major longitudinal study of new graduates by Chang[11] conducted in New South Wales, Australia, both nursing unit managers and graduates believed that the graduates were well prepared in three main areas: (1) communication skills with patients; (2) psychosocial assessment skills; and (3) accountability for their actions.

These areas of strength were consistent with the findings of several other researchers who found that graduates excelled in identifying patients' psychological needs and in communicating with them. Even though more was thought to be needed in the development of technical and clinical skills, both graduates and their managers considered the overall performance to be adequate and felt that their education had been quite adequate in preparing them for the job. Over time, graduates felt more confident and demonstrated significant improvement in performance. This may well have been expected, but strong significant improvement was observed across all areas of their role. In addition, nursing unit managers rated the overall performance of the graduates more positively compared with hospital-trained nurses. The graduates had mostly positive feelings about their tertiary program, and perceived that it had provided them with a theoretical background to care for the multidimensional needs of their patients – not only physical needs but economic, spiritual and psychosocial needs as well.[11,30,53,54]

Other research studies[31,38] show that, over a period of time, graduates were working more autonomously, establishing relationships with their clients and coping with their new role. They saw the importance of their professional role, including being a health teacher, a provider of care, a communicator, an advocate, a coordinator of care, a decision maker and making suggestions for change in practice. These values are consistent with findings from studies in Australia and overseas which have examined the professional or value systems of graduates.[11,30,55,56] There is also evidence of greater skill acquisition in relation to assessing clients more quickly and in giving advice to other staff (p 41).[31] Skill acquisition was an important issue for many graduates as they progressed from novice to advanced beginner.[15]

STRATEGIES TO FACILITATE TRANSITION

Several strategies have been shown to be of use in easing the transition from student to new registered nurse. Cooperation between service and education plays a key role in the success or otherwise of many of these strategies. Many experts in nursing believe that:

> the key to bringing respective expectations [i.e. those of providers of BNE and clinical nursing services] into line with each other … [is] the establishment of a more cooperative framework in which higher education and health agencies both contribute to improvements in clinical practice and in the graduate's transition to work (p 5).[13]

In relation to specific strategies, a positive preceptor relationship, adequate support systems and assignment congruence have been shown to have positive outcomes in the first 6 months of employment as a new registered nurse.[57] Preceptorship programs are one practical strategy offered to reduce culture shock and to assist new registered nurses in the integration of theory and practice. There is extensive literature on pre-ceptorship programs.[29,58–62] One version of this strategy is called the professional nurturance preceptorship program, which can be jointly sponsored by healthcare and tertiary institutions. Reports of graduate nurse preceptorship programs have demon-strated that these programs are an effective means of facilitating the transition process for new graduates, including clinical learning. Such programs could also be incorpo-rated as a subject in the final year of undergraduate nursing courses. During the preceptorship experience, the student is guided by the registered nurse preceptor in caring for appropriate patients. Initially, preceptor and student work closely together; as students develop greater confidence and competence, they are given more auton-omy in patient care. A similar approach can be used with the experienced nurse preceptor and the new registered nurse.

Many important variables make the work environment either positive or negative for graduates. The key factors that appear to facilitate successful transition include a supportive environment which accommodates incremental development in clinical skill acquisition and patient management skills.[14] A graduate nurse who is assigned too many patients within a short timeframe may not be proficient enough to provide for patients' physical and psychosocial care. It is crucial that the workload is structured to provide opportunities for newly registered nurses to see the effective outcomes of their work.

In the practice environments that accept new graduates in nursing there needs to be ready recognition of, and support for, the fact that learning, especially clinical learning, is a lifelong process. Another positive influence on transition is preparedness and commitment by experienced registered nurses to value and nurture new registered nurses as they move through the transition process. The first national review of nurse education carried out in Australia (in 1994) made specific recommendations about transition support for beginning graduates of nursing. Relevant recommendations include that:

> graduates be provided with employer-funded assistance for transition to employ-ment, including appropriate induction and orientation activities, peer support and mentoring as appropriate, and introduction to specific clinical requirements … [and] … where relevant infrastructure is not available (for example in rural and remote areas), funds be made available to provide appropriate levels of support (p 21).[13]

Some employers appear to be high performers in the way they manage new graduates entering employment. Consequently, a number of hospitals and community settings appear to function as 'magnets' for new registered nurses on the basis of the reputa-tion they have built up for supporting and developing new graduate nurses. Other research has found that the attitudes of staff and a welcoming and positive environ-ment also encourage graduates to adjust to the workplace.[63,64]

Knowing how to provide patient care is not enough for new graduates, although this, in itself, is a complex process requiring appropriate exposure and clinical learn-ing. It is important that nurses are able to manage job stressors successfully. Health professionals, including nurses, need to learn how to care for themselves in order to care effectively for their patients. This requires a balanced approach to all facets of life and stress management skills.[2]

It is important to raise issues of concern during transition with appropriate colleagues and support systems. Discussion of these issues will lead to the identification of appropriate ways of managing problems early. This approach can be invaluable in reducing anxiety and stress, and facilitating successful adjustment to nursing practice.

Quality of worklife is a concept that is gaining currency, and health service providers need to address it to ensure adequate recruitment and retention of nursing staff. Sources of dissatisfaction in clinical nursing have been found to include inadequate staffing patterns, conflict with other healthcare providers, lack of support in dealing with death and dying, unresponsiveness in leadership, poor communication among staff and poor administration.[65,66] There is a clear need for leaders in nursing education to work with leaders in nursing service to develop short- and long-term strategies to promote and ensure sustainable nursing. This will require attention to a number of factors and processes that influence commitment to nursing; for example, socialisation programs affect the general satisfaction of staff and their feelings of autonomy and personal influence.

Other factors known to facilitate transition include:

- formal unit orientation programs that incorporate realistic goals[13,64]
- a unit climate of open communication and timely provision of constructive feedback on performance[64,67,68]
- assignment congruence, i.e. not being given tasks beyond the new graduate's sphere of competence[60]
- participative, democratic governance[69,70]
- appropriate guidance from senior staff[71,72]
- continuing staff development opportunities[73]
- the provision of support and counselling for new employees[68]
- using personal strategies such as exercise or recreational activity to reduce stress levels.[52]

It is important that senior students in undergraduate nursing courses and new registered nurses anticipate the issues and challenges associated with transition. By building knowledge and understanding of these phenomena it is possible to plan to manage the transition period.[12] Managing involves the selection of a range of strategies designed to facilitate positive adjustment to the professional registered nurse role.

CONCLUSION

All graduates of nursing courses will experience a degree of culture shock on entry to the world of clinical practice. This experience is complex and multidimensional. Research has uncovered a number of issues and challenges that confront new graduates on entry to the workforce as registered nurses. In addition, a number of strategies have been found to be useful in easing the stress and strain associated with transition. Careful planning and use of resources in the practice environment can also facilitate positive adjustment to employment as a registered nurse. Nursing education and nursing service need to monitor the transition process continually to optimise the number of new registered nurses who manage this phenomenon successfully and go on to enjoy fulfilling, rewarding careers in their chosen profession.

CASE STUDY I.I

Jane, a final-semester third-year student in a Bachelor of Nursing program is preparing a plan to assist her in moving into a registered nurse role. She is apprehensive and anxious to excel in her new role. She knows that she can prepare for transition by drawing on the literature and other resources available to her. In this situation Jane considers the following questions in preparing to develop her transition plan.

REFLECTIVE QUESTIONS

- What do we know and understand from the literature about factors influencing transition?
- What strategies have been found to be successful in enhancing transition to practice?
- What types of resources can be accessed to facilitate individual transition?

CASE STUDY 1.2

Geoff, a nursing unit manager in a cardiac step-down unit, has a number of new graduate registered nurses starting work in his clinical area. He needs to develop an orientation program that will assist them in adjusting to their new roles and responsibilities. What advice could you give him regarding the needs of the new graduates?

REFLECTIVE QUESTIONS

- What specific topics could be covered in the program and why?
- How could Geoff prepare his senior registered nurse colleagues to meet the support needs of the new graduates?

CASE STUDY 1.3

Mary Anne is a new graduate registered nurse, who has worked in an aged care unit for 6 months. She is keen to enhance and extend her level of competence in the area of dementia care.

REFLECTIVE QUESTIONS

- What professional competency frameworks can she access to meet her needs?
- How can she document and validate her learning needs and develop competence for this area of practice?

RECOMMENDED READING

Boychuk Duchscher J, Myrick M. The prevailing winds of oppression: understanding the new graduate experience in acute care. Nursing Forum 2008;43:191–206.

Chang E, Hancock K. Role stress and role ambiguity in new nursing graduates in Australia. Nursing and Health Sciences 2003;5:155–63.

Chang E, Hancock K, Johnson A, et al. Role stress in nurses: review of related factors and strategies for moving forward. Nursing and Health Sciences 2005;7: 57–65.

Chang EML, Daly J, Hancock K, et al. The relationships among workplace stressors, coping methods, demographic characteristics, and health in Australian nurses. Journal of Professional Nursing 2006;22:30–8.

Greenwood J. Critique of the graduate nurse: an international perspective. Nurse Education Today 2000;20:17–23.

REFERENCES

1. Englert J. From the president. NRB Board Works: Newsletter of the Nurses Registration Board of New South Wales. November 2000. Sydney: Nurses Registration Board of New South Wales; 2000.

2. Heath P. National review of nursing education 2002: our duty of care. Canberra: Commonwealth of Australia; 2002.

3. Department of Education, Science and Training. The patient profession: a time for action. Senate Inquiry Report. Canberra: Department of Education, Science and Training; 2002.

4. Australian Health Minister's Advisory Council. National Nursing and Nursing Education Taskforce. Online. Available: http://www.nnnet.gov.au/ 2 April 2007.

5. Clare J, White J, Edwards H, et al. Curriculum, clinical education, recruitment, transition and retention in nursing. Final Report for the Australian Universities Teaching Committee (AUTC). Adelaide: Flinders University; 2002.

6. Theobald K, Mitchell M. Mentoring: improving transition to practice. Australian Journal of Advanced Nursing 2002;20:27–33.

7. Kelly M, Flanagan B. Trends and developments in the use of health care simulation. Collegian 2010;17:101–2.

8. Benner P, Sutphen M, Leonard V, et al. Educating nurses: a call for radical transformation. San Francisco: Jossey Bass; 2010.

9. Health Workforce Australia Workplan December, 2010. Online. Available: www.hwa.gov.au.

10. Preston B. Nurse workforce futures [electronic resource]: development and application of a model of demand for and supply of graduates of Australian and New Zealand pre-registration nurses and midwifery courses to 2010. Burwood, Victoria; 2007. Online. Available: http://nla.gov.au/anbd.bib-an000041213952 2 April 2007.

11. Chang EML. The socialisation of tertiary graduates into the workforce. PhD dissertation. School of Education Administration, University of New South Wales; 1993.

12. Madjar I, McMillan M, Sharke R, et al. Report of the project to review and examine expectations of beginning registered nurses in the workforce. Sydney: Nurses Registration Board of New South Wales; 1997.

13. Reid J. Nursing education in Australian universities: report of the national review of nurse education in the higher education sector 1994 and beyond. Canberra: Australian Government Publishing Service; 1994.

14. Greenwood J. Critique of the graduate nurse: an international perspective. Nurse Education Today 2000;20:17–23.

15. Benner P. From novice to expert: excellence and power in clinical nursing practice. Menlo Park: Addison-Wesley; 1984.

16. Walker K. On philosophy: nursing and the politics of truth. In: Daly J, Speedy S, Jackson D, editors. Contexts of nursing: an introduction. Sydney: Elsevier; 2006. p. 60–72.

17. Conway J, McMillan M. Connecting clinical and theoretical knowledge for practice. In: Daly J, Speedy S, Jackson D, editors. Contexts of nursing: an introduction. Sydney: Elsevier; 2006. p. 317–31.

18. Godinez G, Schweiger J, Gruver J, et al. Role transition from graduate to staff nurse: a qualitative analysis. Journal for Nurses in Staff Development 1999;13: 97–110.

19. Dobbs KK. The senior preceptorship as a method for anticipatory socialisation of baccalaureate nursing students. Journal of Nursing Education 1988;2: 67–71.

20. Fisher JA, Connelly CD. Retaining graduate nurses: a staff development challenge. Journal of Nursing Staff Development 1989;5:6–10.

21. Kramer M. Role conceptions of baccalaureate nurses and success in hospital nursing. Journal of Nursing Research 1970;19:428–39.

22. Jarvis P. The practitioner-researcher in nursing. Nurse Education Today 2000;20:30–5.

23. Myers LC, Arbor A. The socialization of neophyte nurses. Michigan: UMI Research Press; 1979.

24. Corwin R. Role conception and mobility aspirations: a study in the formation and transformation of nursing identities. PhD dissertation. Sociology Department, University of Minnesota; 1960.

25. Kramer M. Reality shock. St Louis, Missouri: Mosby; 1974.

26. Kramer M. Some effects of exposure to employing bureaucracies on the role conceptions and role deprivation of neophyte collegiate nurses. PhD dissertation. School of Education, Stanford University; 1966.

27. Horsburgh M. Graduate nurses' adjustment to initial employment: natural fieldwork. Journal of Advanced Nursing 1989;14:610–7.

28. Perry J. Theory and practice in the induction of five graduate nurses: a reflexive critique. Masters thesis. Palmerston North, Massey University; 1985.

29. Prebble K, McDonald B. Adaptation to the mental health setting: the lived experience of comprehensive graduates. Australian and New Zealand Journal of Mental Health Nursing 1987;6:30–6.

30. Kilstoff K. Evaluation of the process of transition from college student to beginning nurse practitioner. Masters dissertation. School of Education, Macquarie University; 1993.

31. Walker W. The transition to registered nurse: the experience of a group of New Zealand graduates. Nursing Praxis in New Zealand 1998;13:36–43.

32. Troskie R. Critical evaluation of the newly qualified nurse's competency to practise: part 2. Curationis: South African Journal of Nursing 1993;16: 56–61.

33. Dufault M. Personal and work milieu resources as variables associated with role mastery in the novice nurse. Journal of Continuing Education in Nursing 1990;21: 73–8.

34. Kapborg ID, Fischbein S. Nurse education and professional work: transition problems? Nurse Education Today 1998;18:165–71.

35. van Vorst S. New graduate nurses' perceptions of their experience in mental health nursing. Masters dissertation. Faculty of Nursing, Midwifery & Health, Sydney University of Technology; 1999.

36. Speedy S. Theory–practice debate: setting the scene. Australian Journal of Advanced Nursing 1998;6:12–9.

37. Jasper M. The first year as a staff nurse: the experience of a first cohort of project 2000 nurses in a demonstration district. Journal of Advanced Nursing 1996;24: 779–80.

38. Kelly B. Hospital nursing: it's battle! A follow-up study of English graduate nurses. Journal of Advanced Nursing 1996;24:1063–9.

39. Mackay L, Brooke A, Bruni N. The first working year in nursing: an evaluation of a group of college students. Canberra: Commonwealth Tertiary Education Commissioner; 1981.

40. McArthur J, Brooke A, Bruni N. Further comparative evaluation of students and graduates. Canberra: Commonwealth Tertiary Education Commissioner; 1983.

41. Nichols G. Important satisfying and dissatisfying aspects of nurses' jobs. Supervisor Nurse 1974;5:10–5.

42. Rotkovich R. Fifty golden years of education and service: a marriage of convenience or necessity? Journal of Nursing Administration 1973;Sep/Oct:10–2.

43. Crout T, Crout J. Care plan for retaining the new nurse. Nursing Management 1984;15:30–3.

44. Johnson T, Graen G. Organisation assimilation and role rejection. Organisational Behaviour and Human Performance 1973;10:72–87.

45. Lyons F. Role clarity, need for clarity, satisfaction, tension and withdrawer. Organisational Behaviour and Human Performance 1971;6:99–110.

46. Rizzo JR, House RJ, Lirtzman SI. Role conflict and ambiguity in complex organisations. Administrative Science Quarterly 1970;15:1150–69.

47. Kahn R, Wolfe D, Quinn R, et al. Organisational stress: studies in role conflict and ambiguity. New York: Wiley; 1964.

48. Rogers DL, Molnar DL. Organisational antecedents of role conflict and ambiguity in top level administrators. Administrative Quarterly 1976;21:598–610.

49. Szilagyi A. An empirical test of causal inference between role conceptions, satisfaction with work, performance and organisational level. Personnel Psychology 1977;30:43–71.

50. Hardy M. Role stress and role strain. In: Hardy ME, Conway ME, editors. Role theory: perspectives for health professionals. New York: Appleton-Century-Crofts; 1978.

51. McCloskey JC, McCain BE. Satisfaction, commitment, and professionalism of newly employed nurses. Image: Journal of Nursing Scholarship 1987;19:20–4.

52. Chang E, Hancock K. Role stress and role ambiguity in new nursing graduates in Australia. Nursing and Health Sciences 2003;5:155–63.

53. Chang E, Kilstoff K. Implications for professional practice: reflections of issues that impact on nursing education. Paper presented at 6th National Nursing Education Conference, Canberra, Symposium; 1994.

54. Chang EML. Surveying the professional socialisation of tertiary graduates into the workforce. In: Macpherson RJL, Weeks J, editors. Pathways to knowledge in educational administration. Armidale: Australian Council for Educational Administration; 1990.

55. Carroll E, Dwyer L. What kind of crisis? The nursing shortage in NSW. Canberra: Australian Public Policy Case Library; 1988.

56. Goldsworthy A, Pickhaven A, Young W. They seem different. Adelaide: Sturt College of Advanced Education; 1984.

57. Seed A. Crossing the boundaries—experiences of neophyte nurses. Journal of Advanced Nursing 1995;21:1136–43.

58. Allanach BC, Jennings BM. Evaluating the effects of a nurse preceptorship programme. Journal of Advanced Nursing 1990;15:22–8.

59. Brasler ME. Predictors of clinical performance of new graduate nurses participating in preceptor orientation programmes. Journal of Continuing Education in Nursing 1993;24:158–65.

60. Boyle DK, Popkess-Vawter S, Taunton RL. Socialisation of new graduate nurses in critical care. Heart and Lung: Journal of Acute and Critical Care 1996;25:141–54.

61. Santucci J. Facilitating the transition into nursing practice: concepts and strategies for mentoring new graduates. Journal for Nurses in Staff Development 2004;20:274–84.

62. Pickens JM, Fargostein B. Preceptorship: a shared journey between practice and education. Journal of Psychosocial Nursing 2006;44:1–5.

63. Butts BJ, Witmer DM. New graduates: what does my manager expect? Nursing Management 1992;23:46–8.

64. Wootton RM. Orientation of newly registered comprehensive nurses for work in the health care service. Christchurch: Christchurch Polytechnic, Department of Nursing Studies; 1987.

65. Smyth E. Surviving nursing. Menlo Park, California: Addison-Wesley; 1984.

66. Bailey JT. Job stress and other stress-related problems. In: Claus KE, Bailey JT, editors. Living with stress and promoting well-being. St Louis: Mosby; 1980.

67. Hart G, Rotem A. The best and the worst students' experiences of clinical education. Australian Journal of Advanced Nursing 1994;11:26–33.

68. Feldman DC. A practical program for employee socialisation. Organisational Dynamics 1976;5:64–80.

69. Ellis BH. Nurses' communicative relationships and the prediction of organisational commitment, burnout, and retention in acute care settings. PhD dissertation. Michigan State University; 1991.

70. Leveck ML, Jones CB. The nursing practice environment, staff retention and quality of care. Research in Nursing and Health 1996;19:331–43.
71. Vance C. Managing the politics of the workplace. Imprint 1992;39:16–9.
72. Coeling HV. Commentary on supportive communication among nurses—effects on commitment, burnout, and retention. AONE's Leadership Prospectives 1995;3:13.
73. Kiat KT. NYP nursing graduates in the first year. Professional Nurse (Singapore) 1996;23:22–3.

CHAPTER 2

Becoming a competent, confident, professional registered nurse

Jill White

LEARNING OBJECTIVES

When you have completed this chapter you will be able to:

- develop an understanding of the complexity of the development of practice knowledge
- appreciate the deeply contextual nature of professional practice knowledge
- understand the transformation in skill acquisition from novice to expert
- construct a personal plan for reflective practice
- develop a positive perception of yourself as on a career-long journey of refining understandings of nursing practice.

Keywords: competent, competencies, confidence, reflection, professional development

---

INTRODUCTION

On graduation one of the hardest things to come to terms with is the apparent discrepancy between the ways you, as a new graduate, see a clinical situation and the way it seems from the outside to be apprehended by an expert nurse. At university the concentration seemed to be on understanding the signs, symptoms and diagnoses and making decisions through the exercise of 'clinical judgment'. This usually involves breaking the situation down into understandable, 'bite-sized' pieces and then reintegrating them. Experienced nurses rarely seem to do this in their practice. How do I get from where I am now to that sort of confidence and competence? is a question that at times as a new graduate you ask yourself with anguish. Why didn't the university prepare me properly for the real world? And what is this competent/competence/competency anyway?

COMPETENCE IN NURSING PRACTICE

At university, nursing programs focus on the development of competence as meaning the 'skills, knowledge, attitudes, values and abilities that underpin effective … performance in a profession/occupational area' as defined in the Nursing and Midwifery Board of Australia competencies document *National Competency Standards for the Registered Nurse*, commonly referred to as the Australian Nursing and Midwifery Council competencies.[1] These are a set of minimum competencies accepted by the national registration authority in Australia as core standards for registration. They are a means by which expectations of standards of nursing practice can be communicated within the profession, across health professions and to consumers.

There are currently 10 competency standards involving responsibilities related to four domains. These domains are: (1) professional practice (including practising ethically and within the law); (2) critical thinking and analysis (including professional development, and valuing and using evidence and research); (3) provision and coordination of care (including coordination, organisation, comprehensive assessment and the provision and evaluation of care); and (4) collaborative and therapeutic practice (including professional relationships with individuals and groups, and communication and collaboration within interdisciplinary healthcare teams). By now you will be familiar with these as they will have been the benchmarks against which you will be or will have been assessed in the clinical environment to be competent prior to graduation.

University, however, can only do part of the job of preparing a confident, competent professional nurse. It is in the nature of the acquisition of practice understanding that it takes layer upon layer of personal clinical experiences to move towards competence in the practice reality of nursing, as opposed to assessment of 'competence' following graduation from university and the beginning of practice as a registered nurse.

SKILL ACQUISITION

The cardinal work of Patricia Benner[2] provides us with a useful map for understanding the notion of skill acquisition within practice. Benner's work was a refinement and application of the work on skill development by Dreyfus and Dreyfus,[3] who developed this schema by studying airline pilots and chess players. From this study Dreyfus and Dreyfus came up with five levels of skill acquisition: (1) novice; (2) advanced beginner; (3) competent; (4) proficient; and (5) expert. (Yes, there's that word again. It's very confusing when the word 'competent' is used by so many to mean so many different things.)

The novice in Benner's work has no experience of a situation and requires context-free rules to be available in order to make sense of what would otherwise be an impenetrably messy, undifferentiated situation. Remember what it felt like when you approached your first few clinical practice experiences?

The advanced beginner has coped with sufficient clinical situations to have grasped what to do in a global sense and can demonstrate what Benner[2] describes as 'marginally acceptable performance'. It is still difficult for advanced beginners to be really sure of what is important in a situation, and rapidly changing situations or subtle changes often elude them. This time the question is not 'Do you remember this?' but 'Do you recognise this?' Benner suggests that new graduates are advanced beginners and that they remain so until they have spent upwards of a year and a half in one type of clinical setting, at which time they reach Benner's level of skill acquisition of 'competent'.[4] She further states that transferring to a very different clinical environment brings the nurse quickly back to advanced beginner status, despite expertise in another field of nursing.

The biggest jump in practice skill development occurs between the competent nurse and the proficient one, as this represents a move in cognitive grasp from perceiving aspects of a situation to perceiving the situation as a whole. It is at this stage that it becomes easier to tell whether a patient is moving along an expected path, or is moving subtly into difficulties.

The movement through the levels of skill acquisition is characterised by:

a movement from reliance on abstract principles to the use of past concrete experiences; a change in the learner's perception of the demand of the situation, in which the situation is seen as less and less a compilation of equally relevant bits, and more and more as a complete whole in which certain parts are more relevant; and a passage from detached observer to involved performer.[2]

The expert involved performer is defined by Benner[2] as one who:

no longer relies on an analytic principle to connect her or his understanding of the situation to an appropriate action. The expert – with an enormous background of experience – now has an *intuitive* grasp of each situation.

But hang on, isn't intuition the thing that we have without formal education – the 'just knowing' that is demonstrated so well by adolescents?

INTUITION

Two of the most confusing words that are constants of the new environment of work are competence and intuition, and trying to gain a sense of shared understanding about them seems difficult.

'Intuition' is an often used, frequently misunderstood word – we use it colloquially to mean 'undifferentiated gut feeling' and at other times very specifically to mean expert clinical judgment. One of the major confusions in looking at this concept is that we don't often stop to explore and ensure that our use of the word is received with shared meaning.

In a systematic review of the literature on intuition within the discipline of nursing from 1981 to 2006, Rew and Barrow[5] devised the following definition from the literature:

A way of knowing something immediately as a whole that improves with experience, informs their judgements and decisions, and leads them to take action within the caring relationship.

We have all heard people say they 'just knew' something, that they had a 'gut feeling', but what is it that distinguishes the type of intuition ascribed to the expert practitioner and that 'knowing' that we refer to as naive, mystical thinking or simple prejudice? Intuition is not something commonly regarded as descriptive of expert behaviour and yet in the clinical literature it is often seen as the hallmark of expert practice. Perhaps if we look at the practice-focused literature on intuition we may find a clue.

The term 'intuition' appears to have entered the clinical literature in the 1980s with the work on skill development in practice by Dreyfus and Dreyfus[3] and Schon[6] and within nursing by Benner and others.[2,4]

The key aspects that Dreyfus and Dreyfus[3] saw as representing this intuitive judgment were:

- pattern recognition – similarities and links with previous experiences
- similarity recognition – 'fuzzy' resemblances, similarities despite differences
- common-sense understanding – knowing the practice setting and its patterns
- skilled know-how – mastery of the job
- sense of salience – recognition of some events as more important than others
- deliberative rationality – exploring what might stand out as significant if one's perspective were changed.

It is obvious when we look at these aspects of intuitive judgment that they are predicated on deep contextual knowing of a practice situation. So it is time to be kind to yourself, and think of this as an opportunity to look at how you can take best advantage of your new clinical access to begin to gather and mentally file your repertoire of pictures of clinical situations, rather than being harsh with yourself about what you don't know.

If we accept that there is an important component of expert practice that has, for good or ill, been called intuition, I return to the question of how we differentiate this from the more colloquial use of the term. Well, here I think the work of Belenky et al.[7] in *Women's Ways of Knowing* may be helpful. This research was influenced by the work of Kohlberg[8] and Perry,[9] two key figures in our understanding of psychological development, and by Gilligan's[10] critique of these works as gender-distorted, as they were developed studying only men.

As a result of their extensive research with women, Belenky et al.[7] found that the women's positions were better represented as five, rather than Perry's four ways of knowing, and that women have a position previous to Perry's first level. This Belenky called silence, where women perceive themselves as having no voice at all. The five ways of knowing are:

1. silence: nothing worth saying
2. received knowledge: listening to the voices of others and holding them as 'true' – 'black and white' thinking
3. subjective knowledge: the inner voice – personal opinion
4. procedural knowledge: the voice of reason, of what is known
5. constructed knowledge: integrating the voices. Here it is possible to hold a personal opinion, having considered the available literature and being aware of the multiple other positions that might be held on the subject.

The reason for introducing this work here is that it provides us with a strong point of differentiation between the ways in which the word 'intuition' is used. The chapter in *Women's Ways of Knowing* on subjective knowledge begins with the words of a young mother, Inez:

> There's a part of me that I didn't know I had until recently – instinct, *intuition*, whatever. It helps me and protects me. It's perceptive and astute. I just listen to the inside of me and I know what to do.[7]

In this stage of subjective knowledge things cease to be clearcut and personal freedom and personal opinions are asserted. Inez goes on to say:

> I can only know with my gut. I've got it tuned to a point where I think and feel at the same time and I know what is right. My gut is my best friend – the one thing in the world that won't let me down or lie to me or back away from me.[7]

I don't want to denigrate this powerful personal knowing. It is a deep point of inner strength on a journey of knowing, but it is a private knowing and as such has the limitations of 'small sample size and limited generalisability'; it also suffers the inevitable influences of potency of an experience and recency of experience. First-hand experience and the intergenerational stories of those in close private spaces are critical to the development of this knowing. It is the 'feel-right' component of knowing, for example, one's children. It seems not dissimilar to the knowing described by Tanner et al.[11] in their early work on 'knowing the patient', with its indepth knowledge of the patterns of responses and the knowing of the patient as a person. (We return to knowing the patient later.)

Such personal knowing is the agency of maternal authority and is therefore not to be ignored. It is the unwise nurse or doctor who doesn't listen to the mother's report on her child's condition and, particularly, on subtle changes in condition. This mother knows her child but would not be in a position to make a judgment on the child of another mother. The knowing needs to be understood and responded to as highly contextually confined.

As an aside, an interesting difference in the wording of subjective knowledge and Perry's second level, called multiplicity, is the masculine assertion, 'I have a right to my opinion', contrasted with the less confrontational position, 'It's just my opinion'. The qualification 'just' characterises women's description of their intuitions, as does the description of the 'feeling' component.

In moving to procedural knowledge there is a profound shift – a shift to appreciating the fallibility of gut feelings and of the importance of shared knowledge and understanding which can be gained without direct experience of an event. Seeing outside our own frame of reference characterises this stage – setting personal experience within the context of extant knowledge of an informed community.

How then do we gain access to understanding something that we have not or could not directly experience? This is the research and theory base of the procedural knowledge of Belenky et al.[7] and represents the theoretical and research base provided by formal education. It includes work such as the meta-analyses being undertaken by groups like the Cochrane Collaboration with their user-friendly outcome summaries, detailing those practices that reduce negative outcomes, those that appear promising, those that have unknown effects and, most importantly, those that should be abandoned.

The issue for practice and practitioners here is not necessarily the lack of research and theory but the issue of having practitioners incorporate the research findings into practice, particularly those identified as 'should be abandoned'. Procedural knowledge gives the novice-to-competent nurse a basis for determining: What can be wrong? What can go wrong? What can be done? This then allows the nurse to enter the clinical field with a framework of generalised knowledge from which to personalise and contextualise for a specific patient: What should be done for this person, at this time, in this circumstance? Inherent in this is an element that we might call 'knowing the patient'. This, importantly, is where you find yourself now.

KNOWING THE PATIENT

In later refinements of the concept of expert practice, Tanner et al.[11] took Benner's notion of 'involved performer' and explored it further through what they called 'knowing the patient'. They saw this as a precursor to the exercise of intuitive judgments and therefore to moving from the stage of competent to that of proficient or expert nurse. Two specific elements to 'knowing the patient' were found: 'indepth knowledge of the patient's responses' and 'knowing the patient as a person'. Indepth knowledge of the patient's patterns of responses included responses to therapeutic measures, routines and habits, coping resources, physical capacities and endurance, and body typology and characteristics.

This was illustrated by the following clinical exemplar:

you look at this kid, because you know this kid and you know what he looked like two hours ago. It's a dramatic difference to you but [it] is hard to describe that to someone in words.[11]

Knowing the patient as a person, on the other hand, was seen as the need to be able to know the person outside his or her present situation, particularly where the patient was a baby or an unconscious adult.

I had never ever spoken to this man, but I grew to know him because of the family, because I became real close to his wife and son and knew what he was like before.[11]

An extension of this work by Liaschenko and Fisher gave even greater clarity to this notion. They suggest there are three types of knowledge, which they call case, patient and person knowledge. Case knowledge is that generalised knowledge which we were just discussing. The two of particular interest here are patient and person knowledge. These are differentiated as follows.

Patient knowledge includes knowledge of how the individual is identified as a patient, the individual's responses to therapeutics, how to get things done for the person within and between institutions, and a knowledge of other providers involved in the care of the person. This places the person in the context of healthcare and treatment as an individual.

Person knowledge is knowledge of personal biography. Person knowledge is a potent reminder that the life lived is the life of the recipient of care. Nurses use their person knowledge to defend their arguments for an alternative management of disease trajectories and to justify their actions when those actions support an individual's agency, even though this can conflict with established biomedical or institutional courses of action.

Stein-Parbury and Liaschenko[12] took this concept further when exploring the collaborative work of nurses and doctors in the intensive care context. They used the classifications of case, patient and person knowledge to analyse situations in which interprofessional collaboration broke down. They found that 'collaboration broke down when doctors dismissed nurses' concerns because they did not fit into a schema of case knowledge'. Managing the confused patient was seen as a problem to be solved by nurses as it requires 'knowing the patient' in order to be able to respond to the person's particular behaviour and 'making sense' of behaviour is made possible when one could put it in the context of the specific person, i.e. through having patient knowledge.

Liaschenko and Fisher elaborated the importance of social knowledge that links patient knowledge to person knowledge, and here they stressed the importance of understanding illness trajectories beyond the health system and into the world of the person who is the patient. This includes knowledge of:

- the social conditions in which the recipient lives
- the impact of the particular disease on the individual's ability to function and manage his or her disease in a variety of contexts
- the stigma attached to a given disease
- the degree to which the individual takes up the dominant cultural discourse about his or her particular disease.

This type of knowing is helped by providing opportunities to walk in the shoes of the other, and can be accessed through storytelling, by novels or books of accounts of illness experience, through poetry and in movies. These provide us with profound glimpses into the experiences of others, and increase our personal repertoire of knowing and therefore our readiness to interact appropriately with others. This knowing can be elaborated by narrative analysis, and research using a variety of interpretive methodologies.

Understanding culture and its relationship to power, politics, language, identity, family and land connection is an essential part of knowing the person. It includes exploration of whose voices are privileged and whose voices are silenced. It seeks to expose and explore alternative conceptions of reality. Here Ramsden's[13] ground-breaking work on cultural safety developed in New Zealand (kawa whakaruruhau) offers nursing the opportunity to explore its practice in relation to cultural recognition, respect and nurture. This dimension of our nursing knowledge is now being developed in Australia and holds much challenge.[14,15] This challenge is posed to all nurses by the Council for Aboriginal and Torres Strait Islander Nurses. We can enhance our cultural/political understandings through research grounded in critical theory such as action research, by critical ethnography, by feminist studies or by discourse analyses, but the fundamental element of cultural understanding is knowing oneself and challenging 'taken-for-granteds'. Brookfield,[16] although writing over two decades ago now, makes the point in a way I've not seen bettered when he states: 'coming to realise that every belief we hold, every behaviour we cherish as normal, every social or economic arrangement we perceive as fixed and unalterable can be and is regarded by others as bizarre, inexplicable, and wholly irrational'.

Knowing the patient at all three levels of case, patient and person allows the nurse to accrue layer upon layer of clinical pictures and patient responses which, on reflection, enable the nurse to have a body of experience on which to draw 'intuitively' when faced with any of Dreyfus and Dreyfus' aspects of intuition, i.e. pattern recognition; similarity recognition; common-sense understanding; skilled know-how; sense of salience; and deliberative rationality.

This is the experience described by Benner[2] and Schon.[6] It is experience that incorporates reflective practice. They both speak of experience as not simply being time spent in a situation but rather as new understandings that come with a disturbing of the taken-for-granted and expected happenings through reflection in action or reflection on action. In Benner's[2] words, experience results when 'preconceived notions and expectations are challenged, refined, or disconfirmed in the actual situation'[2] or, as she and her colleagues elaborate in a later text:

> Experience, as defined here, is not the mere passage of time but rather is an active transformation and refinement of expectations and perceptions in evolving situations. The nurse shifts from exclusive use of objective characteristics and quantitative measures as guides to understanding and action with particular patients. Clinical reasoning is based on understanding patient changes through time – that is reasoning through transitions.[4]

This work has clear implications for organisational work practices of relevance to new graduates, particularly in terms of consistency of work environment and stable ward staffing to facilitate the development of collegial trust and the authority that comes with trust. It holds implications too for the introduction of models of care delivery that enhance opportunities for continuity of care and carer, a continuity that enables the very thorough 'knowing the person'.

McCormack and McCance[17] have developed a theoretical framework for person-centred nursing which is predicated on the work of Benner, Tanner et al., Liaschenko and others and captures these organisational and staffing issues as well as those of nursing skill acquisition. The framework has four central constructs:

1. prerequisites, which focus on what they call the 'attributes' of the nurse
2. the care environment, which focuses on the care context
3. person-centred processes, which focus on the activities through which care is delivered
4. expected outcomes, which come from effective person-centred nursing.

The attributes of the nurse which form McCormack and McCance's[17] prerequisites include 'being professionally competent; having developed interpersonal skills; being committed to the job; being able to demonstrate clarity of beliefs and values; and knowing self'.

The care environment elements which affect person-centred nursing include: 'appropriate skill mix; systems that facilitate shared decision-making; the sharing of power; effective staff relationships; organisational systems that are supportive; the potential for innovation and risk-taking; and the physical environment'. These elements are heavily dependent on skilled nursing leadership and an open and inquiring organisational culture. They influence the nurse's ability to know the patient and to observe and gain feedback from skilled colleagues.

Person-centred processes require working with the person's beliefs and values, sharing decision making and the provision of holistic care. With the above in place the outcomes should be manifest by the creation of a therapeutic environment within which the patient and family are satisfied with their care.

It is clear then that if the goal of nursing is the creation of a therapeutic environment in which patients receive safe, appropriate and quality care with which they are satisfied, developing the attributes described above are an essential step, that is, becoming a competent, confident, professional registered nurse.

REFLECTIVE PRACTICE

This brings us to perhaps the most potent of all aspects of your continued learning – reflective practice, the key to learning from experience. Much has been written about the importance of reflection to the developing practitioner, most notably by Schon,[6] but it has been elaborated on within nursing by many. Reflective practice is the subject of a chapter of its own (Ch 19) but is referred to briefly here as it is critical to practice skill acquisition and movement towards expert practice. Johns and Hardy[18] provide an excellent example of the transformation of novice to expert learning from practice through reflection by using Belenky et al.'s ways of knowing, as described earlier. This will give you a clear exemplar of this movement in thinking. Rolfe[19] is also helpful here as he provides a framework for different levels of sophistication of reflective thinking. These he calls descriptive, theory–knowledge building and action-oriented reflection. Descriptive reflection asks the question: what? What happened? What was my role? What was the response? Theory–knowledge building reflection asks the question: so what? What does this teach me? What was I thinking? What could or should I have done better? Action-oriented reflection asks the question: now what? What do I need to do to improve care?

There are many texts that will assist you in gaining reflective practice skills. Two of the most accessible 'how to' books are Bev Taylor's[20] *Reflective Practice* and Lioba Howatson-Jones'[21] *Reflective Practice in Nursing,* where the skill development options are extensively laid out. Both books assist you to write, draw, meditate, use a diary – to do whatever will help you look back critically on what you did and how you did it, on how it may have affected people and on what else could have been done, on what you would do differently next time and what you have learnt from the experience.

Deep engagement in clinical practice, deep connection with patients in their circumstances and deep reflection on the process are the essential ingredients of what Belenky et al.[7] call 'constructed knowledge'. Constructed knowledge is the integration of the voices, obliterating the spaces between private and public knowing: 'weaving together the strands of rational and emotive thought and of integrating objective and subjective knowing'. The real learning of artful practice is through the intelligent watching of the practice of ourselves and others and reflecting in and on that practice. This highest level of knowing, necessary for the development of expert practice, allows the very difficult work of the experienced, expert nurse who is often called upon to make judgments with imperfect and often contradictory information and to do so in a time-bound manner.

CONCLUSION

Bringing together intuition from our private life experiences (subjective knowing) and theoretical understanding through research undertaken in the public domain (procedural knowing) in their fullness through practice-based experience gains the other type of intuition (expert clinical practice). But let us call it what it is, the best of constructed knowledge in action – practice wisdom.

Bring forward the best of your theoretical learning as it has been modified and tested through your clinical experiences to date. Bring them together with the layer upon layer of clinical pictures you are beginning to collect and collate, enrich these through reflection on what you have learnt and are learning, deeply engage with your patients and colleagues and be open to changing your current understandings of the meaning of illness, pain and suffering. You are ready. You are at the beginning of the rest of your journey towards being a competent, confident, professional registered nurse. Here's the best bit. The journey can last for as long as you choose to practise. The gaining of wisdom is a never-ending journey. Go well.

CASE STUDY 2.1

Sally is the senior nurse on the general medical surgical ward to which Jane has been allocated for her second new graduate rotation. After dinner one evening, Mr Falter in bed 1 appears unwell and is complaining of epigastric pain but says it's just his heartburn playing up again. Jane reports this to Sally who moves quickly into assessment action and appears to be taking the situation very seriously. And indeed, within a matter of minutes Mr Falter has suffered a heart attack. When Jane and Sally have time to debrief later that shift they discuss the differences in what they saw, what it may have signalled and what action they would have planned.

REFLECTIVE QUESTION

Take a few minutes at the end of a shift to write a brief account of a critical incident in which you were involved that day, one in which an experienced nurse also took part. When you have finished your account, ask the experienced registered nurse to recount his or her recall of the event and what he or she saw as the most significant aspects. How did your account differ? Why might this be so?

CASE STUDY 2.2

Harriet Preacher is a 35-year-old woman from Roseville in Sydney. She was admitted to your hospital last night and is currently in the intensive care unit. She was admitted via ambulance after an episode of lack of consciousness, followed on arousal by complaints of severe neck and head pain. On scan she was diagnosed as having had a small bleed from an aneurysm which was clipped in theatre prior to admission to the ward. Mrs Preacher has a picture of two children beside her bed and they appear to be a boy and girl in their early teens. She is currently being visited by her husband Sean, who tells you that she is very upset at missing the children's school drama production this evening and that she has asked Sean to being her in some food as the hospital food is flavourless.

Which pieces of the above information are case knowledge, patient knowledge and person knowledge?

REFLECTIVE QUESTION

Explore your clinical work on your next shift and note examples of 'knowing the patient' using Liaschenko and Fisher's topology: case knowledge, patient knowledge and person knowledge.

In what way do they each provide different aspects of the information on which you base your care?

CASE STUDY 2.3

Asham has been a registered nurse for 4 years and loves his job. He consistently volunteers to help mentor new graduates and staff who are new to the area. Patients really respond well to him and the feedback the nursing unit manager receives is always that he is such a nice person and an excellent communicator. He leads the 'essentials of care' team in the values clarification exercises, having already completed the facilitator's course, of which introspection and personal values clarification are inherent parts.

Assess Asham in terms of his attributes to engage in person-centred nursing. What other information would you want to know before completing this assessment?

REFLECTIVE QUESTION

In McCormack and McCance's[17] patient-centred nursing framework, give yourself a score out of five for the 'prerequisites' or 'attributes' of the nurse:

1. professional competence
2. interpersonal skills
3. commitment to the job
4. clarity of beliefs and values
5. self-knowledge.

Studying these results, what actions might you take to increase your score so that it is closer to 5 out of 5.

RECOMMENDED READING

Benner P. From novice to expert: excellence and power in clinical nursing practice. Menlo Park: Addison-Wesley; 1984.

Benner P, Tanner C, Chesla C. Expertise in nursing practice. 2nd ed. New York: Springer; 2009.

Howatson-Jones L. Reflective practice in nursing. Exeter: Learning Matters; 2010.

McCormack B, McCance T. Person-centred nursing: theory and practice. Oxford: Wiley Blackwell; 2010.

Taylor B. Reflective practice. Berkeley: Open University Press; 2006.

REFERENCES

1. Australian Nursing and Midwifery Council. National Competency Standards for the Registered Nurse. 4th ed. Canberra: Australian Nursing and Midwifery Council; 2006. Available: http://www.nursingmidwiferyboard.gov.au/Codes-and-Guidelines.aspx.

2. Benner P. From novice to expert: excellence and power in clinical nursing practice. Menlo Park: Addison-Wesley; 1984.

3. Dreyfus H, Dreyfus S. Mind over machine: the power of human intuition and expertise in the era of the computer. New York: Free Press; 1986.

4. Benner P, Tanner C, Chesla C. Expertise in nursing practice. 2nd ed. New York: Springer; 2009.

5. Rew L, Barrow E. State of the science: intuition in nursing, a generation studying the phenomenon. Advances in Nursing Science 2007;30:E15–E25.

6. Schon D. The reflective practitioner. New York: Basic Books; 1983.

7. Belenky M, Clinchy B, Goldberger N. Women's ways of knowing. New York: Basic Books; 1986.

8. Kohlberg L. The philosophy of moral development. New York: Harper & Row; 1981.

9. Perry W. Forms of intellectual and ethical development in the college years. New York: Holt, Rinehart & Winston; 1970.

10. Gilligan C. In a different voice: psychological theory and women's development. Cambridge: Harvard University Press; 1982.

11. Tanner C, Benner P, Chesla C. The phenomenology of knowing the patient. Image 1993;25:273–80.

12. Stein-Parbury J, Liaschenko J. Understanding collaboration between nurses and physicians as knowledge at work. American Journal of Critical Care 2007;16: 470–7.

13. Ramsden I. Kawa whakaruruhau: cultural safety in nursing education in Aotearoa. Wellington: Ministry of Education; 1990.

14. Adams K. Indigenous cultural competence in nursing and midwifery practice. Australian Journal of Nursing 2010;17:35–8.

15. Van der Berg R. Cultural safety in health for Aboriginal people: will at work in Australia. Medical Journal of Australia 2010;193:136–7.

16. Brookfield S. Developing critical thinkers. Milton Keynes: Open University Press; 1987.

17. McCormack B, McCance T. Person-centred nursing: theory and practice. Oxford: Wiley Blackwell; 2010.

18. Johns C, Hardy H. Voice as metaphor for transformation through reflection. In: Johns C, Freshwater D, editors. Transforming nursing through reflective practice. 2nd ed. Oxford: Blackwell; 2005. p. 85–98.

19. Rolfe G. Models and frameworks for critical reflection. In: Rolfe G, Jasper L, Freshwater D, editors. Critical reflection in practice. 2nd ed. Basingstoke: Palgrave MacMillan; 2010. p. 31–51.
20. Taylor B. Reflective practice. Berkeley: Open University Press; 2006.
21. Howatson-Jones L. Reflective practice in nursing. Exeter: Learning Matters; 2010.

CHAPTER 3

Becoming part of a team

Mary FitzGerald, Annette Moore and Alison Natera

LEARNING OBJECTIVES

When you have completed this chapter you will be able to:

- identify realistically the challenges facing new graduates of nursing
- identify the significant characteristics of a nursing team and match them to personal and professional values and career aspirations
- recognise the importance of clarifying responsibility, accountability and authority within role boundaries
- understand the importance of self-awareness in order to assess reliably one's contribution to the team
- know the appropriate sources of critical feedback on performance.

Keywords: teamwork, team profile, reflective practice, performance management, mentorship

---

INTRODUCTION

Introducing the concept of 'becoming part of a team' is hard without resort to platitudes, rhetoric and, frankly, more of the same old stuff. Ideals and theories surrounding teamwork abound; they sound moral (create and maintain mutual respect), sensible (choose the team carefully) and supportive (have a preceptor) – yet the reality is not so clear for many who join a team for the first time as registered nurses. Graduate nurse transition programs (GNTPs) of one type or another are the norm in Australia. While the GNTP nurse may be assigned a mentor or preceptor, there is no guarantee of how often they will work together; and, in order to gain a range of experience, new graduates may be allocated to teams as temporary members, rendering the notion of 'choosing your team' obsolete.

This chapter is written for both the GNTP and the first-year post-GNTP nurse. Following the program, with experience and more confidence, registered nurses are in a good position to find a team to suit their career aspirations and settle down to nurse successfully.

We write here about some of the 'old stuff' but hopefully it is with a measure of common sense born of experience in the health system. There is plenty of evidence (both anecdotal and research-based) that the first year can be both 'tough' and 'tremendous'.[1-7] We hope to write in a way that prepares the reader to dodge or ride the tough and appreciate and capitalise on the tremendous. This involves:

- considering the make-up of any team, beginning with overt and covert values held by the team
- defining the new role, responsibilities and accountability mechanisms
- learning to assess as accurately as possible one's contribution to the team
- planning and organising in order to maximise chances of success in the new team.

In short, the process of transition from nursing student to registered nurse is one of socialisation.[8] The new member of the team learns the knowledge, skills and behaviours of the group in order to become part of the team.[7] The process is not automatic, and wise graduates will approach the transition with healthy amounts of common sense complemented by an ability to draw on prior learning, question the status quo and assess their place within the team.

CAREER OR JOB ASPIRATIONS

During the years of undergraduate study the goal is crystal clear – to register as a nurse and graduate from university. Longer-term plans may seem unreal but it is expedient to spend some time questioning and clarifying career aspirations. If nurses have social priorities, they may ultimately choose an area that offers regular hours or one that is conveniently situated for travelling to work. Some nurses may have plans to travel. For these nurses experience in areas that would make them a valuable casual employee overseas is the right choice. A few may want to become academics in the future and begin this course by enrolling in a GNTP that offers an Honours degree and later work in areas where they have a clinical research interest.[9] Many will know of an area of specialisation that they would like to work in and should seek advice on the best experience that will make them attractive employees in that specialist area. For example, theatres may prefer new team members to have had experience in a surgical ward; a nursing home may prefer staff to have worked in a general medical ward. Some nurses may want to be leaders in nursing and choose areas where there is the likelihood of early promotion.

Although not specifically relating to teams, Glover et al.,[10] in a survey of newly registered nurses, found that the reasons for choosing hospitals related to the following: the hospital's reputation, the location of the hospital, the conditions of employment, personal preferences and familiarity. Since that survey was conducted there has been a change in nurse labour force numbers and opportunities for newly registered nurses to capitalise on projected nursing shortages do exist, particularly in rural, mental health and elderly care.[11] Be aware that there are very different versions of GNTPs across the country.[12]

Clear aspirations may help nurses to make convincing applications for a particular type of experience, even where managers allocate places. Acknowledgement of such aspirations may also help nurses to locate their own frustration in a particular, and possibly unwanted, allocation and to accept that the fault does not lie with the new team. Nurses who find themselves in an area that does not suit their plans are well advised to recognise that there is a range of generic nursing technologies that need to be practised and there is always something to be gained during an allocation. Any postregistration experience is considered valuable, and reports that nurses collect describing their ability to adapt and work well within a team are likely to impress future selection committees.

THE TEAM PROFILE

Some teams have readily available information that describes the area, the service, the people (clients and multidisciplinary team), work systems, evaluation techniques, goals, values and beliefs about nursing. The information may be found in printed mission/philosophy statements and locally prepared documents and protocols.[13] It is possible for new nurses to judge from these documents the degree to which the team matches their own ideas and ideals of how nursing should be and the degree to which they might 'fit in'.

Surveys of new nursing graduates have shown that they tend towards having strong professional ideals[5,14] which may or may not wane as they become socialised. These ideals also appear high in more experienced staff when they are asked about nursing as it should be.[14,15] However, it may be difficult for both new and experienced nurses to translate ideals into practice in contemporary health service organisations. This particular point is shown in a study by Pearson et al.[15,16] of patterns of nursing care in a fairly typical large Australian hospital. Comparisons were made between:

- stated philosophies
- verbal accounts of beliefs, values and work practices
- actual practice.

In theory the teams espoused current nursing ideology such as care of the individual, holistic nursing, preserving human dignity, advocacy and health promotion. The nurses' practice was observed using a work-sampling technique that showed that ideals, in terms of time allocated to various aspects of nursing work, were not on the whole translated into practice. Proportionally, little time was spent in health promotion or social care of patients, and continuity of care was provided through reporting mechanisms rather than allocation of nurses to the same patients each day. Direct patient care time was spent predominantly in physical care of patients rather than attending to social or psychological problems with either the patients or their families. When challenged, the nurses, quite reasonably, argued that with increasing acuity and shorter stays in hospital physical care is a priority for both nurses and patients.

From the taste of practice that most newly qualified nurses have had during undergraduate clinical placements they realise that it is not always possible to achieve idealistic standards of nursing. Philosophies and mission statements are indicators that allow new members to know how the team would like practice to be and the way towards improvement through change. New team members will not be popular if they are openly critical of custom and practice, especially before they have some experience of working in an area. They do, however, bring a fresh view to the area and their impressions may remind the team of their stated values and purposes. It is possible to adopt small changes, in line with the stated philosophy, to make improvements; for example, asking to look after the same group of patients, getting to know their families and improving discharge planning. Once individual nurses are established as permanent, trusted and respected members of the team it is more likely that they will be able to influence substantial change.

Nursing is hierarchical and it is worth working out who the different members of the team are and how much experience they have, so that it is known which staff member can help in specific circumstances and to whom the new team member should account. One GNTP nurse from the intensive care unit said:

> but the thing I found good in the first few weeks was the support from senior staff. I felt comfortable really from day one, in knowing, that if I was in trouble, I could just sing out, and there would be someone. And I asked a lot of questions.[3]

In the early days some kind of preceptorship or mentorship is essential. Whilst traditional methods of one-to-one preceptorship continue, new models of preceptorship are emerging as clinical areas are faced with periods of instability. Workplace staff shortages, differing skill levels and increased patient acuity all have an impact on the success of individual preceptorship.[17] The lack of structure and continuity between a preceptor/allocated nurse and novice/graduate nurse can have a negative impact upon the novice nurse's experience of the environment and can affect patient–nurse rapport, critical care skill development, clinical competence and confidence.[18,19] Effective preceptorship models must be implemented to ensure nurses in transition to practice remain appropriately supported.[20] Clinical areas may adopt the use of a team preceptorship model to support nurses new to clinical practice. Nurses in transition to practice can benefit from the support of expert nurses as well as less experienced preceptors who are often able to demonstrate support and empathy for the new nurse due to their own recent postgraduate experience.[21] Newly registered nurses gain exposure to a broader and more diverse range of resources by different nurses within the team approach to preceptorship.[21] In turn the novice nurse new to preceptorship can learn from experienced practitioners as they work in a collaborative relationship.[21] Team preceptorship can facilitate effective socialisation of new nurses as it engenders a more supportive environment.[21]

Some areas are a lot better than others at providing this type of support and some preceptors are better than others. Determine what you want of the preceptor, make sure to capitalise on the shifts worked together and determine how to get essential support if your preceptor is not on every shift that you work. It is worth remembering that a great deal is learnt when working alone. This forces the practitioner to work things out and to watch carefully to see the results of any decisions taken. Reid,[22] drawing on the work of Daloz,[23] contends that too much support can impede progress while a few challenges can promote progress.

In any organisation where there are obvious power differentials between staff there is the possibility that the more powerful will make the less powerful feel uncomfortable. The behaviour of some team members may intimidate new staff members and this will adversely affect their experience in the team. Much seemingly unreasonable behaviour is more understandable if there is a fair attempt to see the incident from the other person's perspective. Remember that the pace of work in some areas of nursing, coupled with the acuity of the patients and the added responsibility that comes with seniority, makes nursing stressful for more experienced nurses too. In these situations, think through the incident carefully and try not to take it personally – unless, that is, it was meant personally!

Madeline demonstrates how she settled down after she found confidence:

> I found the first two or three months really, really stressful. Um, I found staff – half the staff, to be really supportive, and the other half of the staff didn't want to have a bar to do with you. So I found that really upsetting and what not. Umm … but the last three months, when everything started to fall into place, I really enjoyed myself.[3]

More than 10 years later new graduates are saying similar things.[7] However, when people are encountered who abuse their power, a practical response is to find a neutral person who will talk through the situation with either party or both parties. There is evidence that bullying is rife in the nursing profession, and most worrying is that one's response is to become acculturated and in time mimic the bullying behaviour oneself.[24,25] Griffin[26] has studied bullying in nursing and offers practical advice to nurses about what constitutes bullying behaviour and how to respond assertively. Formal complaint processes are cumbersome, have serious repercussions and can be extremely stressful for the complainant. Nevertheless, if the behaviour amounts to bullying, a formal process should be pursued. The longer it takes for corrective measures to be taken, the worse the behaviour is likely to become. Bullies typically pick on people in the organisation who are perceived to have no power, and this makes the new nurse particularly vulnerable.

KNOWLEDGE FOR PRACTICE

Deborah Mitchell wrote about her first placement after graduating that 'the learning curve went straight up!'[2] Predominantly, learning will be from experience. The opportunity to rehearse new skills until they become almost like second nature is extremely rewarding. The techniques of critical reflection on practice, learnt in most undergraduate schools of nursing and detailed in Chapter 18, should help the new graduate to make sense of what is going on and to gain confidence.

Routines and procedures in any area of nursing are essential early learning because supervision is required until they are mastered. Although it sounds obvious, until new nurses know where stocks are kept they will have to interrupt other people's work to be shown, or waste time looking for themselves. Most nurses are busy and it will be appreciated if the new nurse is considerate and tries to save others time, but this has to be balanced against the risk of being perceived slow and/or inefficient if you don't ask – it is a fine balancing act!

Watson[27] describes the core and trim of nursing. Core nursing comprises those elements relevant to nursing, irrespective of specialty, and is organised by Watson into 12 carative factors. These elements of nursing will be familiar to new graduates for they are the very substance of most nursing curricula. Trim, on the other hand, 'refers to the practice setting, the procedures, the specialised clinical focus, and the techniques and specific terminology surrounding the diverse orientations and preoccupations of nursing'. New members of any team need to concentrate on trim skills and knowledge for, once they have mastered the specialist knowledge, they will be more confident to refine and extend their expertise in core skills such as nursing assessment, establishing and maintaining therapeutic relationships, health promotion and communication.[28]

Nursing is becoming so specialised these days that there are bound to be equipment or procedures in each new area that have not been encountered before. Describing her early experiences, Mitchell[2] wrote:

> I had never encountered central lines and many of the oncology drugs and procedures mentioned in that first ward report. During the next few weeks I experienced stress as high as any I'd known … I am relieved to report that by week seven and eight, I was no longer overwhelmed. I knew enough to be reasonably confident, cheerful and more relaxed.

It will be time to reopen the books and read about physiology and pathophysiology, medical treatments, pharmacology and best practice in the form of systematic reviews of available research and summary sheets available on the evidence-based practice sites listed. Watch the experienced clinicians as they perform procedures, ask questions and relate their practice to theory in order to understand the processes. The following extract is from a GNTP nurse in the intensive care unit talking about her early experiences:

> you follow other nurses around, watch what they do, get their habits, and do the same thing … how someone might do this, or do a turn, or how someone might do suction, and how someone might check the ventilators … any little procedure, CVC [central venous catheter] lines, using the pumps.[3]

The multidisciplinary team members are also valuable sources of knowledge and expertise. Mitchell[2] advises other nurses on graduate nurse programs to ask questions and to make frequent notes in a journal.

RESPONSIBILITY AND ROLES

Although hierarchies are thought by some to obstruct the autonomy required for professional practice, in the early days of practice it is probably an advantage to be part of an organisation with predetermined spheres of work and authority.[29] Newly registered nurses may retain a degree of control by determining their specific role in the team and thereby confidently decide what they should be doing and what there is to be learnt. There are formal and informal clues to the precise nature of the role. Informally, nurses who are new team members but with slightly more experience can be valuable in terms of sharing experiences and giving advice about team membership and cooperative working. The ward clerk or administrative assistant in any unit can be a mine of information, as can some of the longer-term patients who will 'look out for' the new nurse.

Formally, the senior nurse in any team should agree with new team members what their job involves and how they fit into the routine. By delegating these duties the senior nurse is offering certain responsibilities to the new nurse. The senior nurse is accountable for this decision. In turn the new nurse makes a decision to accept the responsibility and is then accountable for actions and decisions that he or she makes in the specified area of practice. The important factor is that both decisions (the delegator's and delegatee's) are reasonable in light of each individual delegatee's experience and knowledge to date. The Australian Nursing and Midwifery Council decision-making framework[30] is an invaluable resource regarding scope of practice for all clinicians.

Two hypothetical situations may demonstrate this: a new graduate is asked to receive a patient back to the ward following cardiothoracic surgery; the patient arrests while the monitors are being set up and recognition of ventricular fibrillation and consequent defibrillation is delayed. It is not reasonable for the new nurse to be delegated this responsibility and the senior nurse will be held accountable for the decision. There is an onus on all nurses to refuse a responsibility for which they are not qualified. On the other hand, if a new nurse who was asked to take and record the observations of a patient with congestive heart failure failed to report that the patient's blood pressure had dropped from 120/80 to 85/40 mmHg, this nurse would be accountable for the error. The person who gave the nurse the responsibility should not have a problem convincing people that, in light of the nurse's education and training to date, it was reasonable to ask the new nurse to undertake this task and to expect her to report a significant change.

There is a degree of autonomy in the role of the new nurse as long as the freedom is exercised within the boundaries of the role. The definition of autonomy is: 'freedom to make discretionary and binding decisions consistent within one's scope of practice and freedom to act on these decisions'.[31] 'Discretionary' refers to decisions made based on wisdom, 'binding' refers to accountability and 'scope of practice' refers to the role within specific boundaries. It is not necessary for newly registered nurses to defer to seniors on every matter. There are areas of practice where they have been assessed and deemed competent. As new nurses gain experience and confidence, autonomous decision making within their role will become both challenging and very rewarding. It will increase independence and thereby the contributions made by the nurse to the team's work.

The job description is the document that is used to define roles, responsibilities and boundaries. Some of these documents are precise and extremely helpful, while others are frankly obtuse. Irrespective of the standard of the documentation, it is important to talk with someone senior about the job and what is expected from the new team member. New nurses who demonstrate an appreciation of their role and work well within its boundaries may quickly gain the trust and respect of the rest of the team.

ASSESSING PROGRESS

I was looking after this dialysis, while this guy was out at lunch. And, he had, sort of, explained it all to me, umm … beforehand. Which way the fluid was going, which way that fluid was going. And, umm … I seemed to be doing really well. As long as it didn't really beep, I was fine. [smiles] He thought I did really well.[3]

It is not difficult to pick up from others whether you are 'doing OK' or not and this is an important daily marker for the new nurse. However, as can be seen from the quotation above, this kind of feedback is not particularly reliable and depends, to some extent, on the personalities involved and the way the day is going generally. New nurses need constructive critique of their work and progress in order to know how they are doing, what next to learn and what new responsibilities they may reasonably be able to accept. Van Hooft et al.[32] remind readers that critique is not criticism; rather, it is a rational examination of, in this case, the new nurse's work and may or may not produce praise. Critique, because it is a rational process, provides reasons for judgments and this lends authority to appraisals. Remember that it is as informative and helpful to receive negative feedback on performance as it is to receive positive information. The new nurse can encourage others to provide constructive feedback by receiving it in a professional manner. Floods of tears or loud remonstrations, either face to face or behind a person's back, are difficult to handle and some people will avoid the future possibility of such episodes by saying nothing when improvement is needed in the future. Johns[33] writes of the myth of the 'harmonious team' in which problems are never approached for the sake of keeping the peace. He recommends that professionals learn to give and receive rational feedback in order to maintain high standards of nursing work in any nursing team.

The obvious person to provide new nurses with constructive feedback is the preceptor. Both parties may find it tempting, if things feel as if they are going 'well enough', not to bother. At the end of a shift all people want to do is go home. One nurse who experienced this laissez-faire attitude said:

I think feedback should be a regular thing … I didn't know what stage I was at. I thought I was progressing. The other[s] [graduate nurses] that I talked to felt the same way as I did. They were having trouble, struggling, things like that … once I started applying myself, I ended up really loving it there. I didn't want to leave. My attitude towards the nurses changed and I was much happier within myself.[3]

Times for detailed feedback and planning do need to be arranged with transition nurses, clinical nurse educators or the nursing unit manager so that this important process is not ad hoc or hurried. Some type of framework helps. The performance appraisal processes used by health services differ; however, we would recommend that regular formal written feedback and plans for professional development are recorded. Using the appraisal system means that it may be more likely that nurses once they have completed a transition program will continue to ask for a performance agreement each year. Whatever the framework, both parties need to know about it beforehand. At the end of the session the main points should be summarised and agreement on these reached. Together, decide what the targets are for the next period of practice and how these might be achieved. The experience and the study required to meet the targets should also be discussed and planned.

Patients are a source of feedback. It is not always spoken but observant nurses watch carefully to gauge the impact their nursing has had. The man who sleeps because he has been positioned comfortably after the administration of pain relief, the discharge that has gone smoothly because it was planned well and the elderly woman who is dry because she was walked to the toilet on time are indicators of good nursing.

Colleagues who work alongside the new nurse on a shift, or take over their patients on the next one, are seldom used to provide critique and yet they are in an excellent position to judge the work of all members of the team. In particular, they can tell how the nurse is blending into the team. Peer review is a well-known but little-used form of performance appraisal in Australia.[34] Of course, this appraisal or critique is not exclusively one-way. The new nurse will be capable of judging the behaviour of team members, particularly in terms of their ability to help new graduate nurses settle into the team. It is probably wise, however, to wait until constructive feedback is solicited before giving it. When members of the team have been helpful it is appropriate to give them positive feedback on their behaviour and acknowledge their help to the rest of the team.

An ability to make a sound estimate of one's own strengths and weaknesses is something everyone should consciously work towards. Pearson et al.[35] were told by a range of nurses in their study, intended to identify indicators of continuing competence, that nurses with performance problems commonly have a problem with insight. They simply cannot see where their work is substandard. The reverse is probably true of nurses who lack insight into their strengths, as they are likely to be less confident than they might be and probably slower to reach their full potential.

Maintaining a journal is one way to practise critical reflection and to learn from experience. If this is too laborious, then some time after a shift should be taken for critical thinking about the decisions and actions that have occurred at work and the contribution the individual is making to the work of the team.

PLANNING AND MANAGEMENT

To keep control of progress and to optimise opportunities, systematic planning is essential. With the help of the preceptor, or a number of the more experienced nurses in the team, it is quite possible to plan specific learning opportunities to help new nurses gain the experience they require to become confident level-one nurses. There are several methods that can be used to help with this planning process. A written plan will enable nurses to pace their learning and experience and ensure that these are comprehensive. This type of learning is proactive, but of course a great deal of learning from experience is reactive in so far as it is opportunistic. That is, opportunities arise without warning and the astute nurse will make the most of them. For example, a patient who has been cared for over several shifts by a new nurse dies when she is on duty. It may be quite appropriate that, with the right support from a senior nurse, this nurse breaks the bad news to the family. The preceptor and the new nurse may not have planned for this experience but at the time it seems to be appropriate for both the nurse and the family. Remember that these opportunities are as valuable in terms of learning as those that are planned.

Time management is another skill that, once acquired, will make the new nurse feel a part of the team. Almost by definition nurses are busy and a feeling of constant pressure to get through tasks is extremely stressful.[36] An analysis of the routine tasks undertaken each day and some estimation of the time required to do them will allow nurses to calculate how much time there is to deal with unforeseen tasks and emergencies. An ability to prioritise demands on time and to ask for help when it is all getting too much is worth acquiring. The difficulty is that the day the new nurse is busy is likely to be the day when the whole team is just as stretched.

Good time management practice is as valuable as it is difficult to develop. Worse still, it is difficult to apply consistently to nursing work because so much of what occurs during the day is not predictable. However, it is possible to reduce work by being organised. Truthful nurses will admit that when they spend their day just responding to the next request a great deal of work does not get done. Even though routines and rituals are lampooned by some, in terms of managing busy nursing schedules they have some merit.[37] Once routine physical care is given the nurse can be assured that all the patients are safe and comfortable. There is then time for some of the work that can be neglected such as psychological support, health promotion and discharge planning.

CONCLUSION

At the beginning of the chapter we referred to long-term plans and careers in nursing. However, most of the learning in the first year is necessarily focused on the job and the acquisition of specialist knowledge, language and skills. To become accepted as part of the team, new nurses are usually required to demonstrate to members of the team that they can do the job or, in other words, be useful and take a share of the workload. Mastering a set of skills for which the employer remunerates the new nurse is a requirement of employment. Experiences in the first year are likely to elicit a mixture of emotions – stress, distress, frustration, pride and satisfaction. The more positive emotions tend to dominate as confidence and a feeling of belonging to the team develop.

Our advice is similar to Mitchell's:[2]

- Be honest: admit your mistakes.
- Ask questions: no question is a dumb question – it is better to ask beforehand than to blunder in, then try to fix up a mess afterwards.
- Make frequent notes in a journal to improve your problem-solving skills.
- Spend a few minutes of quality time with your patients at the beginning of the shift – this can make them your allies and not your opponents.
- Practise friendly assertiveness.
- Try hard not to make enemies.

Beyond Mitchell's good advice, we reiterate that it is possible to control the situation from a position of limited power by good planning and by getting agreement from team members to the plan. This is a time to appreciate knowledge and to become aware of the synergy there is between the intellectual training you received at university and the problem-solving skills required in practice; the evidence generated from research and applied in practice; and the theories that explain and make sense of nursing.

CASE STUDY 3.1

Tina had been on her new ward for around 3–4 weeks when information started to filter through the nursing team to the transition office that she was not 'coping' or at the 'expected level' in her clinical practice that the team thought she should be. A performance management plan was set in place between Tina, her preceptor and the certified nurse educator from the transition office to facilitate Tina's learning needs and to provide her with extra clinical support.

REFLECTIVE QUESTION

- How would you assist Tina with her performance management plan?

CASE STUDY 3.2

Despite the performance plan, Tina's development progressed very slowly and at times it seemed that, as hard as she tried, she could not do a thing right. Although Tina did have some areas of clinical practice that required improvement, it became evident that her cultural background was a factor interfering with two-way communication and acceptance into the ward culture. A way forward was chosen to ensure that Tina was culturally safe and to help her to learn more about different ways of working and communicating. Tina attended cultural diversity workshops and she was moved to another clinical area. Workshops were set up and well attended by staff from the wards and nurse educators. There were no preconceived ideas about Tina when she moved to her new ward; she assimilated into the team very quickly and as her confidence grew so did her standards of practice. Tina is now a valued and respected team member of her ward and has secured employment to remain there beyond her graduate placement.

REFLECTIVE QUESTIONS

- How would the areas of clinical practice that required improvement be communicated effectively to Tina, taking into account her cultural background and the ward culture?
- How would Tina have benefited from attending these cultural diversity workshops and what would she be able to take back to the workplace?

CASE STUDY 3.3

Jenny burst into tears during the first week of orientation. She was very disappointed about her placement in the aged-care assessment wards. She wanted to learn to nurse in the acute hospital and to become a confident practitioner. She was surrounded by friends who had places in intensive care, emergency and cancer services and she felt she was being left behind.

After some sound advice from the transition office staff and her family, Jenny started work on the ward. She put on a brave face and was pleasantly surprised at the welcome she received from both patients and the ward staff. She very quickly began to appreciate how the different skill mix on the elderly care ward meant that she was challenged to take a leadership role much earlier than some of her friends. The work that she was asked to do related well to the preparation she had had at university and every day she felt as if she had really stretched herself. Soon she found herself offering advice to enrolled nurses and enjoyed taking responsibility for a team of nurses. The patients were very complex and she learnt a great deal about discharge planning and the realities of social and physical support for people with continuing care needs in the community. When after 6 months she began work on a general medical ward, she found she was more confident than her peers at leading a team, supervising the practice of enrolled nurses and providing holistic care to patients with complex needs. She would advise any new nurse to start work on the elderly care assessment unit.

REFLECTIVE QUESTIONS

- How could Jenny have overcome her initial disappointment with regard to her placement?
- What processes could Jenny put into place once she was capable of leading a team of her peers in this area to assist future staff who are experiencing these difficulties?

EXERCISE 3.1

1. Write a career plan for the next 10 years. Start with the general objective and then plot the steps you will need to take to get there. In particular, make a note of the opportunities you require in the first year of practice to set you on track. Remember that when you go for interviews it is always impressive if you can refer to things that you have achieved.
2. Take a trip to the library in the institution in which you work. Locate and browse through the specialist journals relating to the types of patients you are nursing. Ask the librarian for help if you are unfamiliar with the library.
3. At the end of each shift make some time to reflect and note down at least five things that you have learnt during the day.

RECOMMENDED READING

FitzGerald M. Meeting the needs of individuals. In: Daly J, Speedy S, Jackson D, editors. Contexts of nursing: an introduction. 2nd ed. Sydney: MacLennan & Petty; 2006. p. 240–51.

Joanna Briggs Institute for Evidence Based Practice. Best Practice Information Sheets. Online. Available: www.joannabriggs.edu.au

Levett-Jones T, Bourgeois S. The clinical placement: an essential guide for nursing students. Sydney: Elsevier; 2007.

Malouf N, West S. Fitting in: a pervasive new graduate nurse need. Nurse Education Today 2011;31:488–93.

Pearson H. Transition from nursing student to staff nurse: a personal reflection. Paediatric Nursing 2009;21:30–2.

REFERENCES

1. Maben J, Macleod J. Project 2000 diplomates' perceptions of their experiences of transition from student to staff nurse. Journal of Clinical Nursing 1998;7: 145–53.
2. Mitchell D. Riding the learning curve roller-coaster. Nursing Review 2000; June:44.
3. Amadio J. The experience of being a new graduate nurse in intensive care [MNSc]. Adelaide: Adelaide University; 1997. p. 92.

4. Kelly B. Hospital nursing: it's a battle! A follow-up study of English graduate nurses. Journal of Advanced Nursing 1996;24:1063–9.

5. Boyle D, Popkess Vawter S, Taunton R. Socialization of new graduate nurses in critical care. Heart & Lung: The Journal of Critical Care 1996;25:141–54.

6. Cubit K, Ryan B. Tailoring a graduate nurse program to meet the needs of our next generation of nurses, Nurse Education Today 2010;31:65–71.

7. Malouf N West S. Fitting in: a pervasive new graduate nurse need. Nurse Education Today 2011;31:488–93.

8. Goslin D. Handbook of socialization theory and research. Chicago: Rand McNally; 1969.

9. Hawes C, Schmitz K. A model for the future integration of the Bachelor of Nursing 33. 33. Honours Degree with the Graduate Nurse Program. Collegian: Journal of the Royal College of Nursing Australia 2000;7:10–3.

10. Glover P, Clare J, Longson D, et al. Should I take my first offer? A graduate nurse survey. Australian Journal of Advanced Nursing 1998;15:17–25.

11. Australian Institute of Health and Welfare, 2006. Nursing Labour Force 2004. Canberra: AIHW (National Health Labour Force Series); 1999.

12. Levett-Jones T, FitzGerald M. A review of graduate nurse transition programs in Australia. Australian Journal of Advanced Nursing 2005;23:40–5.

13. FitzGerald M. A unit profile. In: Vaughan B, Pillmoor M, editors. Managing nursing work. London: Scutari Press; 1989. p. 81–95.

14. McCloskey J, McCain B. Variables related to nurse performance. Image. Journal of Nursing Scholarship 1988;20:203–7.

15. Pearson A, FitzGerald M, Walsh K, et al. Patterns of nursing care, Vol. 5. Adelaide University: Department of Clinical Nursing; 1999.

16. FitzGerald M, Pearson A, Walsh K, et al. Patterns of nursing: a review of nursing in a large metropolitan hospital. Journal of Clinical Nursing 2003;12:326–33.

17. DeWolfe J, Laschinger S, Perkin C. Preceptors' perspectives on recruitment, support, and retention of preceptors. Journal of Nursing Education 2010;49: 198–206.

18. Proulx DM, Bourcier BJ. Graduate nurses in the intensive care unit: an orientation model. Critical Care Nurse 2008;28:44–52.

19. Myer E, Lees A, Humphris D, et al. Opportunities and barriers to successful learning transfer: impact of critical care skills training. Journal of Advanced Nursing 2007;60:308–16.

20. Scott E, Smith S. Group mentoring: a transition-to-work strategy. Journal for Nurses in Staff Development 2008;24:232–8.

21. Beecroft P, Hernandez A, Reid D. Team preceptorship: a new approach for precepting new nurses. Journal for Nurses in Staff Development 2008;24: 143–8.

22. Reid B. The role of the mentor to aid reflective practice. In: Burns S, Bulman C, editors. Reflective practice in nursing: the growth of the professional practitioner. 2nd ed. Oxford: Blackwell Science; 2000. p. 79–102.

23. Daloz L. Effective teaching and mentoring. London: Jossey-Bass; 1986.

24. Randle J. Bullying in the nursing profession. Journal of Advanced Nursing 2003;43:395–401.

25. Hutchinson M, Vickers M, Jackson D, et al. Workplace bullying in nursing: towards a more critical organizational perspective. Nursing Inquiry 2006;13: 118–26.

26. Griffin M. Teaching cognitive rehearsal as a shield for lateral violence: an intervention for newly licensed nurses. Journal of Continuing Education in Nursing 2004;35:257–64.

27. Watson J. Nursing—the philosophy and science of caring. Colorado: Colorado Associated University Press; 1985.

28. FitzGerald M. Educational preparation for primary nursing. In: Ersser S, Tutton E, editors. Primary nursing in perspective. London: Scutari; 1991. p. 49–61.

29. Singleton E, Nail F. Role clarification: a prerequisite to autonomy. Journal of Nursing Administration 1984;October:17–22.

30. Australian Nursing and Midwifery Council. National framework for the development of decision-making tools for nursing and midwifery practice. Canberra: Australian Nursing and Midwifery Council; 2007.

31. Batey M, Lewis F. Clarifying autonomy and accountability in nursing service: part I. Journal of Nursing Administration 1982;September:13–7.

32. van Hooft S, Gillam L, Byrnes M. Facts and values: an introduction to critical thinking for nurses. Sydney: MacLennan & Petty; 1995.

33. Johns C. Ownership and the harmonious team: barriers to developing the therapeutic nursing team in primary nursing. Journal of Clinical Nursing 1992;1: 89–94.

34. Wainwright P. Peer review. In: Pearson A, editor. Nursing quality measurement: quality assurance methods for peer review. Chichester: John Wiley; 1987. p. 15–25.

35. Pearson A, FitzGerald M, Borbasi S, et al. Study to identify the indicators of continuing competence in nursing, final report. Adelaide: Australian Nursing Council; 1999. p. 139.

36. Huber D. Leadership and nursing care management. Philadelphia: WB Saunders; 1996.

37. Ford P, Walsh M. New rituals for old. Oxford: Butterworth Heinemann; 1994.

CHAPTER 4

Understanding organisational culture in the community health setting

Amanda Johnson, Deborah Hatcher and Kathleen Dixon

(adapted from the original chapter by Gay Edgecombe and Keri Chater)

LEARNING OBJECTIVES

When you have completed this chapter you will be able to:

- identify the meaning of organisational culture and apply it to your own setting
- define the general structure and role of the healthcare system in which you work
- recognise the primary healthcare and health promotion principles that frame community nursing practice
- demonstrate an understanding of evidence-based nursing practice in the community setting
- demonstrate your understanding of community nursing culture.

Keywords: culture, community nursing, primary healthcare, health promotion, research/evidence-based practice

---

INTRODUCTION

In this chapter we will introduce you to organisational culture and illustrate what we mean by taking examples from community nursing practice and community health services (CHSs). But first we need to come to an understanding about the meaning of culture.

CULTURE

Culture has been described as the values and rules of communities; in other words, their shared common understandings and beliefs.[1] Research and writings on culture have predominantly come from the fields of anthropology and social sciences. More recently, leaders in management and organisations have examined culture from an organisational perspective.[2] For organisations, culture represents a set of shared values and customs that can be seen as a unifying factor for a group of people who have a common language and belief system of the agency where they work. These shared values allow the group to function cohesively and also to protect itself. The shared values and beliefs, both implicit and explicit, may create a type of insider/outsider division.

Community nurses work in organisations that have their own sets of values and beliefs. Within the community, development of a community culture happens gradually over time.[3] However, culture is also dynamic and may change slowly or quickly in response to external influences or events. If you are about to start work as a community nurse or are contemplating a change to community-based nursing practice, learning about the new organisation's culture is important in understanding how your role and practice function within this context.

ORGANISATIONAL CULTURE

In order to locate community nursing practice within its context and to gain an understanding of the community health setting, it is necessary to have an understanding of the global and national influences that frame the practice of community nursing. Australia and New Zealand, like all nations, do not create healthcare policy in a vacuum. Both countries seek direction from organisations that provide international expertise and leadership, including the World Health Organization (WHO), the World Bank and the International Nursing Council. At a national, state and territory level, professional organisations networked for policy advice include the Public Health Association Australia and the Royal College of Nursing Australia; and in New Zealand, the Nursing Council of New Zealand.

There have been a number of major policy influences on community health nursing policy and practice. Three seminal examples are the WHO technical report on community health nursing,[4] the WHO Alma Ata declaration[5] and the Ottawa Charter[6] and, subsequent to these, the 1998 WHO report on primary health care in the 21st century[7] and the 2008 WHO annual report *Primary Health Care, Now More Than Ever*.[8] The Alma Ata declaration refers to the primary healthcare approach and the Ottawa Charter to health promotion. In order to understand the culture of community nursing you need to be familiar with some of the key documents that continue to guide the practice of community nurses around the world. We recommend that you read these documents in full.

The federal government of Australia, through the Department of Health and Ageing (and in New Zealand through the Ministry of Health), formulates policies in relation to community health. These policies are then supported through federal, state/territory and local governments (Australia) or federal and regional areas (New Zealand), and then implemented throughout Australia and New Zealand in a multitude of practice settings. Community health nurses play a key role in the implementation of new community health policy.

Organisational culture in the local community health context is based on history, geographical location, the community it serves, government policy (federal, state and local government) and the availability of general health services. There may be special features in the organisational culture that include regular multidisciplinary meetings, issue-based teams, regular community networking meetings for all local agencies (i.e. hospitals, police, schools), all levels of government and non-government organisations (e.g. Rotary or religious groups).

A strong focus of community nursing culture is the ongoing support for universal services (population-based services such as maternal and child health and school health services) and targeted services designed to meet the needs of vulnerable families with young children or older people living alone. More recently services have been expanded to include chronic disease programs focused on early intervention, education and support for self-management:

> Universal health services are usually free at the point of access and are intended to promote equal access to all individuals and families (p 278).[9]

Other features of contemporary community nursing culture, not as prominent in the acute-care setting, are the inclusion of health promotion principles throughout the lifespan,[10] the use of a multidisciplinary approach to managing care[11] and the integration of complementary and alternative therapies as modalities of care in their own right.[12]

WHO MANAGES THE COMMUNITY HEALTH FACILITY WHERE YOU WORK?

CHSs in Australia are diverse in their development and organisation.[13] This diversity has been exacerbated by the federal government no longer providing dedicated funds for community services but rather requiring competition with acute hospital care from central funds.[13] The implication of this changed funding process can be reflected in the way community-based services are managed, the type of services they provide and the sources of funding they can access to support these services. This variance may now exist both within and between Australian states and territories. For example, in Victoria maternal and child health services are usually funded by local and state government, and the maternal and child health nurses (who are usually sole workers working in this area) are accountable not only to their community but also to their local municipality and the Department of Human Services. Local government provides the day-to-day management support while the Department of Human Services develops the statewide policies. Similarly, the Royal District Nursing Service in Victoria will have its own nursing management structure with district nurses accountable through that structure. However, the Royal District Nursing Service is also accountable to its funding body in Australia, which includes both federal and state governments.

CHSs have a more complicated management structure than the two services described above. They may receive funding from a range of sources that support a variety of different services provided by each CHS centre. For example, the general running of the CHS may be funded by the government in each state, but the podiatry or occupational therapy component of the service may be funded by the Federal Home and Community Care program. The CHS is accountable to each body that provides funding.

What makes CHSs different is the structure of the management. CHSs are usually managed by what is known as a community-based committee of management. The responsibility of these community committees of management is to have direct management and control over programs and finances.[13] Generally these committees meet on a monthly basis to discuss and oversee the delivery of programs and services to their community, as well as to discuss new initiatives that may need to be instituted. You will see how this structure can be traced to the Declaration at Alma Ata.[5]

The unique aspect of community-based committees of management is that they work hard to reflect the population base and key agencies in the area where the service is located. For example, if the service is located near an area of public housing that has a culturally diverse resident base, then the CHS will attempt to get community representation from both the public housing aspect (e.g. tenant associations) and representatives from the resident cultural groups. Community-based committees of management may also have representatives from local welfare, religious, school or senior citizens groups.

The rationale for including this diverse range of people on the committee of management is twofold. First, the philosophy underpinning this is primary healthcare. In other words, the diverse committee representation reflects the diversity of the community where they live and the service is located. Concomitant to this the committee members can represent the specific needs of their community or interest group. This primary healthcare approach supports the cultural competence of the organisation in that staff can become aware of healthcare beliefs that are affected by language and culture.[14] In this regard, primary healthcare in community health is both a philosophy and an activity.[3,15] Second, the empowerment process in primary healthcare involves encouraging and supporting community committee members. The implication here is that the individual committee member may not feel that he or she has the skills to participate constructively or may feel nervous or anxious about being on the committee. Staff members and other committee members can then support this person to increase their knowledge and skill potential.[16]

COMMUNITY NURSING AND THE MULTIDISCIPLINARY TEAM

Traditionally, CHSs are made up of multidisciplinary teams, of which community nurses are an important component.[17] Team members may include doctors, social workers, physiotherapists and financial counsellors, to name a few. Where possible, CHSs will employ bilingual staff to ensure that key language groups in the community are reflected in the community health team. This can help prevent misunderstandings and miscommunications about health issues.[18] Such teams work collaboratively and focus on both the individual and the population as a whole.[19] The individual or community is located within a specific geographical context which usually includes remote, rural, regional and urban (inner-city) areas. Each of these geographical contexts requires integrated teams to ensure that services are equitably provided to all community members. Single-issue groups will continually lobby community health teams for more services for their needs. Examples include the special needs of single parents, frail aged living at home and people with a chronic physical or mental health condition.

CHSs always have a number of ongoing programs (e.g. postnatal depression groups, men's health, drug and alcohol programs, adolescent support groups), but need to be flexible enough to respond to issues that arise, including natural disasters and disease outbreaks.

To work within an institutional setting, the community nurse needs to know the language and rituals of that setting. A newly graduated nurse will not be expected to know the rituals or language of the practice domain at first, but over time and with experience will learn the cultural norms of this work setting. During this adjustment to the work setting the new community health nurse will be exposed to other nursing practice settings with differing organisational cultures. The nurse may have the opportunity to undertake outreach home visits from an acute hospital setting, and decide to apply for a position in a community health centre, school or domiciliary nursing organisation (e.g. Royal District Nursing Service in Victoria, Australia, or the Royal New Zealand Plunket Society).

THE CULTURE AND PHILOSOPHY OF COMMUNITY HEALTH NURSING

Prior to the early 1970s, community-based nurses in Australia were known by a range of titles, including public health nurse, school health nurse, maternal and child health nurse. The latter two titles remain to this day. However, the WHO 1974 technical report on community health nursing[4] and the introduction of community health centres and services by the Whitlam government in the early 1970s greatly influenced state and territory health departments across Australia. It was at this time that the title 'public health nurse' was changed to 'community health nurse'. These changes also had an impact on the new tertiary-based schools of nursing, which began offering courses in community health nursing. The terms 'community health' and 'community health centre' gradually became the norm across the country.

Community health nursing culture is based on a set of shared beliefs which include access and equity, community participation, cultural competence,[20] empowerment of the individual,[21,22] family and group, advocacy, social support and being a well-prepared and current professional nurse.[23] Community nursing is practised within the primary healthcare model.[19] Primary healthcare can be practised by the sole nurse but is also located within an integrated team where the community is also the partner. It includes healthcare, education and health promotion and is framed within a social view of health.

Community health nursing today has a strong professional and organisation culture which is influenced by professional continuing education and professional bodies (e.g. the Royal College of Nursing, Australia, and the Public Health Association of Australia). Community nursing is characterised by a health promotion approach, multi-disciplinary team work, collaboration and flexibility. The focus of community nursing, however, is changing as a result of spiralling hospital costs, leading to an unsustainable healthcare system, an ageing population and a greater prevalence of people living with chronic illness.[24] This changing focus has also meant that the role and scope of the community nurses' practice are being transformed.[24] However, it is the health promotion approach across the lifespan that has had an enduring impact on the culture of community health nursing.

The following original principles of health promotion were prepared by the WHO in *Health Promotion: Concepts and Principles. Report of a Working Group*[25] and have had an enduring impact on the policy and practice culture of community health and community nurses worldwide.

1. Health promotion involves the population as a whole in the context of their everyday life, rather than focusing on people at risk for specific diseases. It enables people to take control over, and responsibility for, their health as an important component of everyday life; both as spontaneous and organised action for health. This requires full and continuing access to information about health and how it might be sought by all the population using all dissemination methods available.

2. Health promotion is directed towards action on the determinants or causes of health. Health promotion, therefore, requires a close cooperation of sectors beyond health services, reflecting the diversity of conditions that influence health. Government, at both local and national levels, has a unique responsibility to act appropriately in a timely way to ensure that the total environment, which is beyond the control of individuals and groups, is conducive to health.

3. Health promotion combines diverse, but complementary, methods or approaches, including communication, education, legislation, fiscal measures, organisational change, community development and spontaneous local activities against health hazards.

4. Health promotion aims particularly at effective and concrete public participation. This focus requires the further development of problem-defining and decision-making life skills, both individually and collectively.

5. While health promotion is basically an activity in the health and social fields, and not a medical service, health professionals – particularly in primary health care – have an important role in nurturing and enabling health promotion. Health professionals should work outwards, developing their special contributions in education and health advocacy.[25]

Community health nurses have been involved in health promotion programs for many decades. Nutbeam et al.[26] point out, however, that not all health promotion programs are successful. They are of the view that successful programs are those where social determinants of health are well understood and the problem issue is examined with the community participants in the program. So what are the determinants of health? Wilkinson and Marmot[27] list the research-based social determinants of health as:

1. the social gradient
2. stress
3. early life
4. social exclusion
5. work
6. unemployment

7. social support
8. addiction
9. food
10. transport.

COMMUNITY NURSING ROLES AND EXPECTATIONS

In Australia community nurses' practice is dependent upon the demographic location of their community and their needs.[24,28] They fall into two key groups: (1) population-based roles (e.g. maternal and child health nurses and school nurses); and (2) individual client-focused roles (e.g. home-based acute nursing for the aged, recently discharged patients, palliative care). The generalist community nurse responsible for a metropolitan or remote geographical area may provide a range of services for communities and families. Such generalist services may include both population-based services (immunisation, health screening, illness prevention and health promotion) and individual-based services (domiciliary midwifery and aged care).

Community needs assessment

In order to undertake your role in any community setting you first need to undertake a community needs assessment.[29] If you are new to community nursing this will probably already have been undertaken by a community nurse and you will continue to do this routinely each year because populations and their needs change. However, for the new community nurse, it is vital that you have an understanding of the current community needs.

In order to undertake a community needs assessment you will need to make contact with all relevant agencies in your area. You can build up a community profile and needs analysis while making yourself known to the people in the area and allowing them to get to know you. In addition, you will need to know the population size, density, migration patterns and the geographical area, paying particular attention to issues that include water, pollution, industry and climate. Added to this you will need to understand the sociocultural breakdown, in relation to employment, housing and family types (for example, single parents or nuclear families). Finally you will need to know about other available services, including transport, health and education facilities, council services and health services.[30]

Having undertaken your community needs assessment you are now in a position to analyse the data gathered. This information will help you to work with the community health team to develop programs that are tailored to the needs of your community. The programs you wish to develop or the changes and recommendations you make will then be taken back to your committee of management (representing your community). Your findings may also be distributed to the wider community for feedback and clarification.

This is a vital stage of the needs assessment because the whole focus of community health is on participation and partnership with your community. The success or failure of your proposed changes or introduction of new programs rests with community acceptance of these proposals. If the community does not have the opportunity to give feedback then your proposals may be doomed to failure.

Health promotion and illness prevention constitute the end product of your community needs assessment. In relation to illness prevention, epidemiological information and health screening provide the best indicators of what interventions are needed. Older models of epidemiological data focused on infectious diseases, which is still of vital importance today depending on which community you are working in. More recently epidemiology has focused on the lifestyle or chronic health conditions that may affect populations. This may include chronic health issues. Examples are diabetes, cardiovascular disease, mental health issues, cancer and arthritis.[31]

Having an understanding of the epidemiological profile of your community is very important. For example, if the epidemiological data suggest that diabetes or cardiovascular disease is common in your area, then the nurse may routinely screen for signs of these conditions.[32] Health screening is of benefit as it can detect underlying symptomatology in people who appear to be healthy. Then the community nurse can, with the client, devise a health plan to prevent the condition worsening.

This part of community nursing is located within the health teaching framework and relates directly to epidemiology and health screening. Health teaching and learning take place at all levels: national health promotion campaigns to prevent obesity and promote exercise; local community campaigns that focus on a particular issue, for example effects of pollution on asthma; and finally, family and individual health teaching and learning.

Whilst there is debate about the efficacy of such health promotion campaigns they are still an integral part of community nursing. The nurse needs to have knowledge about the sociocultural and migration history of the person or group being targeted. This can indicate what level of health literacy the person has. Health literacy refers not just to the ability of the individual to read (many cannot), but also to having the personal skills and knowledge to achieve healthy change.[10,16,23,33] This is directly in keeping with the position of WHO on empowerment for healthy changes.[26,34]

As well as health screening, illness prevention and participation in state or federal health promotion campaigns, the community nurse may also develop programs or groups that relate directly to the community where the local community health centre is located. These groups and activities are established based on the needs of the local community. Some groups and activities may have a long duration whilst others may run for a short period of time.

So how does this all fit together? How does the community nurse get to the point of organising and running community groups? The fundamental principle is that there is community participation and support. As with community-based committees of management, health development groups and activities need to be organised in partnership with the community and respond directly to the needs of the community.[34] The programs and activities not only address the gaps in services identified by the community needs assessment, but also build on the strengths in that community and the health organisation. Valuing and building on strengths is known as capacity building.[35]

COMMUNITY PARTICIPATION AND PARTNERSHIP

The idea of community participation and partnership in health and health promotion is not new and has been advocated since the 1980s.[36] Indeed, community health has as one of its central tenets patient/client-centred services that not only reflect the needs of the community but are also responsive to community needs as they arise.

However, community participation and involvement have two different but inter-linked facets. First, the community facility must provide client-centred services where the recipients of that care is not passive but actively engaged in partnership of their care. Decisions about care become joint decisions. The care providers must be accountable back to the community for the type and range of care models delivered. This is achieved through community forums, community-based committees of man-agement and regular community needs assessments. The community centre must also work within the parameters set down by local communities, including other local agencies. Examples include local government, schools and community groups (e.g. church and social welfare groups).[37] These partnerships all operate from within state, federal and international policy guidelines.

Second, there is a need for community health workers to participate in empower-ing the community so that individuals and groups have the skills and the confidence to be able to participate. In order to do this the WHO has recognised the need to create supportive and empowering environments.[38]

COMMUNITY NURSE AS RESEARCHER AND EVALUATOR

So far in this chapter we have examined the organisational culture of community health agencies and different models of management. We have focused on the com-munity as a partner in not only managing the centre but also working in partnership with individuals, groups and the community to support positive health outcomes. We have examined the different roles and functions of the community nurse from health screening through to health promotion and program planning. In particular, we have discussed the need for all community nurses to undertake a needs assessment.

In this next section we aim to bring this all together by giving a practical example of community development and participation in health promotion from the field. First, though, we need to examine evidence-based practice.

Evidence-based practice

There has been a growing worldwide trend[39] linking healthcare practice with sound evidence of the efficacy for healthcare interventions. This is known as 'evidence-based practice'. Evidence-based or 'best-practice' nursing in Australia is supported by the Joanna Briggs Institute. The Institute follows the Cochrane Collaboration model developed in the UK whereby a systematic review of the literature pertaining to a particular nursing intervention is undertaken. This is then examined for levels of evidence to support the intervention claim, and then graded accordingly.

Although evidence-based practice is growing, it is not without its critics. Wollen and St John[40] point out that the 'gold standard' of evidence – randomised controlled trials – may not be attainable in the community setting. They also point out that randomised controlled trials do not take into consideration an individual's personal and sociocultural background which influences health choices.

How does evidence-based practice operate in the community nursing setting? Whilst understanding the limitations of trying to achieve the 'gold standard' in evidence-based practice, community nurses can still achieve high standards through undertaking nursing research. In planning health promotion strategies we need to research the health issue of concern and what will work for our particular community, as well as plan, implement and evaluate our intervention.[28]

So how can health promotion research be undertaken? Hockenberry et al.[41] explain one approach using the evidence-based model which is cyclical and comprises five steps that follow closely the nursing process of: (1) assessment; (2) diagnosis; (3) planning; (4) implementation; and (5) evaluation. Coopey et al.[42] support this approach and propose the following steps:

- Gathering a body of evidence: this can be done by undertaking a literature review and incorporating this knowledge into your community needs assessment.
- Synthesis of the evidence: this is akin to the diagnostic aspect of the nursing process whereby data from all relevant sources are systematically reviewed.
- Translating the evidence into actions: this is the planning stage where guidelines and quality measures are drawn up based on the identified health promotion outcomes that you want to achieve.[43]
- Implementation: at this stage of the process the guidelines or quality measures based on the evidence are put into practice.
- Evaluation.

The evaluation of any program (intervention) is integral to the entire process. Primarily you want to know if the program worked. If the program was successful and there is clear evidence of this, then the continuation of the program is justified. This is solid evidence for your committee to continue to support the program. If the program did not meet all the desired outcomes, then it may need to be modified to meet the outcomes; alternatively, the outcomes need to be revisited.

Another aspect of the evaluation of any project is the dissemination of your findings, successful or not. Remember you started your evidence-based research by doing a literature review of your chosen area as well as a community needs assessment. You need to write up the whole process and the outcomes of your program so that this information can be shared with other nurses and community groups. Also remember that you are in partnership with your community and the program participants. To continue this partnership you may consider inviting the participants from the program into a writing group so that you become joint authors. Once your results are published, your research findings may then become part of the evidence-based cycle of reviewed literature, and your findings will help inform other, similar programs. Box 4.1 contains some useful web addresses for evidence-based practice.

Box 4.1 Websites for evidence-based research

Cochrane Collaboration: www.cochrane.org
Joanna Briggs Institute: www.joannabriggs.edu.au
University of NSW Centre for Primary Health Care and Equity: http://www.cphce.unsw.edu.au/

In the next section of this chapter your understanding of the organisational culture of community-based services and the role of community health nursing is applied to three case studies.

CASE STUDY 4.1

Max is a 35-year-old Australian Indigenous man with a known history of diabetes. He has been brought to the clinic by an elder. Although he previously attended the community clinic regularly, staff had not seen him for over a year. Max's health records show he has a history of ischaemic heart disease, asthma and retinal degeneration. Max currently reports feeling in 'good health' but the elder is concerned because Max is always tired, and has been experiencing shortness of breath and chest pain on exertion. Max recently took up smoking. On assessment of his vital signs, Max's blood pressure is 170/105 mmHg, blood glucose level 18.2 mmol/L and total cholesterol is 6.81 mmol/L.

REFLECTIVE QUESTIONS

- What are the barriers to Australian Indigenous people accessing health services for health assessment? (Use the social determinants of health as a starting point.)
- When undertaking a community needs assessment with an Australian Indigenous community, what aspects would you need to consider?
- As a community nurse, how might you engage Max in community service and health promotion programs?
- How does the presence of comprehensive, community-based services support bridging the gap between the health status of non-Indigenous and Indigenous Australians?
- What knowledge and skills would a nurse need to perform in the role of a community nurse within an Indigenous community? How might you acquire this knowledge and skill?

CASE STUDY 4.2

Smithville in the state of NSW has an abnormally high incidence of sexually transmitted infections among schoolchildren aged 13–17 years. The local media have given a voice to this issue, parent bodies in the local secondary schools have held meetings and local churches have held a combined forum with their parishioners. Collectively the local community is seeking assistance from the community health team on how to manage this issue as they are concerned about the health of their young people and the effect of the stigma associated with having a high incidence of sexually transmitted infections on the community as a whole.

REFLECTIVE QUESTIONS

- What five primary issues can you identify following a community needs assessment?
- Why is it important to have a multidisciplinary team approach to manage this issue?
- How might you involve various community groups and partners as part of the solution?
- What types of health promotion principles would you perform in your community nursing role?
- What types of health promotion programs may be usefully implemented in Smithville?

CASE STUDY 4.3

A CHS is located in the midst of a large, high-density housing estate. The estate comprises several tower blocks ranging from 12 to 20 storeys in height, as well as low-level terrace-style home units. Accommodation varies in size from one- to four-bedroom flats. The estate has a mix of single older people and young family groups comprising Australian-born residents and residents who have more recently arrived from other countries, in particular South-East Asia.

The residents of the estate come from diverse cultural backgrounds. A range of languages are spoken and the ability to understand and communicate in English is varied. Most residents on the estate have little knowledge of the local healthcare system. There are many and varied social and health problems experienced by people living on the estate, and at times there have been hostility and episodes of violence. These factors have a significant impact on the community health nurses' caseload.

Meetings were called of residents, community health workers, local council workers and housing workers so that people could voice their concerns and find solutions to the problems. One of the solutions proposed by the residents was to have resident-managed activities that would create a safe and non-threatening environment in their community hall.

REFLECTIVE QUESTIONS

- What role/s does a community nurse have in managing the diversity of need present in this case study?
- Which principles of primary healthcare would staff in the CHS adopt to support residents in this community?
- Following a community needs assessment, identify the health promotion programs that might assist the residents.
- How would a community nurse evaluate the effectiveness of these programs?
- Why is it important to involve the wider community in seeking a solution for these residents?

CONCLUSION

This chapter provides you with an overview of the organisational culture of community-based healthcare. We introduced you to the role of the community health nurse as well as the underlying philosophy and policies that guide community nursing practice. We have explained the importance of the links between healthcare and the community, and explained why it is so important to embrace the concepts of community participation and partnerships.

We invite you to become involved early in evidence-based research, community needs assessment and ongoing program evaluation. We urge you to write up the findings of your projects so that you too can become part of the evidence-based research process. Armed with this knowledge you will be well grounded in the culture of community health and be able to participate actively in your community health team.

RECOMMENDED READING

Edelman CL, Mandle CL. Health promotion throughout the life span. 7th ed. St Louis, Missouri: Elsevier Mosby; 2010.

McMurray A, Clendon J Community health and wellness: primary health in practice. 4th ed. Sydney: Elsevier Churchill Livingstone; 2010.

Nutbeam D, Harris E, Wise M. Theory in a nutshell: a practical guide to health promotion theories. 3rd ed. Sydney: McGraw-Hill; 2010.

Rosen A, Gurr R, Fanning P. The future of community-centred health services in Australia: lessons from the mental health sector. Australian Health Review 2010;34:106–15.

St John W, Keleher H, editors. Community nursing practice theory, skills and issues. Australia: Allen and Unwin; 2007.

REFERENCES

1. McMurray A, Clendon J. Community health and wellness: primary health in practice. 4th ed. Sydney: Elsevier Churchill Livingstone; 2010.

2. Dubrin AJ. Leadership research findings, practice, and skills. 6th ed. OH,USA: South-Western; 2010.

3. Talbot L, Verrinder G. Promoting health the primary health care approach. 3rd ed. Sydney: Elsevier Churchill Livingstone; 2009.

4. World Health Organization, Community Health Nursing. Report of an Expert Committee, Technical Report Series, No. 558. Geneva: WHO; 1974. Online. Available: http://whqlibdoc.who.int/trs/WHO_TRS_558.pdf 9 March 2011.

5. World Health Organization, Declaration of Alma Ata. Geneva: WHO; 1978. Online. Available: http://www.who.int/publications/almaata_declaration_en.pdf 9 March 2011.

6. World Health Organization, Ottawa Charter, 1986. Online. Available: www.who.int/hpr/NPH/docs/ottawa_charter_hp.pdf 9 March 2011.

7. World Health Organization, Primary health care in the 21st century is everybody's business. Press release WHO/89; 27 November 1998. Online. Available: http://www.who.int/inf-pr-1998/en/pr98-89.html 9 March 2011.

8. World Health Organization, World Health Report 2008 Primary health care, now more than ever. Online. Available: http://www.who.int/whr/2008/whr08_en.pdf 9 March 2011.

9. Edgecombe G, Stephens R. Healthy communities: the evolving roles of nursing. In: Daly J, Speedy S, Jackson D, editors. Contexts of nursing. 3rd ed. Sydney: Elsevier Churchill Livingstone; 2010. p. 274–86.

10. Smith B. Health promotion. In: Willis E, Reynolds L, Keleher H, editors. Understanding the Australian health care system. Chatswood: Elsevier Churchill Livingstone; 2009. p. 107–17.

11. James A, Mitchell G, Bissett M, et al. Role of the interdisciplinary/multidisciplinary team. In: Chang E, Johnson A, editors. Chronic illlness and disability. Principles for practice. Chatswood: Elsevier Churchill Livingstone; 2008;14–32.

12. Twohig J. The complementary and alternative health care system in Australia. In: Willis E, Reynolds L, Keleher H, editors. Understanding the Australian health care system. Chatswood: Elsevier Churchill Livingstone; 2009. p. 155–65.

13. Labonte R. Power, participation and partnerships in health promotion. Melbourne: Victorian Health Promotion Foundation; 1997.

14. Omeri A, Raymond L. Diversity in the context of multicultural Australia: implications for nursing practice. In: Daly J, Speedy S, Jackson D, editors. Contexts of nursing. 3rd ed. Sydney: Elsevier Churchill Livingstone; 2010. p. 287–300.

15. Koch T, Black J, Rogers M, et al. Nursing leadership and management in the community: a case study. In: Daly J, Speedy S, Jackson D, editors. Nursing leadership. Sydney: Churchill Livingstone; 2004. p. 207–20.

16. Patterson E. Health teaching. In: St John W, Keleher H, editors. Community nursing practice theory, skills and issues. Australia: Allen and Unwin; 2007. p. 157–70.

17. Palmer G, Short S. Health care and public policy an Australian analysis. 4th ed. South Yarra Melbourne: Palgrave Macmillan; 2010.

18. Johnstone M, Kanitsaki O. Culture, language and patient safety: making the link. International Journal for Quality in Health Care 2006;18:383–8.

19. Jackson CL, Nicholson C, Doust J, et al. Integration, co-ordination and multi-disciplinary care in Australia: growth vs optimal governance arrangements. Australian Primary Health Care Research Institute. Canberra: Australian National University; 2006.

20. Warner JR. Cultural competence immersion experiences. Nurse Educator 2002;27:187–90.

21. Kickbusch I. The contribution of the World Health Organization to a new public health and health promotion. American Journal of Public Health 2003;93: 383–8.

22. Wright S, Cloonan P, Leonhardy K, et al. An international programme in nursing and midwifery: building capacity for the new millennium. International Nursing Review 2005;52:18–23.

23. Productivity Commission. Australia's health workforce. Research report. Canberra: Commonwealth of Australia; 2005.

24. Brookes K, Davidson P, Daly J, et al. Community health nurisng in Australia: a critical literature review and implications for professional development. Contemporary Nurse 2004;16:195–207.

25. World Health Organization, Health Promotion: Concepts and Principles. Report of a Working Group. Copenhagen: WHO Regional Office for Europe; 9–13 July 1984. Online. Available: http://whqlibdoc.who.int/euro/-1993/ICP_HSR_602__m01.pdf 9 March 2011.

26. Nutbeam D, Harris E, Wise M. Theory in a nutshell: a practical guide to health promotion theories. 3rd ed. Sydney: McGraw-Hill; 2010.

27. Wilkinson R, Marmot M, editors. The social determinants of health: the solid facts. 2nd ed. Copenhagen: WHO Regional Office for Europe; 2003. Online. Available: www.euro.who.int/document/e81384.pdf 27 January 2007.

28. Laffrey SC, Dickenson D, Diem E. Role identity and job satisfaction of community health nurses. International Journal of Nursing Practice 1997;3:178–87.

29. Houston AM, Cowley S. An empowerment approach to needs assessment in health visiting practice. Journal of Clinical Nursing 2002;11:640–50.

30. St John W, Keleher H, editors. Community nursing: practice theory, skills and issues. Australia: Allen and Unwin; 2007.

31. Johnson A, Chang E. Chronic illness and disability: an overview. In: Chang E, Johnson A, editors. Chronic illness and disability. Principles for practice. Chatswood: Elsevier Churchill Livingstone; 2008. p. 1–13.

32. St John W. Health Screening. In: St John W, Keleher H, editors. Community nursing practice theory, skills and issues. Australia: Allen and Unwin; 2007. p. 117–35.

33. World Health Organization. The WHO Health promotion glossary. Geneva: WHO; 1998. Online. Available: www.who.int/healthpromotion/about/HPG/en/pdf 9 March 2011.

34. Huang CL, Wang HH. Community health development: what is it? International Nursing Review 2005;52:13–7.

35. Gandelman A, DeSantis L, Reitmeijer C. Assessing community needs and agency capacity: an integral part of implementing effective evidence-based interventions. AIDS Education and Prevention 2006;18:32–45.

36. Naidoo J, Willis J. Public health and health promotion: developing practice. 2nd ed. Edinburgh: Bailliere Tindall; 2005.

37. Ryan C, Shaban R, St John W. Working in a community-based organisation. In: St John W, Keleher H, editors. Community nursing practice theory, skills and issues. Australia: Allen and Unwin; 2007. p. 309–30.

38. Haglund B, Pettersson D, Tillgren P, editors. Creating supportive environments for health. Geneva: WHO; 1996.

39. Fleming ML, Parker E. Health promotion principles and practice in the Australian setting. 3rd ed. Australia: Allen and Unwin; 2007.

40. Wollen J, St John W. Research and evidence for community nursing practice. In: St John W, Keleher H, editors. Community nursing practice theory, skills and issues. Australia: Allen and Unwin; 2007. p. 184–204.

41. Hockenberry M, Wilson D, Barrera P. Implementing evidence-based practice in a pediatric hospital. Pediatric Nursing 2006;32:371–7.

42. Coopey M, Nix M, Clancy C. Translating research into evidence-based nursing practice and evaluating effectiveness. Journal of Nursing Care Quarterly 2006;21:195–202.

43. Nutbeam D. Evaluating health promotion-progress, problems and solutions. Health Promotion International 1998;13:27–44.

CHAPTER 5

Understanding organisational culture in the hospital setting

Gary Day and Claire Rickard

LEARNING OBJECTIVES

When you have completed this chapter you will be able to:

- explain the three common organisational designs found in healthcare organisations: functional, divisional and matrix
- describe the traditional bureaucratic organisation and the development of the professional bureaucratic organisation in healthcare
- understand the internal complexity of the social/task relationships in and between organisational subsystems
- understand the influences on nursing practice within healthcare organisations
- discuss the structure of authority in nursing services and its influence on the culture and areas of potential conflict within a health service.

Keywords: organisational culture, organisational structures, functional design, bureaucracy, learning culture

---

INTRODUCTION

This chapter illustrates three common organisational designs found in healthcare organisations in Australia: the functional, divisional and matrix designs. We give an overview of the traditional bureaucratic organisational structure and examine the development of the professional bureaucratic organisational structures found in health services. We discuss the structure of authority in nursing services and its subsequent influence on the organisational culture of a health service. Finally, we look at a range of issues, including conflict management strategies.

DESIGNS OF HEALTH SERVICES ORGANISATIONS

'Organisational design' refers to the manner in which the building blocks of the organisation – the authority, responsibility, accountability, information and rewards – are arranged to ensure efficient and effective use of resources. The specific design options used by an organisation depend on environmental demands, the organisation's strategic objectives, how various activities within the organisation are grouped and how decision making will occur.[1] Common designs found in health services organisations are the functional, divisional and matrix designs.

Functional design

The functional organisational structure groups together departments and areas whose workers perform the same function or task[2] (Fig 5.1). This design is commonly found in smaller facilities such as general hospitals of fewer than 100 beds or aged care facilities. As Figure 5.1 shows, hospital administrative services are separated from clinical services, and functional departments are formed with a departmental manager responsible for each department. The functional design is extremely hierarchical in nature and allows decision making to be centralised. This design is found to be most appropriate when the organisation is small and simple in function, and the environment is reasonably stable with few changes taking place. Functional organisational designs also have the benefit of economies of scale for like disciplines and greater efficiency of service through repetition and the refinement of tasks.[2] When an organisation is large and operating in a dynamic changing environment, the functional design has difficulty coping. A dynamic changing environment may include changes in service profiles; models of care or changes to regions or districts within which these hospitals operate. In these cases, functional organisational structures may not be able to handle urgent information requirements and response time can be too slow. Additionally, functional organisational structures have the potential to compromise communication between functional units as well as promote lack of accountability for achievement of organisation-wide objectives at the expense of departmental goals.[2]

Divisional design

The divisional design may be found in larger tertiary teaching hospitals that operate in an environment of uncertainty (Fig 5.2). The utilisation of modern and complex technologies together with the complexities of medical and nursing training creates an environment that requires fast responses to a variety of inputs throughout the organisation. This design is found to be useful where clear divisions or groupings can be made within the organisation. Such divisions were originally grouped according to traditional medical specialties such as medicine, surgery, pathology, radiology and psychiatry. More recently, hospitals are beginning to group divisions based on 'product lines' – for example, those organised around target groups of patients such as the elderly, or around body organs such as the liver (by grouping internal medicine and surgery and endocrinology together). Ideally, these structures should facilitate a more multidisciplinary, collaborative approach to patient care.[2]

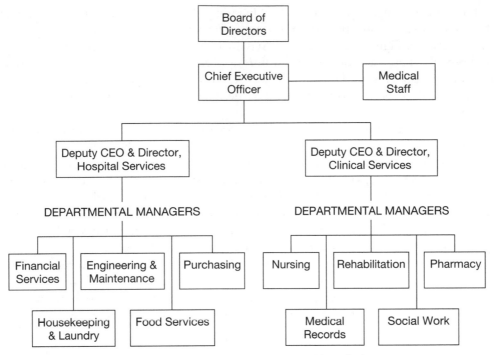

Fig 5.1 A functional design: 100-bed community general hospital.

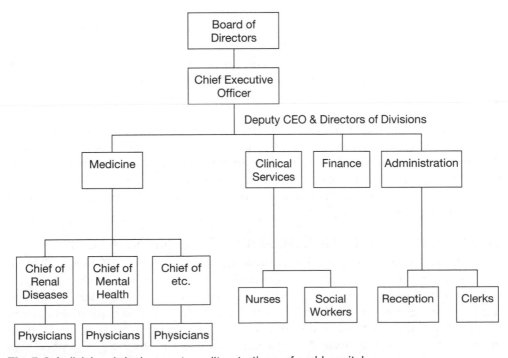

Fig 5.2 A divisional design: metropolitan tertiary referral hospital.

From management's viewpoint, the divisional design allows for decentralisation of decision making and provides those with the key expertise more autonomy to make decisions. Figure 5.2 illustrates a divisional design used in a metropolitan teaching hospital where each division has a nursing director, a manager of administrative services and also a financial officer or manager, who all report to the divisional executive officer. Various other types of divisional design can be found within health service organisations.

The decentralisation of decision making in the divisional design model is said to enhance the ability of the specialised unit to respond to the dynamic changing environment and to handle relevant elements of the environment directly, so as to improve the organisation's ability to develop strategies tailored to the specific 'product line' of the organisation. However, difficulties with the divisional design can occur when higher organisational levels set priorities for resource allocation. It may be difficult for divisional managers to see the perspective of the whole organisation as they focus only on their own divisional needs and fail to gain an understanding of the needs of the organisation as a whole. While divisional structures promote faster decision-making processes and greater clinician accountability for resource utilisation, there is often competition between departments for resources and the additional added cost of each division having its own decentralised management structure.[2]

Matrix design

The matrix design was developed originally in the aerospace industry, and is characterised by a dual-authority system of decision making. The matrix design has evolved in an endeavour to overcome some of the difficulties of functional and divisional designs, as outlined earlier, and combines elements of both functional and divisional organisational designs. A typical matrix design is found in a very highly specialised technological environment where innovation is paramount. Functional and program (or product line) managers report to a common chief executive officer (Fig 5.3).

This design facilitates the formation of work teams and gives team members the opportunity to contribute their key expertise as required. However, difficulties can arise from the dual-authority lines of the model. Conflicting expectations and ambiguity for individual workers can occur as they may perceive they have two bosses: the functional manager as well as the program manager. In these structures success is heavily reliant on good communication as the reporting lines are not always evident. Additionally, a matrix organisational structure may be costly to maintain due to increased management costs.[2]

THE EVOLUTION OF THE BUREAUCRATIC ORGANISATION

Generally acclaimed to be the father of organisational theory, Max Weber, a German social scientist, developed the most comprehensive formulation of the characteristics of a bureaucracy during the 1920s. The bureaucracy was an ideal weapon to routinise the energy of production during the Industrial Revolution. However, Weber's work did not consider the complexities of managing a dynamic organisation in the 21st century. He wrote during a time when the motivation of workers was taken for granted, and his simplification of manager and employee roles did not

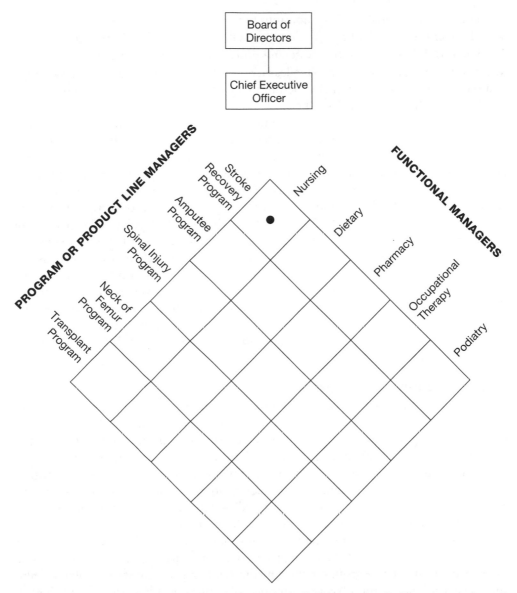

Fig 5.3 A matrix design: rehabilitation centre. An individual worker in this example is part of the stroke recovery program as well as a member of the nursing department.

examine the complexities of the bilateral relationships found between employee and manager in the majority of organisations today.[3]

In his ideal bureaucracy Weber[3] describes five main characteristics of the bureaucratic type of organisation:

1. They have a high degree of specialisation.
2. They have a hierarchical authority structure with limited areas of command and responsibility.

3. There is impersonality of relationships between organisational members.
4. The recruitment of officials is based on ability and technical knowledge.
5. There is differentiation of private and official income and fortune.

We find that modern managers have learnt about human behaviour, and now design and redesign their organisational structure in an effort to reduce rigidity and increase flexibility for their individual workers.

The other theorist who had a major impact on the early structure of organisations was Frederick Taylor. Taylor supported the system of bureaucracy but, in contrast to Weber, he was not so much interested in the organisational problems of society's power structures (general administrative management), but in the practical problem of efficiency (scientific management). His main unit of analysis was not society as a whole, but the individual workplace and the organisational productivity related to this workshop level. Taylor[4] (p 23) states that: 'the principal object of management should be to secure maximum prosperity for the employer, coupled with maximum prosperity for the employee'. Taylor believed that, for every process, every task in industry, there is one best way of performance. To discover this unique way, one has to examine the parts of the organisation in a scientific way. When they are known, they can be applied in the working situation to regulate the various activities and other factors of production in such a way that maximum productivity is achieved. Thus, scientific knowledge replaces intuition and the rule-of-thumb method in organisational behaviour.

Traditional bureaucratic organisations

The traditional bureaucratic organisation is found to have a hierarchy of authority and a dependence on rules and regulations. Rules govern most official business, leaving little opportunity for creativity or discretion in decision making. The repetitive and highly predictable nature of the work means it can be easily monitored. The organisation functions through coordination of work and tasks and, as the organisation grows and becomes more complex, the administration also grows to support and maintain the organisation's systems. A middle-management layer is necessary to oversee and monitor the specialised work of the core business.

In healthcare organisations there are many organisational objectives. The major objective is patient care and there are professional participant groups who contribute to the patient care. These groups include medical, nursing, administrative, allied health and other staff. Each group has its own body of professional knowledge and they all interpret organisational objectives according to their own value systems. Such issues can be problematic in terms of the coordination and integration of work, as what arises are competing and different groups exercising legitimate authority in the same organisation with no line of authority between them. A complex organisation like a healthcare facility requires coordination through the standardisation of the skills of its employees. Such a configuration is known as a professional bureaucracy.[5]

Professional bureaucratic organisations

Professional bureaucratic organisations can lead to conflict. In the Australian health industry conflict has been evident between the medical and other health professions, and hospital managers. Professionals have extensive training designed to enable them to undertake complex and uncertain tasks independently. This leads to the view that professionals need the freedom to apply the appropriate skills to any given situation. Managers, however, in exercising their responsibility for the overall performance of their organisation are required to coordinate, direct and control the professionals who perform the tasks. Ultimately, managers are brought into conflict with 'professional' resistance to control.[6] In order to achieve their goals, professionals tend to focus on their individual clinical contribution and their treatment of the patient, while managers focus on the organisation as a whole and endeavour to ensure that all parts of the organisation are coordinated.

The demand for healthcare and the costs of providing it have increased significantly in Australia over the last decade. Efforts to control the costs, coupled with advances in medical technology, have had an impact on health organisational structures and the organisational subsystems. Advances in medical technology have resulted particularly in increasing diversification, based on intensive training and subspecialisation in all professional disciplines. Such diversity and specialisation of activities necessitate an extensive division of labour which, coupled with an already complex organisational structure, requires an elaborate system of coordination of tasks, functions and social interactions. Coordination by means of organisational hierarchy (traditional bureaucracy) is difficult. Administrative rules and procedures serve to coordinate routine events, but for non-routine, complex patient care problems one of the primary means of integration must be the voluntary coordination and willingness of the participants to work effectively together to deal with unusual events. The value system emphasising patient care is the basic factor influencing voluntary coordination.

In many healthcare systems, this has led to the development of a matrix-type organisation, with both hierarchical (vertical) integration through departmentalisation and formal chain of command, and lateral (horizontal) integration across departments. These complex organisations have, as workers, sophisticated specialists or professionals who are required to combine their efforts in project teams coordinated by mutual adjustment. Here, coordination is achieved by mutual adjustment because line management and staff functions, as well as a number of other distinctions, tend to break down. Some matrix designs express themselves as 'divisionalised' structures with semiautonomous units or sections responsible and accountable for their own budgets. In some matrix organisations, the functional (vertical) divisions retain most of the control so that the teams are set within a bureaucratic structure from which it is often difficult to break free. However, there have been cases where innovation and efficiencies have been achieved.

Public versus private hospital environment

It is important to recognise that the organisational environments outlined above may differ in Australia between the public and private hospital systems. Private organisations have tended to be more traditional in the bureaucratic sense. That is, they are more hierarchical and often have traditional authority positions. This is partly due to the complexities of the relationships and the ownership of some of the organisational issues. In the public sector, most, although not all, medical staff are salaried employees. In the private system, fewer specialist medical practitioners are employed: most work on a private basis, thereby making them a key 'customer' of the organisation which brings in revenue by choosing to admit patients to any one hospital over other potential institutions in the geographical region. As long as access to facilities and equipment is provided by the hospital to enable medical practitioners to complete their required tasks in an efficient and coordinated manner, clinician interest in, and ownership of, the organisational issues can vary considerably. This is often because 'the organisation' is not the only or even the major affiliation they have with healthcare institutions. The medical practitioner's income and livelihood, although connected to the organisation, is basically the relationship with the patient (depending on the specialty) and can be satisfied outside the organisation. However, structural designs in private hospitals are changing. As private hospitals move from being stand-alone cottage industries to networked conglomerates of private businesses, the organisational structures have become more business-like. Private hospitals have become larger, more highly specialised, complex and offering tertiary services and, as such, their organisational structures are beginning to look like those in the public sector.

Boundaries of work environment

No matter how an organisation is structured, the boundaries between work groups act to reinforce the relationships and accomplishment of the work within groups. They also act to hinder the development and maintenance of relationships among people and the accomplishment of work that crosses the boundaries of different groups. In complex organisations like healthcare organisations there is no perfect structure.[7] As a newly qualified professional functioning in such systems, it is important to understand the complexities of the relationships and work boundaries that will influence the achievement of either your work or your unit's work.

INFLUENCES ON NURSING PRACTICE IN HEALTHCARE ORGANISATIONS

Many authorities govern and influence nursing practice in Australia. These range from the internal organisational structures to the professional bodies, registering authorities, educational and training institutions and nursing unions. All these bodies have an important role to play in the way nursing is practised and developed.

Career structures

The 1980s saw significant changes in Australian nursing structures. During this decade nursing began to move from hospital-based training to university-based training. There was a shortage of nurses in many states and most Australian states adopted a formal career structure for nursing. Career structures are seen to be important for several reasons. They provide acknowledgment of differing areas of expertise in nursing, such as clinical expertise or administration or education expertise. This acknowledgment allows advancement and remuneration opportunities that assist work satisfaction and help retain nurses within the profession. More recently, there has been a need to redefine nursing roles in the context of their contribution to healthcare reform, cost containment and improved clinical outcomes. Nurses are in a key position to influence many of these changes, and appropriate career structures provide a mechanism to recognise this contribution.[8] Career structures are a way of providing status and economic incentives to nurses who contribute to both the profession and the organisation through direct clinical care or by other means.

Role of nursing unions

Nursing in Australia has a long history of high uptake of trade union membership. The nursing unions assist in negotiating employment conditions with government, and continue to play an important part in advocating and negotiating conditions of work, including career structures for the nursing profession. Unions have traditionally been involved in the issue of award conditions, such as remuneration, hours of work and rostering practices. Enterprise bargaining is undertaken collectively at a state or national level for all nurses employed in the public, private or aged care sectors. Recent changes to industrial laws in Australia are perceived by some to reduce the power of unions and their role in collective bargaining; however, unionisation has a strong history in Australia and it is anticipated unions will continue to have a role in negotiating working conditions for nursing for many years to come. Unions also assist individual nurses who may require representation and help negotiating with management over employment issues.

Role of professional colleges

Professional colleges, such as the Royal College of Nursing, Australia, are the collegial affiliations of the profession and aim to advance the profession through reviewing and setting nursing standards, influencing state and national policy that has an impact on nursing, promoting research, disseminating new and up-to-date information and acting as spokespersons for the profession.[9] The professional colleges also play a role in continuing education and run numerous contemporary education activities and forums that are designed to assist and support nurses in their practice. Numerous specialty groups and colleges exist, with one of the largest being the Australian College of Critical Care Nurses.

Professional colleges are an important part of professional life in nursing, and all nurses are encouraged to join and benefit from participation. It is important for the colleges to represent the profession as a whole and new graduates and junior nursing staff, being the future of the profession, should be involved as early as possible in their careers.

Role of registering bodies

The registering bodies perform the function of ensuring that the regulations and standards governing the nursing profession are upheld. They have an important role to play in ensuring the community can feel confident about the conduct of nursing professional practice. There have been a number of significant changes to nursing and midwifery registration and practice recently. National bodies have been established in a move to centralise functions to ensure consistent practice and registration.

The Nursing and Midwifery Board of Australia (NMBA) is the national body whose role it is to facilitate a national approach to nursing and midwifery education in developing appropriate and effective standards to meet the needs of the community. In 2009, the newly formed NMBA provided a national approach[10] to:

- developing standards, codes and guidelines for the nursing and midwifery profession
- handling notifications, complaints, investigations and disciplinary hearings
- assessing overseas-trained practitioners who wish to practise in Australia
- approving accreditation standards and accredited courses of study.

The NMBA plays a significant role in assisting individual professionals who are having difficulty with their professional practice, due either to illness and/or a genuine error of judgment, to rehabilitate and return to work.

From 2010, the NMBA, supported by the Australian Health Practitioners Regulation Agency, has taken over the role of the state and territory registering bodies to provide a central organisation for the registration of nurses across Australia.

STRUCTURE OF AUTHORITY IN NURSING SERVICES

All healthcare organisations have some form of hierarchical structure that coordinates the delivery of nursing services to patients. Depending on the complexity of the organisation, there will be a director of nursing and, reporting to the director of nursing, a further one or two levels of nursing hierarchy between the director and the nurses providing direct patient care. Most wards (or patient care units) have one position on the ward that is responsible for standards of care and for coordinating the delivery of care to patients. In larger organisations a further position is usually responsible for coordinating care for a group of patient care units. Even in a divisional matrix-type structure, a nurse is commonly involved at this level as, often, the medical clinician manager undertakes half-time clinical practice and the responsibilities for managing a division are shared.

Nurses work in the hospital system 24 hours a day, 7 days a week. Therefore, traditionally, they have the after-hours coordinating role of replacing staff on sick leave, ensuring human resources are evenly allocated on any one shift, dealing with any organisational problems that may arise, organising retrievals and transfers of patients and dealing with clinical or other crises.

Recent changes in the health industry have also influenced nursing structures within organisations. In contemporary Australian healthcare, the structure of the line of authority for reporting day-to-day issues associated with budgets, staffing and the general running of the ward or patient care area may not be directly to a more senior nurse. However, for professional nursing practice issues the reporting line should always be directly to a nurse.

Role of the senior nursing authority

The role of the senior nursing authority in a hospital is to ensure that standards of nursing practice are upheld, to use nursing resources efficiently, to advocate on behalf of the profession, to promote nursing research and to monitor and maintain nursing standards and conduct. A director of nursing has a professional responsibility to deal with professional practice issues and to notify registration boards of breaches in professional conduct. In fact, any nurse has the responsibility to notify the appropriate person if there is a breach of standards or conduct.

ORGANISATIONAL CULTURE OF A HEALTH SERVICE

The design of an organisation can shape the institution's culture. Organisational culture can best be described as enduring attributes such as values, assumptions and beliefs that are unique to each organisation. Scott-Findlay and Estabrook[11] suggest that organisational culture gives 'a sense of what is valued and how things should be done in an organisation'. Marquis and Huston[3] define it as the total of an organisation's values, language, history, formal and informal communication networks, rituals and 'sacred cows'. Hemmelgarn et al.[12] argue that these beliefs and expectations are the basis for socialising co-workers in how to behave within an organisation, and create a social climate that shapes the tone, content and objectives of work accomplished within the organisation. Simply put, new members to the organisation are taught through observation, modelling and personal experiences the 'way things are done around the organisation', as well as the rewards, punishments and expected outcomes that follow from one's work behaviour (p 77).[12]

Types of organisational culture

Culture can be categorised or described in a number of ways. Cameron and Quinn[13] argue that any organisation's culture is based on competing values and the 'tension' between an organisation's (or department's) flexibility over control and internal focus over external focus creates certain cultural characteristics.

Cameron and Quinn categorised culture as being one of four types:

1. clan culture
2. adhocracy culture
3. hierarchy culture
4. market culture.

Gifford et al.[14] discuss these four cultural groupings in terms more helpful to health-care. The authors account for clan culture as group culture; adhocracy culture as developmental culture; market culture as rational culture; and hierarchy culture remains unchanged.

Group (or clan) culture can best be described as an organisation (or department) that values cohesion and high morale with an emphasis on the training and development of its staff. This culture is alternatively described as a human relations model.

Developmental (or adhocracy) culture is best described as an organisation that values growth, resource acquisition and external support. This type of culture is highly adaptable and ready for change. The culture can be best described as an open systems model.

Rational (or market) culture describes an organisation that values productivity and efficiency. The key attribute of this type of culture is a focus on planning and goal setting. This type of culture can be categorised as a rational goal model.

Hierarchical culture describes as organisation that values stability and control. Organisations with this type of culture are driven by information management and communication processes. This type of culture can be categorised as an internal process model.

How is an organisational culture spread?

There are several views about how organisational culture is spread, reproduced or changed within an organisation. The most favoured view is that there exists within an organisation a single culture that is developed or imported by its organisational members. Similar values, beliefs and perceptions are said to be shared by the members of the organisation.

Sovie[15] believes that a positive and constructive hospital culture is essential to achieve organisational goals and thus is too important to be simply left to chance. To move to a constructive culture, the leader of the organisation must take an active role in building the type of organisational culture that will bring success to the organisation.

CREATING A LEARNING CULTURE WITHIN A HOSPITAL

While nurses' learning needs are ultimately their own professional responsibility, there are many ways these can be achieved within their employing organisation.

In-service education

Many health service organisations arrange in-service sessions in wards during the day/ evening shift changeover period. These sessions usually last about 30 minutes and nurses attend during their afternoon tea break. In-service sessions are usually prepared by the ward staff and are informal. One or more nurses are usually responsible for organising in-service sessions, and ideally they seek input from the other staff on desirable topics. Some wards expect all staff to give regular in-service sessions, which can provide very good learning opportunities.

Organisation-based education courses

Short courses are often made available to nursing staff at no or minimal cost. These courses are an excellent opportunity to access updates on various aspects of clinical practice, and also provide an opportunity for employees to display to the employer their interest in further opportunities and responsibilities. Staff undertaking these short courses should be mindful not to limit themselves to organisation-based courses as, inherently, these are biased to the beliefs and values of the institution. A balanced approach should be made and more formal university- or profession-based qualifications should also be sought.

Support for external courses

Most hospitals offer financial support for staff members who wish to undertake formal university-based courses. Surprisingly, there are often few applicants for these grants. For those who do apply, emphasising the knowledge and skills that will be acquired as a future resource for the organisation is usually the key to achieving support. Some organisations offer support to staff who undertake courses that the employer considers desirable; for example, graduate qualifications in specialty areas such as mental health, midwifery or critical care.

Developing a learning culture

A key element to retaining and recruiting nursing staff is to create a culture that values and empowers nurses to develop professionally and personally. It means creating a culture where learning is valued, where everyone is making improvements. By creating such a facilitating culture it should be possible to develop a learning organisation.[16]

Learning organisations also promote the notion of lifelong learning amongst their staff. There are two elements to creating lifelong learning. One is the need for organisations to ensure staff are oriented, have opportunities for professional development and are adequately prepared to implement and use new equipment and technology. Second, the organisation needs to build the capacity for staff to seek out development opportunities independently throughout their careers. This approach demonstrates an organisation's professional duty to support and nurture new graduates, new staff and undergraduate students. While it is accepted that human capital investment in health or education is the key to future prosperity and economic growth,[17] the final responsibility for learning rests with individuals themselves, a function of their current work needs and interests in their longer-term career aspirations.[18]

Performance management systems

The employment of registered nurses is generally governed by a formalised performance planning and review (PPR) system that takes place annually. This PPR system involves registered nurses meeting with their supervisor, documenting their performance goals and establishing a plan to achieve their identified performance goals. This process should not be seen as a pointless bureaucratic activity, but as an opportunity to achieve learning goals. Specific learning goals that may be included in a PPR are presented in Figure 5.4.

Performance plans should be relevant to employer expectations and service focus. Attending a course on diabetes will not be seen as desirable if the ward does not care for such patients. Documentation of learning goals not only makes the employee

---

In the next 12 months I will fulfil my role as a registered nurse by:

Clinical

Observing cardiac angiography and cardiac angioplasty

Attending the hospital 2-day program 'Managing diabetes'

Education

Giving in-service sessions on angiography, angioplasty and managing diabetes

Acting as preceptor to a new staff member

Management

Discussing 'in charge of shift' role with clinical nurse consultant

Undertaking 'in charge of shift' role 'buddied' with a senior nurse on three shifts

Research

Discussing current ward research with nurse researcher

Reviewing a research article for journal club

Fig 5.4 Performance planning and review (PPR) learning goals.

responsible for achieving the goals but, importantly, also places a responsibility on the supervisor and the organisation to assist the staff member to achieve the goals by providing educational sessions.

Educators and other resource people

Nurse educators are employed in hospitals to facilitate staff education. Registered nurses should approach their nurse educator and supervisor to discuss their learning needs. However, there are many other ways to improve knowledge. There is usually only one educator allocated to several wards and the educator's workload may be largely dictated by broad organisational needs. For example, hospital standards usually require all nurses to undertake a cardiopulmonary resuscitation competency annually, which is a time-consuming responsibility for the educators. Nurse colleagues and other healthcare professionals can be consulted informally as matters arise, although care should be taken to back this up with formal documents such as procedure manuals, resource manuals, online journals and evidence-based practice guidelines published by reputable professional groups; these are usually located at the nurses' station in the ward.

NURSING ORGANISATIONAL ISSUES AND POTENTIAL CONFLICT SITUATIONS

Clinical nurses are concerned mainly with giving care and providing for the needs of their patients. However, nursing executives tend to focus on the overarching organisational issues that involve the governing of the hospital as a whole. There are thus many organisational and administrative issues that have an impact on the everyday working lives of clinical nurses and have the potential to lead to conflict situations. We now look at some examples of these issues.

Balancing the budget

As healthcare costs continue to rise, government health budgets are increasingly being stretched, and hospital departments and service areas are required to compete among themselves for the limited funding now available; for example, the medical division competes for funds with the surgical division. Clinical departments have budgets for nursing wages, equipment and disposables and the distribution of funds between various departments and service areas can become a source of much conflict across divisions within hospitals.

Human resources management

The processes of employing staff, providing orientation, managing performance and resignations are all regulated by government legislation and organisational bureaucratic structures and systems (e.g. the Nursing Act in the relevant jurisdiction and hospital orientation programs). These requirements may sometimes be seen to conflict with the ability of the organisation to bring about change.

Organisational performance

Healthcare organisations are required to evaluate the extent to which they deliver quality care. Formalised processes such as quality assurance programs and accreditation exist to fulfil this function. Performance is also measured in terms of the cost of services performed. Clinical staff are expected to collect data on patient/nurse dependency ratios to help justify spending and plan for future services. However, the collection of such data may seem unnecessary or take time away from the delivery of patient care.

Variation of policies and procedures

Healthcare organisations have developed a variety of documents to guide staff in their provision of quality, consistency and external justification of care. These documents may be very specific and apply only to one ward, or they may be more generically applicable to the whole hospital. The documents may be clinical in nature (e.g. how to undertake a dressing) or more administrative (e.g. how to apply for annual leave). Because these policies/procedures are so parochial, there is the potential for dissatisfaction for registered nurses who move around the same or different hospitals. Official hospital policies and procedures should be adhered to in the same manner as a legal guideline.

Unfortunately, policies often become out of date and the informal culture within an organisation may be such that it is acceptable not to follow the official policy because it is out of date. These situations should be brought to the attention of the clinical nurse consultant (or similar) so that the policy can be reviewed and reissued to reflect current practice and research. It is common for junior nursing staff to assist in the development and review of policies with assistance from their supervisor and this can be an excellent learning opportunity.

Informal and unofficial practices

Because hospitals consist of people, the element of informal, unofficial mores and procedures will exist. These can be confusing for a newcomer to the ward or organisation, as these practices are not explicit and are not included in official orientation manuals. Preceptors or co-workers may be helpful in enlightening new colleagues on these matters. However, it is more likely such practices will be learnt through observation at best, and trial and error at worst. Perceptions of competency or seniority among ward staff are often linked to familiarity with the unofficial culture.

CONFLICT MANAGEMENT

Conflict is a natural and unavoidable aspect of any setting of human life. Conflict occurs when individuals have different needs or desires or when they have different ideas about the best way to meet goals. Conflict can be useful and lead to positive change or, at least, allow discussion of issues so that some sort of resolution can be achieved. Unfortunately, conflict can also be destructive, causing personal anguish as well as decreased productivity.

Types of conflict

Registered nurses regularly experience conflict during the course of their work, whether it is during their day-to-day work practices or secondary to larger organisational conflict. The three major types of conflict that occur within healthcare organisations are intrapersonal, interpersonal and intergroup conflict.

Intrapersonal conflict occurs within an individual rather than between individuals.

CASE STUDY 5.1: INTRAPERSONAL CONFLICT

After Hiong had finished her graduate year on an oncology ward she felt unsure of the next step to take in her career. A lot of her fellow graduates were going overseas on a working holiday – something she had always wanted to do. On the other hand, she felt that perhaps she should consolidate her experience a little more before she went. After all, she had only worked on one ward; she should probably move to another area to increase her confidence and experience. She did like her ward though, and that was another problem. The nurse educator and charge nurse were really nice and they were strongly encouraging Hiong to take a place in the Graduate Diploma in Oncology. Hiong did like oncology but she wondered if it was only because she had not tried anything else.

REFLECTIVE QUESTIONS
- What if Hiong left and then decided she wanted to return?
- What are some of the intrapersonal conflicts Hiong may be experiencing?

Interpersonal conflict occurs between individuals in the work environment. If two people are on an equivalent power level, interpersonal disagreements may simply cause annoyance. However, if one person has real or perceived authority over the other, the situation has the potential to lead to conflict.

CASE STUDY 5.2: INTERPERSONAL CONFLICT

As a new graduate, Zarina was assigned a preceptor called Darryl. At first Zarina was grateful for his help, but as she grew more confident she started to think that Darryl didn't always know as much as he made out. She wanted him to treat her the same as any registered nurse on the ward, but he just wouldn't leave her alone and kept giving her long, boring lectures that slowed her up when she was trying to get her work done and made her look silly in front of her patients. Zarina didn't know how to deal with it. She wanted to brush him off but she worried that he would turn nasty – after all, he was often in charge of the shift. What if he started allocating her the hardest patients or told the charge nurse that she wasn't performing well? Zarina dreaded going to work when she knew that Darryl was also rostered on.

Intergroup conflict occurs between professional groups or different departments.

CASE STUDY 5.3: INTERGROUP CONFLICT

One thing Matt felt quite confident in when he graduated was stoma care. He had undertaken quite a few placements where patients had stomas, but when he got a job in a surgical ward he was surprised to find there was a nurse employed in the very grand-sounding job of stomal therapy consultant. One day, as he was educating a patient about his stoma care, the charge nurse apologised for interrupting but asked him to come to her office straight away. When he arrived, he found the stomal therapist there also. Matt sat there in disbelief as the two senior nurses told him that he was not to perform stoma care or education with his patients, as this was not in his role. When he protested that he felt it was within his abilities they became quite short with him. Didn't he appreciate how lucky he was to work in a place with such a resource? It was people like him who were jeopardising professional opportunities and specialised nurses, they said. Matt went home that night feeling so angry that he wanted to resign.

Conflict resolution strategies

Various options exist for conflict resolution:

- Compromise/collaboration: the conflicting parties work together to reach a mutually satisfactory outcome.
- Competition: one party attempts to defeat any opposition.
- Cooperation/accommodation: in this case one party gives in or smoothes over the conflict.
- Avoidance/withdrawal: the individual avoids any attempts to resolve the conflict or pretends it does not exist.

Deciding which strategy to choose can become a challenge, and depends on the following:

- the urgency with which the conflict must be resolved
- the power/status of the person you are experiencing conflict with
- how important you perceive the issue to be
- previous experience and comfort within conflict situations
- personal factors such as being tired and having other worries on your mind.

Conflict resolution in the healthcare organisation

Conflict may not always be able to be resolved to the satisfaction of all parties but, if patience and willingness to appreciate another's point of view and a focus on shared goals are present, there is a good chance that at least an acceptable compromise can be reached. Conflict for nurses in the workplace should always be resolved with the emphasis on patient safety and quality care first, and then with regard to what is the best outcome for the majority of staff.

Compromise for a 'win–win' situation is often promoted as the preferred option of conflict management, but this should be carefully considered. In situations where patient care is jeopardised, an urgent and even non-consultative decision must be made. In these situations the authority of the nurse leader/s should be sought. However, more minor grievances should be resolved by those involved.

CONCLUSION

This chapter presents an overview of the traditional bureaucratic organisational structure and examines the way in which professional bureaucratic structures have evolved within health services in Australia. Illustrations are provided of three common organisational designs, namely the functional, divisional and matrix designs, as well as a discussion on the differences between the public and private hospital environment in Australia. Understanding the structure, design and purpose of healthcare organisations gives staff an awareness of how organisations operate and how organisational culture is developed. In addition to providing an understanding of organisational structures, the chapter outlines the role and function of registering bodies, professional colleges and nursing unions in setting standards, conditions of employment and approaches to initial and ongoing nursing education. The chapter concludes with a discussion on key elements of organisational climate and the areas of potential conflict in healthcare organisations.

CASE STUDY 5.4: ORGANISATIONAL CULTURE

After graduation, Jessica worked on a surgical ward in a large city hospital which was committed to evidence-based practice. Policies for wound dressings were updated regularly to reflect the latest research. After a few years Jessica returned to her home town and started work at the local hospital. During orientation she was shocked to learn that wound care policies differed for each surgeon. For example, laparotomy wounds were washed in the shower for surgeon A, with antiseptic for surgeon B and with saline for surgeon C. The nurses seemed to have little idea or interest in what wound research had been done.

Jessica tried to discuss her frustrations with her colleagues but could not convince them to work towards a standardised best-practice approach. 'You'll never get the surgeons to agree' and 'We don't have much infection, so it probably doesn't matter which way we do the dressings' were common statements. After a while Jessica just gave in and learnt each surgeon's preference. She had succumbed to the ward culture.

REFLECTIVE QUESTION

• Why did Jessica succumb to the ward culture?

CASE STUDY 5.5: HUMAN RESOURCES MANAGEMENT CONFLICT

At a ward meeting, the nursing staff decide they would like to trial 12-hour shifts, which would mean working only 3 days per week. The nurse manager is supportive and agrees to look into the matter. There is excitement in the ward until the nurse manager reports back that the Nurses Act prohibits 12-hour shifts and that the Nursing Union is against any change to this. Ward staff express frustration and disbelief that they are to be stopped doing something that they all want because of what they see as 'red tape'.

REFLECTIVE QUESTION

• Can you think of other examples of human resources management conflict?

RECOMMENDED READING

Daly J, Speedy S, Jackson D, editors. Nursing leadership. Sydney: Churchill Livingstone; 2004.

Malloch K, Porter-O'Grady T. The quantum leader: applications for the new world of work. Boston: Jones and Bartlett; 2005.

Marriner-Tomey A. Guide to nursing management and leadership. St Louis: Mosby; 2000.

Mick SS, Wyttenbach ME, editors. Advances in health care organization theory. San Francisco: Jossey-Bass; 2003.

Porter-O'Grady T, Malloch K. Quantum leadership: a textbook of new leadership. Boston: Jones and Bartlett; 2003.

REFERENCES

1. Shortell SM, Kaluzny AD. Health care management: organisational design and behavior. New York: Delmar; 1994.
2. Maddern J, Courtney M, Montgomery J, et al. Strategy and organisational design in health care in managing health services: concepts and practice. 2nd ed. Sydney: Elsevier Mosby; 2006.
3. Marquis BL, Huston CJ. Leadership roles and management functions in nursing: theory and application. 5th ed. Philadelphia: Lippincott; 2006.
4. Taylor FW. The principles of scientific management. New York: Harper; 1911.
5. Mintzberg H. Organisation design: fashion or fit? Harvard Business Review 1981;Jan–Feb:103–16.
6. Southon G. Health service structures, management and professional practice: beyond clinical management. Australian Health Review 1996;19:1–5.
7. Charns MP. Changing health care organisations for increased effectiveness. Australian Health Review 1984;7:98–105.
8. Shapiro M. A career ladder based on Benner's model. Journal of Nursing Administration 1998;28:13–9.
9. Royal College of Nursing, Australia. Memorandum of Association and Articles of Association. Canberra: Royal College of Nursing, Australia; 1994.
10. Nursing and Midwifery Board of Australia. Online. Available from: http://www.nursingmidwiferyboard.gov.au/About-the-Board.aspx 20 December 2010.
11. Scott-Findlay S, Estabrook CA. Mapping the organizational culture research in nursing: a literature review. Journal of Advanced Nursing 2006;56:498–513.
12. Hemmelgarn AL, Glisson C, James LR. Organizational culture and climate: implications for services and interventions research. Clinical Psychology: Science and Practice 2006;13:73–89.
13. Cameron KS, Quinn RE. Diagnosing and changing organizational culture. Reading: Addison-Wesley; 1999.
14. Gifford BD, Zammuto RF, Goodman EA, et al. The relationship between hospital unit culture and nurses' quality of work life. Journal of Healthcare Management 2002, 47:13–26.
15. Sovie MD. Hospital culture—why create one? Nursing Economics 1993;11: 69–75.
16. Chapman L, Howkins E. Developing a learning culture. Nursing Management 2001;8:10–3.
17. Calpin-Davies PJ. Management and leadership: a dual role in nursing education. Nurse Education Today 2003;23:3–10.
18. Legge D, Stanton P, Smyth A. Learning management (and managing your own learning). In: Harris MG, editor. Managing health services: concepts and practice. 2nd ed. Sydney: Elsevier Mosby; 2005.

CHAPTER 6

Preparing for role transition

Kathleen Milton-Wildey and Suzanne Rochester

LEARNING OBJECTIVES

When you have completed this chapter you will be able to:

- understand the influence of social processes on nursing role acquisition
- demonstrate an awareness of the elements of role stress
- examine ways of reducing role stress
- appreciate the importance of positive role models and a positive self-concept to successful transition
- undertake a number of activities in preparation for transition and during transition that will enhance coping.

Keywords: transition, role acquisition, work relationships, role stress, coping

---

INTRODUCTION

Role theory provides student nurses with a useful theoretical perspective from which to consider their beginning practice. In this chapter we will explore the following aspects of role theory in relation to transition:

- roles and society
- role acquisition – primary, secondary and tertiary
- role stress – incongruity, conflict, ambiguity
- maintenance of role relationships and a positive self-concept.

In your new role as a nursing graduate you will face a period of transition when your university-acquired values, ideals and behaviours will require some adjustment in order to meet the expectations of the clinical setting.[1–5] Transition from nursing student to registered nurse is a challenging process that you will find both exciting and rewarding. During this period you will experience rapid growth as a person and as a professional nurse, and as a result of this process you are likely to experience emotional highs and lows. It is likely that you will feel some anxiety and apprehension about how well you will function in your new role and whether or not you will meet the expectations of the institution, your colleagues and your patients.[6] No amount of prior learning or experience can completely prepare you for role transition but thoughtful preparation can help to ease the stress and strain.[7] In this chapter we focus on furthering your understanding of the role of the registered nurse and how you can prepare yourself to meet the organisational expectations of your role performance during transition by utilising role theory as the underlying perspective.

ROLES IN SOCIETY

Roles are assigned to individuals and groups in society because they describe predictable and patterned behaviour. In other words, each recognisable role has certain behaviours that are associated with it. This process makes it easier for us to function because we know what to expect from others. Each member of society can hold a myriad of roles at any one time; our immediate role may change from one situation to the next; and we can play numerous roles across the course of our life. Furthermore, the way we regard ourselves is highly dependent on the roles we hold and how they are valued by the people that interact with us. Learning to conform to role expectations starts when we are very young because most people seek the approval and acceptance of others: the approval of others is a strong motivation to conform throughout our lives. The feeling that one does not fit in can be uncomfortable and can influence us to adapt our behaviour very quickly in order to be accepted by the group to which we want to belong.[8] To resist the pressure to conform can be difficult; however, in some situations if the behaviour change required by the group is so great that we feel our behaviour is no longer acceptable to ourselves, or if it requires more effort to maintain our behaviour than we are willing or able to give, this can prove to be just as uncomfortable. Such feelings may lead to role relinquishment and group abandonment.[8]

One way of looking at your behaviour is to see yourself as an actor playing a part and following scripts that direct your performance. The first notions that led to the development of role theory were generated in this way.[9–11] Our role scripts contain the rules about how others in society expect us to behave. Many of our roles come to us because of our abilities, education and training and these are more likely to be formal, in that they have an identifying role name and are tightly controlled – that is, they are more tightly scripted by society. The registered nurse role is a good example as the practice of registered nurses is regulated and subject to codes of conduct, ethics and standards.[12,13] All professional groups experience this type of role control. However, there remain many aspects of a professional role, no matter how formal, that are not always clearly scripted or accessible. These aspects can be situation- and/ or context-dependent. Expectations of the registered nurse role can therefore differ according to whether the nurse is working in a hospital ward or in the community. Even experienced nurses will talk about the challenge of meeting set expectations when moving from one specialty area to another.[14] Most nurses will never fully understand their professional role until they are experiencing or acting their part. Furthermore, script expectations may not become clear to an actor until the person transgresses the role boundaries or does not fully address what is expected by inter-dependent others. When expectations are not met, fellow actors exert pressure to control an actor's behaviour in order to bring it into line with expectations. Resisting the pressure to conform takes a good deal of effort and resolve on the part of an actor.

A word of advice: even though acceptance by nursing colleagues will be crucial to your professional development and comfort in the clinical setting, it should not come at the cost of losing the values you developed at university.[1] Furthermore, the responsibility to make role expectations 'right' is not a task for the new graduate alone. The tertiary sector and industry are also responsible and need to work towards removing the incongruity between sector expectations that can make beginning practice for the new graduate more stressful than necessary.[15]

Learning the role of the registered nurse, like other formal roles in society, involves not only acquiring knowledge about the role and all its dimensions but also an aware-ness that there are aspects of the role that are only accessible through experience. Careful preparation is essential to a smooth transition, and of equal importance is the acceptance that your conception of the nursing role now will be altered to some degree by exposure to the expectations of others in the workplace.

Primary and secondary role acquisition

As mentioned above, role acquisition is a social process. Your decision to become a registered nurse has evolved over time and can be divided into primary, secondary and tertiary phases.

During the primary phase of socialisation you internalised values, beliefs and behaviours from significant others that motivated you to become a nursing student.[16] This motivation is in part related to an internalised set of expectations about the nursing role, expectations that have probably been altered in many ways by your education. Exercise 6.1 will allow you to compare your earlier expectations of nursing with the ones you hold now; it will be interesting to consider how your perceptions have changed over time.

EXERCISE 6.1 CHANGING IMAGES OF THE NURSING ROLE

- If you had been asked on your first day of university to draw an image of a nurse, what would you have drawn? How would the nurse have looked? What would the nurse have been doing? In what role situation would you have depicted the nurse?
- What aspects of the above picture would you like to change? What parts do you feel should stay the same? Consider the ways in which your image of nursing and the nursing role has changed over the course of your studies.
- Discuss these findings with your study group.

Secondary socialisation has to do with acquiring knowledge, skills and dispositions such as those you have learnt during your university program.[16] Your present image of the nursing role has been shaped by this process, and this is probably evident from your reflection in Exercise 6.1. It is during this phase that your professional values and standards are formed and integrated with a developing understanding of the nursing profession's scope of practice and variety of service. Despite an almost completed undergraduate education, however, you may still feel somewhat unclear about what the registered nurse role fully encompasses. A good place to begin to increase your understanding is by reviewing the various codes and standards that apply to practice as a registered nurse.

An understanding of the codes and standards that apply to the professional behaviour of registered nurses is essential for student nurses who are preparing for transition. Australian undergraduate nursing programs aim to address the standards developed by the Australian Nursing and Midwifery Council (ANMC) within its curricula, and this then forms the basis for curriculum approval by the registration board. In addition, universities and health facilities use these standards for the clinical assessment of students and new graduates.[12] The ANMC has also developed codes of professional[17] and ethical[18] conduct for nurses in Australia.

The competencies address not only the expected standards for registered nurses, but also the competencies related to enrolled nursing.[19] It is important that enrolled nurses who upgrade their qualifications to become registered nurses understand that there are higher expectations of professional behaviour in the new role. As is often the case when you have been successfully working in an associated role, elements such as a sense of responsibility and accountability can be underestimated or discounted in regard to the new and more responsible role and result in increased stress.[5] For graduating students who entered their Bachelor of Nursing with enrolled nurse qualifications it may be beneficial to discuss with registered nurses from similar educational backgrounds the challenging aspects of their transition to the workforce. This process allows graduates to 'reframe their practice' within the realities of the work setting.[6] Simulated learning experiences may also serve to provide a feeling of the responsibility and accountability associated with the new role that is not achievable through clinical practicum because the nurse is always in the student role.

Exercise 6.2 suggests that you review the ANMC standards for the registered nurse and compare these competencies with those that guide the practice of the enrolled nurse. By undertaking this activity you will become clearer about your role in relation to a closely associated role. This activity will provide you with a clearer understanding of the competencies of a group of health workers that you will often supervise in practice and to whom you will delegate responsibilities.

EXERCISE 6.2 UNDERSTANDING ROLE DIMENSIONS THROUGH THE ANMC COMPETENCY STANDARDS

- Review the ANMC standards (www.anmc.org.au/professional_standards) for registered and enrolled nurses.
- Identify how the standards differ between the two levels of nursing.
- Discuss the implications of these differences for the registered nurse's role.

While Exercise 6.2 will broaden your understanding of the registered nurse role, your understanding will be greatly enhanced by exploring with a clinical nurse the application of these standards in practice. Exercise 6.3 explores how the national competency standards are expressed by a registered nurse in the workplace.

EXERCISE 6.3 EXPLORING HOW THE ANMC COMPETENCY STANDARDS ARE INTEGRATED IN NURSING PRACTICE

- Interview a second- or third-year graduate nurse or nurses.
- Explore with the nurse/s the meaning of the ANMC competency standards.
- Ask the nurse/s how the ANMC competency standards are addressed in their present role.
- Compare the responses of the registered nurse/s interviewed.
- Discuss the factors that promote or hinder integration of the ANMC competency standards in practice.

Tertiary role acquisition

Tertiary socialisation takes place when you enter specific work situations as an employee.[20] At this point you will be required to demonstrate the expected behaviours associated with your professional role. It is often the case that the beliefs, values and behaviours developed through primary and secondary socialisation do not fit easily or exactly into the institution in which you have chosen to work. As role acquisition is a lifelong process, you have entered a new and important phase of learning that focuses on acquiring the values and norms relevant to the clinical context. A nursing identity is formed during this phase and the values and attitudes learnt in other phases of socialisation may be changed or modified.

Your role set will have a significant influence on your behaviour during your transition. A role set is made up of role partners who have an interdependent role relationship with you, for example medical staff, your nursing unit manager, other nurses and your patients.[21] It is important that you have a clear idea of who your role partners are and their areas of responsibility and skill. This knowledge will help you function more effectively as a group member.

Each member of your role set will be affected in some way by what you say or do, and will have attitudes and beliefs about what to expect from you in your role as a registered nurse. Sometimes these attitudes and beliefs will differ from your own expectations of your role and you will experience role conflict. Part of successful preparation for practice should include an exploration of the role of interdependent others in your prospective workplace. Exercise 6.4 assists you in identifying your role set members and what their role responsibilities involve.

EXERCISE 6.4 IDENTIFYING AND UNDERSTANDING YOUR ROLE SET

- List the roles in a typical ward situation that are interdependent with nursing.
- Determine the responsibilities and skills associated with each role, and the lines of authority where applicable.
- Consider the degree of influence these roles can or should potentially exert on your practice.

ROLE STRESS

It is almost impossible for graduates to avoid some level of role stress when you consider the complex socialisation processes involved in learning how to work competently as a registered nurse.[14] Furthermore, new graduates often report that they feel unprepared for the workload, shift work and managerial responsibilities associated with the role of the registered nurse.[6,7,22–25] Many studies also indicate that graduates have difficulty maintaining what they consider to be excellence in nursing care in the face of workload expectations, and that this can result in strong feelings of stress, inadequacy, guilt and disillusionment.[2,7,14,22,25] It appears that the ideals and values new graduates learnt at university can often set them apart from other staff.[7,15,22,26]

A lack of effective collaboration between the university and the clinical institutions in regard to undergraduate nursing education is partly responsible for the role difficulties that may arise during transition. While universities focus on educating student nurses in relation to the ANMC competencies in their fullest sense, and embrace the theoretical and ideological aspects of nursing, the clinical sector continues to expect proficient 'hands-on' practitioners upon graduation.[15,24,26] Students attending clinical practicum as part of their university study are allocated to a mainly supernumerary role where they have time to consider their theoretical knowledge and how this informs their clinical actions. However, as graduate nurses they still need time to adjust these values to the reality of the hospital workplace, which can result in role stress as they attempt to grapple with the level of proficiency needed in the often resource- and staff-constrained clinical settings.[8] Moreover, this high expectation by clinicians in healthcare facilities for all graduates to be competent and accountable for clinical decisions can be even more stressful for those graduates who have an initial qualification.[7] This discontinuity between sectors leads to a general lack of recognition of the graduate as a new practitioner and a misunderstanding of the graduate's educational preparation.[24,26] Pressure is often exerted by a graduate's role set to control and regulate the behaviour of novice nurses in line with the traditional norms set by the clinical sector.

It would be a great loss to the nursing profession if frameworks for practice developed at university, such as critical thinking, reflective practice, evidence-based practice and cultural safety, were abandoned by the graduate in order to 'fit in' with a controlling social environment. There is room to move on both sides; that is, for nurse clinicians and nurse educators to work together to implement innovative programs or strategies to redress the discontinuity. An example of such a strategy can be the design of clinical practicums in the final year of the degree, which provide nursing students with experiences that mirror the reality of the hospital workplace they will encounter on graduation. This can, for example, include the allocation of several patients of different dependency levels so students can learn to plan and complete their caring practices competently within the expected timeframe. Clinical experiences such as this may offer the best opportunity for maintaining the theoretical frameworks for practice while still achieving the requirements of their professional role, especially, if these students are also given adequate support and understanding during this practicum by staff while they learn to cope with the pressures and expectations of the workplace. Role stress can be reduced if tertiary programs endeavour to prepare graduates more realistically for transition, and industry eases the process of transition for new graduate nurses by respecting their achievements and supporting their beginning practice.[7,22,24,26,27]

Types of role stress

Four types of role stress have been identified – (1) role incongruity; (2) role conflict; (3) role ambiguity; and (4) role overload – and it would be unusual for new graduates not to experience some degree of strain on commencing work. Role strain is the outward expression of stress that can be evident in your behaviour.[28] You may feel frustration, tension or anxiety in response to role stress, which may result in distancing, denial and avoidance.[29] These negative effects can eventually have an impact on your patient care and your relationships with others, and so it is important to try and identify the symptoms when they occur.

Role incongruity

This aspect of role stress is largely cognitive and is related to the dissonance in values or self-concept between the nurse and the institution in which the nurse works.[30] Case study 6.1 illustrates role incongruity where the nurse's personal skills or values about the nursing role may not align with the requirements of the role as expected by the health facility. Role incongruity can be lessened in situations where the work environment encourages open communication and reciprocal exchange between staff. Your interpersonal skills, respect for others, a willingness to listen and self-reflection are important considerations here.

CASE STUDY 6.1

During the first few weeks working on his new ward, Graham admitted he felt frustrated and stressed because he was not able to provide patient care at the standard he had been educated to provide. He was resentful of the other staff who he believed did not care that his patient care was being compromised.

REFLECTIVE QUESTIONS

* Do your values about your caring role differ from those of the other nurses working on your ward?
* What could account for the difference in values between nursing staff?
* How can Graham resolve this situation and find a way to work with the other nursing staff, while maintaining his own values?

Many nurses resolve their role incongruity by developing a pragmatic and multi-dimensional understanding of nursing values and their professional self-concept. When this occurs, the nurse is able to integrate the nursing values that incorporate holism and caring for the humanistic needs of the patient with the professional role of nursing, while maintaining loyalty to the institution and its work values, rules and regulations. Others are able to change or adapt to difficult situations by developing resilience.[14] Some nurses, however, are not able to move on and may decide to leave nursing or to capitulate their own values fully to the values of the institution.[31] It is up to each nurse to reflect on the continuing expectations of his or her role. Unless nurses are prepared to reflect honestly on their practice, it is difficult to resist task–oriented and ritualised care based on the bureaucratic ideals of efficiency and conformity. Exercise 6.5 will encourage you to challenge your perceptions and expectations of your clinical role and can be utilised for continuing professional development.

EXERCISE 6.5 REFLECTION ON PRACTICE

- Reflect back on your student role activities during clinical practice.
- Consider what percentage of your time was task-focused.
- Determine in comparison the amount of your time that was spent on professional or holistic patient care activities.
- What are the implications of your findings for transition?

Role conflict

Role conflict involves the recognition of the urge to act in different ways to what one may want, because of different role pressures. Compliance with role pressure from one source will make compliance with another difficult, and affect both behaviour and feelings. This conflict can occur within the nurse or between two or more individuals who have different perceptions of the role to be enacted.[28] One example of role conflict can be encountered when graduate nurses feel pressurised because of competing priorities in the work role. Conflicting situations can arise during times when the ward may have inadequate or less experienced staff. Case study 6.2 demonstrates the conflict a nurse can experience between work and personal role pressures.

CASE STUDY 6.2

During the night Roger's 3-year-old daughter, Lindy, was ill with a high fever and, although her temperature had subsided, she was not well enough to be left at the kindergarten. Roger, a single parent, did not have close family support or friends who could help. He was feeling stressed about his conflict as he would prefer to remain home and care for Lindy. He was 'rostered on' for the day shift and he knew that if he did not go to work his nurse unit manager would be angry. Roger did not want to let his manager and the other staff down but he really wanted to stay at home and be with Lindy.

REFLECTIVE QUESTIONS
- What would you do in this situation?
- How would you approach the nursing unit manager if you found you were unable to work your shift because of a personal matter?
- What could Roger do to avoid a similar situation of role conflict in the future?

If work role requirements are not completed at the set times expected during the shift, then role conflict may develop between the nurse and any other interdependent role set member or group. One way to avoid this type of role conflict is to organise a plan at the beginning of the shift concerning which aspects of the work role need to be actioned within set periods of time. Staff will be more supportive if they see that there is a determined effort to complete aspects of the role within an expected timeframe. Another example of role conflict can be caused by personal demands which have an impact on the work role.

Because of a general misunderstanding of the nursing role, particularly in regard to relatively recent changes in nursing education and career development, nurses often face this type of role conflict. It is in the interest of the nursing discipline that these situations are negotiated in a way that promotes the status of nurses and enlightens the understanding of others.

Role ambiguity

Situations arise for new graduates where expectations by role set members are not clearly expressed, leaving graduates feeling confused and uncertain of their role behaviour.[28] Expectations of the new nurse may be unstated and only found when reflected in the values and behaviour of other staff. These expectations include the impressions that role partners have developed about the position of new staff members and these may be adapted for each new employee. Exercise 6.6 may be useful in determining the unstated role expectations that exist in your prospective workplace.

EXERCISE 6.6 EXAMINING THE INFLUENCE OF ROLE PARTNERS' EXPECTATIONS

- Reflect on an incident during one of your clinical placements where you felt your practice was inconsistent with what other staff expected.
- Describe the people who were in your role set at that time.
- Write a short summary, or illustrate the experience with a diagram.
- In retrospect, what do you feel the expectations of your role partners were?
- Were these expectations stated or unstated norms of the clinical setting?
- Explore the effect of your role partners' expectations on your nursing practice and self-concept during this incident and since.
- What did you learn from this experience?

Role overload

This type of role stress occurs when graduates are unable to meet all of the expectations of their role.[28] Aspects of their work that new graduates often find difficult include time management, adapting to shift work, lack of managerial abilities and getting through the volume of work required in times when staff shortages are a common occurrence in the healthcare sector. Case study 6.3 presents an example of role overload new nurses may experience in attempting to meet time management commitments on the ward.

CASE STUDY 6.3

Joanne, a new graduate nurse, was not enjoying her role as a registered nurse on a busy medical ward. She explained that caring for her patients was very satisfying but sometimes she was not able to complete her work on time. She felt that this affected her relationship with the other nurses and when she asked them questions or needed help they sometimes ignored her.

- If this situation occurred to you, how would you feel?
- How would you respond in a similar situation?
- How could you prevent a similar situation from occurring again?

To prepare yourself for this particular role stress, it may be helpful for you to experience a facilitated clinical block that includes exposure to shift work and managerial responsibilities similar to those undertaken by new graduate nurses.

It is important that you recognise the symptoms associated with the four types of role stress and seek support to balance their negative effects. One important piece of advice is to find out as much as possible about the institution you are joining as this may assist in making your transition much smoother. Of particular note is whether or not the facility offers supportive initiatives such as orientation, supervision and preceptor programs.

If you recognise that you are feeling role strain it is your responsibility to develop a number of personal coping strategies. These may include seeking assistance from other staff, graduate peers and/or family and friends, activating your existing coping mechanisms, or simply having fun and maintaining activities outside the work role.

Maintenance of role relationships and self-concept

Finding support from role models or peers and learning to manage your emotions and relationships more effectively during transition can make a significant difference to your self-concept as a beginning nurse. Your self-concept is the way in which you see yourself: it is related to your emotional and social intelligence and is important because it influences your behaviour towards others. Your beginning nursing self-concept, which is your sense of who you are as a nurse upon graduation, has developed through your interaction with others, principally your nursing lecturers, clinical facilitators, peer group and patients. Once these reactions are internalised they become part of your image of yourself and set up your self-expectations.[5,22,25,31] In your beginning practice you will attempt to meet these expectations.

Self-esteem is enhanced by positive feedback from others that supports and aligns with the expectations you hold for yourself in the role of a registered nurse. If you receive negative responses about your role, your self-concept may be called into question and you may experience a degree of self-doubt. Figure 6.1 presents activities that may assist you in maintaining your self-esteem during times of self-doubt in the nursing role.[32]

Reflect on positive aspects of your practice as a nurse

Search out other nurses who will provide support and encouragement

Involve yourself in work projects that will offer you a sense of achievement

Develop supportive personal affirmations based on your known strengths

Recognise that it is unrealistic to expect to be liked by all your colleagues or to succeed at everything you do

Fig 6.1 Advice for maintaining positive self-esteem.

A positive self-concept can only be maintained over time if your role partners and peers acknowledge your contribution.[32] A strategy that will help you in this regard is to find a supportive role model. A role model is someone you admire and identify with, someone whose professional characteristics you value.[26,31,33] If you are able to form a relationship with this person you could approach your role model for advice and support in times of stress. Role models can also act as mentors and assist you in achieving your career goals.[30,31,33] This relationship should be positive, constructive, developmental and grounded in reality. It should enhance your self-esteem and make you feel more accepted as a nurse. A good mentor can contribute to your role satisfaction.[31,33,34,35]

Also, a support network made up of your peers can be a useful asset in maintaining a healthy self-concept during transition.[29] In most instances, when you commence employment you will attend an orientation program with other new graduates. This is an opportune time to discuss with these colleagues the notion of forming your own support network. By meeting on a regular basis, either face to face or online, this group could help you cope with your new role and the changes you will have to face in adapting your self-concept to the reality of the workplace. Mutual sharing of the highs and lows can be extremely useful in relieving role stress. In addition, forming a new-graduate group can be helpful in raising issues with management and lobbying for change within the institution that would be of benefit to new graduates.

As you are well aware, how you feel and relate to others is closely aligned to your emotions; and as transition is often a period of heightened emotions, developing your emotional intelligence is another invaluable means of coping and of managing your relationships with members of your role set. Emotional intelligence, as defined by Goleman,[36] is characterised by five attributes: (1) self-awareness; (2) self-regulation; (3) motivation; (4) empathy; and (5) social skills. These attributes allow us to recognise the early signs of emotional stress in ourselves and control subsequent behaviour with others, and this is particularly useful when our self-concept is under threat. Emotional intelligence helps us understand the emotions of others and behave towards them with this understanding in mind.[29] You can become more emotionally intelligent by critically reflecting on your behaviour and focusing on the part your emotional reactions played in motivating that behaviour.[29,37] This reflection, in light of further reading on emotional intelligence, will heighten your self-awareness.

CONCLUSION

This chapter has discussed aspects of role theory that will help you in preparing for transition. The acquisition of the nursing role is a social process that undergoes primary, secondary and tertiary phases. During the primary phase, significant people in your life were influential in shaping the values and beliefs within you that motivated you to study nursing. You are now almost at the end of your secondary phase of socialisation where a university program has provided you with the knowledge, skills and dispositions appropriate for practice as a registered nurse. During this phase your ideals and values about the nursing role have been enhanced through academic study and clinical exposure. The primary and secondary phases of role acquisition have been synthesised to form your nursing role expectations. Your expectations will now undergo another stage of development during transition.

Transition is a period of highs and lows when the realities of the clinical setting and the expectations of your role partners will exert pressure on your present image of yourself as a nurse. Transition is not an easy process, but the role stress that may occur can be moderated by thoughtful preparation, formal and informal support strategies, developing and maintaining a positive self-concept and personal resources, including emotional intelligence. We hope that this chapter has provided you with useful strategies to improve role stress and strain and smooth your personal experience of transition.

RECOMMENDED READING

Duchscher J, Myrick F. The prevailing winds of oppression: understanding the new graduate experience in acute care. Nursing Forum 2008;43:191–206.

Fox K. Mentor program boosts new nurses' satisfaction and lowers turnover rate. Journal of Continuing Education in Nursing 2010;41:311–6.

Hayes B, Bonner A, Pryor J. Factors contributing to nurse job satisfaction in the acute hospital setting: a review of recent literature. Journal of Nursing Management 2010;18:804–14.

Latham C, Hogan M, Ringl K. Nurses supporting nurses. Creating a mentoring program for staff nurses to improve the workforce environment. Nurse Administration 2008;32:27–39.

Wangensteen S, Johansson I, Nordstrom G. The first year as a graduate nurse – an experience of growth and development. Journal of Clinical Nursing 2008;17: 1877–85.

REFERENCES

1. Duchscher J. A process of becoming: the stages of new graduate professional role transition. Journal of Continuing Education in Nursing 2008;39:441–50.
2. Duchscher J, Myrick F. The prevailing winds of oppression: understanding the new graduate experience in acute care. Nursing Forum 2008;43:191–206.
3. White J. The client and the healthcare environment. In: Crisp J, Taylor C, editors. Potter and Perry's fundamentals of nursing. 3rd ed. Sydney: Mosby/Elsevier; 2009.
4. Beecroft P, Dorey F, Wenten M. Turnover intention in new graduate nurses: a multivariate analysis. Journal of Advanced Nursing 2008;62:41–52.
5. Mooney M. Facing registration: the expectations and the unexpected. Nurse Education Today 2007;27:840–7.
6. Hodges H, Keeley A, Troyan P. Professional resilience in baccalaureate-prepared acute care nurses: first steps. Nursing Education Research 2008;29:80–9.
7. Kelly J, Ahern K. Preparing nurses for practice: a phenomenological study of the new graduate in Australia. Journal of Clinical Nursing 2008;18:910–8.
8. Milton-Wildey K, O'Brien L. Care of acutely ill older patients in hospital: clinical decision-making. Journal of Clinical Nursing 2010;19:1252–60.
9. Michener H. Social psychology. Toronto: Wadsworth; 2004.
10. Goffman E. Presentation of self in everyday life. New York: Anchor Books; 1959.
11. Harre R, Secord P. The explanation of social behaviour. Oxford: Blackwell; 1972.

12. Wilson V. Introduction to nursing, midwifery and health. In: Dempsey J, French J, Hillege S, et al., editors. Fundamentals of nursing and midwifery. A person-centred approach to care. Sydney: Wolters Kluwer/Lippincott, Williams & Wilkins; 2009.

13. Australian Nursing and Midwifery Council. ANMC National competency standards for the registered nurse. Canberra: ACT; 2006. Online. Available: http://www.nursingmidwiferyboard.gov.au/Codes-and-Guidelines.aspx

14. Duddle M, Boughton M. Intraprofessional relations in nursing. Journal of Advanced Nursing 2007;59:29–37.

15. Parry J. Intention to leave the profession: antecedents and role in nurse turnover. Journal of Advanced Nursing 2008;64:157–67.

16. Poole M. Socialisation and the new genetics. In: Germov J, Poole M, editors. Public sociology. An introduction to Australian society. Australia: Allen & Unwin; 2007.

17. Australian Nursing and Midwifery Council. ANMC Code of professional conduct for registered nurses. Canberra: ACT; 2006 Revised. Online. Available: http://www.nursingmidwiferyboard.gov.au/Codes-and-Guidelines.aspx

18. Australian Nursing and Midwifery Council. ANMC Code of ethics for the registered nurses. Canberra: ACT; 2002 Revised. Online. Available: http://www.nursingmidwiferyboard.gov.au/Codes-and-Guidelines.aspx

19. Australian Nursing and Midwifery Council. ANMC National competency standards for the enrolled nurse. Canberra: ACT; 2006 Revised. Online. Available: http://www.nursingmidwiferyboard.gov.au/Codes-and-Guidelines.aspx

20. Roy C. Introduction to nursing: an adaptation model. 2nd ed. New Jersey: Prentice Hall; 1984.

21. MacGuire J. The function of the 'set' in hospital controlled schemes of nurse training. In: Smith J, editor. Sociology and nursing. Edinburgh: Churchill Livingstone; 1968.

22. Duchscher J. Transition shock: the initial stage of role adaptation for newly graduated registered nurses. Journal of Advanced Nursing 2009;65:1103–13.

23. Lavoie-Tremblay M, O'Brien-Pallas L, Gelinas C, et al. Addressing the turnover issue among new nurses from a generational viewpoint. Journal of Nursing Management 2008;16:724–33.

24. Romyn D, Linton N, Giblin C, et al. Successful transition of the new graduate nurse. International Journal of Nursing Education Scholarship 2009;6: article 34.

25. Newton J, McKenna L. Uncovering knowing in practice during the graduate year: an exploratory study. Contemporary Nurse 2009;31:153–62.

26. Morrow S. New graduate transitions: leaving the next, joining the flight. Journal of Nursing Management 2009;17:278–87.

27. Burns P, Poster E. Competency development in new registered nurse graduates: closing the gap between education and practice. Journal of Continuing Education in Nursing 2008;9:67–73.

28. Hardy M, Conway M. Role theory. USA: Appleton & Lange; 1988.

29. Stein-Parbury J. Patient and person. Interpersonal skills in nursing. 4th ed. Sydney: Elsevier Australia/Churchill Livingstone; 2009.

30. Benner P, Benner R. The new nurse's work entry: a troubled sponsorship. New York: Tiresias Press; 1979.

31 Young M, Stuenkel D, Bawel-Brinkley K. Strategies for easing the role transformation of graduate nurses. Journal for Nurses in Staff Development 2008;24: 105–10.

32 Price S. Becoming a nurse: a meta-study of early professional socialization and career choice in nursing. Journal of Advanced Nursing 2009;65:11–9.

33. Niven N. The psychology of nursing care. 2nd ed. New York: Palgrave Macmillan; 2006.

34. Murray T, Crain C, Meyer G, et al. Building bridges: an innovative academic-service partnership. Nursing Outlook 2010;58:252–60.

35. Weng R, Huang C, Tsai W, et al. Exploring the impact of mentoring functions on job satisfaction and organizational commitment of new staff nurses. BMC Health Services Research 2010;10:1–9.

36. Goleman D. Emotional intelligence: why it can matter more than IQ. London: Bloomsbury; 1996.

37. Akerjordet K, Severinsson E. The state of the science of emotional intelligence related to nursing leadership: an integrative review. Journal of Nursing Management 2010;18:363–82.

CHAPTER 7

Processes of change in bureaucratic environments

Patrick Crookes, Kenneth Walsh and Angela Brown

LEARNING OBJECTIVES

When you have completed this chapter you will be able to:

- examine a realistic yet constructive introduction to the culture of innovation in contemporary nursing
- understand the imperative of developing effective nursing leaders in the years to come
- reflect upon practical and theoretical knowledge regarding ways in which one can function and actively participate in decision making in rapidly changing environments
- identify ways of dealing with the stresses involved in working in rapidly changing environments
- devote time to thinking now about being a leader of the future.

Keywords: transformational leadership, transactional leadership, oppressed group behaviour, self-empowerment, change management

---

INTRODUCTION

This chapter discusses the forces that operate within bureaucratic environments and the impact upon individuals and groups within them. It also discusses some of the positive movements towards assisting innovation and change in these environments.

Change can be likened to a fast-flowing river: it continues remorselessly and it is very easy to get caught up in its currents. Once you are within a context where change is happening all around you, it becomes very difficult to do anything other than work extremely hard to keep your head above water. This is the situation for many nurses when they take up their first position in health services. However, as we shall see, it is not a situation that is peculiar either to nursing or to relatively inexperienced people.

WHAT IS AN ORGANISATIONAL BUREAUCRACY?

This section will discuss briefly the nature of the environment in which most nurses work before going on to discuss the spirit of innovation that may or may not exist within it. Whatever setting, large or small, urban or bush, nurses work in an organisation. Despite differences in size and complexity, they are all organisations.

Major organisation theorists and writers on organisations[1,2] agree that, despite differences in perspective, organisations exist in order to fulfil goals and they do so by carrying out defined, consciously coordinated activities. In other words, they exist for specific purposes, such as the provision of healthcare, and are structured to fulfil that purpose.

Ideally, the goals of organisations are clearly defined, though unfortunately this is not always the case. Many organisations have mission statements and other means of communicating their goals to staff but these may only be actively referred to during orientation or times of accreditation. However they are communicated, meeting these goals requires people with specialised skills and knowledge who are prepared to work for and be loyal to the organisation. So, ideally, organisations have specific goals and the efforts of people in those organisations are aimed at meeting them as effectively as possible.

In an effort to ensure this is so, people working in organisations are typically managed in relatively systematic ways and their efforts coordinated by fairly formal leadership structures.[3] A major influence on our understanding of the shape and functions of organisations in the 20th century was Max Weber, via his notion of the 'bureaucratic organisation'.[2] It was Weber's view that interaction can be seen to be more objective if people are separated from each other, technically specialised and formally evaluated. In bureaucratic organisations, goals are achieved by grouping together employees who carry out similar work, overseen by individuals who have been placed in positions of authority. Submission to this rule of authority is due to a set of related beliefs. Weber believed that a position of authority should be achieved as a result of individuals acquiring, and being viewed as possessing, specialist technical knowledge. In such a system, obedience is due not to the person who holds the authority but to the impersonal order that has granted the person this position.

This view is neatly summarised by Adrian Carr[4]:

> This technical orientation … encourages managers and administrators to view organisations as abstractions from their environment, and their roles as managers and administrators as being one of responsibility for controlling any disturbances to the status quo. Bureaucracies are, of course, archetypes of such an orientation. The organisation is conceived as largely a control mechanism. The emphasis is on formality, rules and regulations. People are regarded as atomistic, passive and rational in their responses; and assessments of results/outcomes are based on technical efficiency (p 289).

BUREAUCRACIES IN HEALTHCARE

Given this description, it can be seen that traditional hospitals consisting of groups of wards and clinical departments, designed for a specific function such as surgical and medical nursing or radiography services, are clear examples of bureaucratic structures. The same can also be said for health services provided in community and other non-institutional settings, in that they are all managed by professionals who possess the relevant qualifications and experience. These managers are attributed with defined levels of authority to enforce the rules and policies of the organisation. In turn, they are themselves expected to abide by the same rules and policies. In terms of change and its management, the main implications of this are that, in such organisations, the impetus for change and its direction are invariably mandated from above; and, due to the fact that the division of labour is based on roles or structures, insufficient action is taken to ensure ownership by the workforce. According to Charles Handy,[5] the chosen route to efficiency via concentration and specialisation in a bureaucratic culture has reached a dead end because it restricts flexibility and runs counter to the cultural preferences of most of the people it needs to work. It is interesting therefore to note that health services are still managed predominantly through bureaucratic management structures. The management of change is thus affected because, in addition to the above, there rarely exist the multidisciplinarity, mutual respect, trust and sense of self-worth that are required to allow agreement and cooperation across the whole organisation.

According to Hodson,[6] workers and organisations are constantly engaged in a simultaneous ballet of cooperation and resistance. Under overly controlling or overly chaotic work regimes, workers establish systems of self-worth through resistance activities. Under more permissive and inclusive work models, workers establish systems of self-worth through citizenship activities. Workers will always seek meaning in their work and citizenship activities are more likely to develop by working with workers in respectful ways that support meaningful work, and worker dignity. Hodson defines dignity as 'the ability to establish a sense of self-worth and self-respect and to appreciate the respect of others' (p 3). Understanding and supporting patient dignity has long been an important ingredient of high-quality healthcare.[7] However, the notion of worker dignity, its application to nursing and its place in healthcare reform and innovation have been less well understood. Karl Marx[8] wrote that dignity is lost when workers are alienated from: the products of their labour (that is, they no longer determine what is to be made or how it is to be used); the process of work (someone else controls the pace, techniques and processes of work and workers become emotionally separated from their work); the ability to be creative (when workers' capacity for self-directed creativity is denied); and finally when workers are alienated from others (when group interactions are dictated by rigid hierarchies which determine who can relate to whom).

To a lesser or a greater extent these factors can be seen in the complex healthcare systems where patients and healthcare workers are turned into the object of 'worker' or 'patient'. According to Hodson,[6] successfully addressing these threats to dignity can result in the development of worker 'agency', that is, 'the active and creative performance of assigned roles in ways that give meaning and content to those roles beyond what is institutionally scripted' (p 16).

When we do this we are more likely to be able to tap into the social and intellectual capital that is staff, patients and community. This may help us finally stop committing the hubris that only certain elites in our health services have the knowledge and capacity to design and implement solutions to the complex problems we face in health.[9,10]

Thus, despite the work of Carr,[4] Handy[1] and Hodson,[6] the majority of organisations providing healthcare still retain a predominantly bureaucratic structure. As a result, newly graduating nurses, as fairly lowly placed members of the organisation, may find themselves feeling relatively powerless and inconsequential. In part this is due to the factors outlined above, reinforced by the processes of line management with its typically 'top-down' approach to running its business (including the management of change) and an emphasis on adherence to policy. In such circumstances in some organisations, there may be little opportunity for staff to participate in change in anything other than a passive role. There is a tendency from the outset, therefore, for newer members of the nursing team to continue with this passivity to the degree that it translates into a state of learnt helplessness.[11] This is defined as the behavioural state of a person who believes control over the environment has been lost and his or her efforts are ineffectual or futile.[12] It has been said that professionals such as nurses can be socialised into such a mindset.[13-15] Such writers argue that, quite quickly after entering the workforce (within a few months), many nurses can be seen to have adopted a bureaucratic orientation to their work whereby decisions are made very much with the rules and regulations of the employing institution in mind. They do so as a means of minimising the risk of contravening policy or custom and practice. This is opposed to legitimising actions and decisions from a service perspective (where the emphasis is on the dignity and humanity of the patient) or a professional perspective (where the emphasis is on occupational standards, transcending institutional policies and practices). Furthermore, it is these authors' view that nurses do so because this appears to help them to avoid conflict with supervisors and peers and so 'fit in'[16] as quickly as possible.

'OPPRESSED GROUP BEHAVIOUR' IN NURSING: ITS IMPLICATIONS FOR INNOVATION

The situation described above can be reinforced even further in nursing by the presence of what has become known as 'oppressed group behaviour'. According to Roberts,[17,18] this model of behaviour was developed from literature on colonised Africans, Latin Americans, African Americans, Jews and, more recently, women.[19] These groups are said to have been oppressed by virtue of being controlled and exploited by forces external to themselves.

In his seminal text *The Pedagogy of the Oppressed* (1971), Paolo Freire[20] explains how, over time, the norms and values of the dominant group come to be accepted as the 'right' ones by all concerned. In turn, the leaders of the oppressed group, as they emerge, tend to identify with the characteristics of the dominant group (e.g. white people, landowners, those guarding them, men) as a means of 'fitting in' and being accepted. This typically includes their coming to view those they have 'left behind' with a degree of cynicism and even disdain. Meanwhile, those who have been left behind are said to behave in a submissive–aggressive manner[21] whereby malice or even aggression felt towards the oppressor(s) is not expressed towards them but rather at easier targets – others within their group, usually those even lower down the pecking order. Fanon calls this 'horizontal violence'.[22]

Nearly 30 years on from Roberts' article,[17] horizontal violence as a symptom of oppressed group behaviour is still seen as a major issue in contemporary nursing.[18,23,24] However, the term most widely used today is 'bullying'. Bullying may take the form of personal attacks, erosion of professional competence and reputation and attack through work roles and tasks[25]; it does not include being asked to undertake legitimate tasks or to take instruction from a legitimate authority. In contemporary nursing there is a recognition that bullying exists and most organisations have measures in place to deal with it.

The amalgamation of all the above is that the leaders emerging from oppressed groups may not value the views of their subordinates, while those same subordinates tend not to make their views known because they see no point in doing so. A catch-22 scenario thus often exists.

Whilst this may seem to be a bleak picture, there are examples of health services trying to utilise the expertise of all their staff to ensure provision of the best possible care via initiatives such as patient-centred hospitals and clinical governance. However, many newly graduating nurses will find themselves working in a bureaucracy where work will tend to be guided by adherence to policy and procedure. Changes to those policies will almost inevitably occur as a result of top-down initiatives and will do so via the processes of line management. As such, the socialising tendency will be to adopt a bureaucratic, as opposed to a social or professional, orientation to their work. They will do this along with peers and supervisors who will exhibit, to some degree, oppressed group behaviour, which has been indicated to lead to a tendency to stifle change and innovation from the bottom up.

Some solutions?

So, given that most nurses will work within a bureaucratic structure, how can they position themselves so as to be able to deal constructively with change, participate in it and perhaps even initiate it?

Part of the answer to this requires change to the nursing profession as a whole. Susan Jo Roberts published her seminal work on the theory of oppressed group behaviour and its application(s) to nursing back in 1983.[17] She and her colleagues[18] updated this work in 2009 through a review of the literature. Roberts provides a history of the concept, and goes further to provide useful and practical suggestions on how to avoid or diminish the oppressed group behaviour. In essence, this amounts to the need for:

* an acceptance among nurses that oppression and its related behaviour exist within its ranks
* a recognition that such behaviours are not due to the fact that nurses are inherently inferior, but rather that they have come to feel so within a wider culture that does not value them properly
* the development of nursing leaders who do not subscribe to the view that the rank and file are to be viewed with disdain

- the rediscovery, under the guidance of such leadership, of the cultural heritage of nursing.

Together, Roberts believes, such initiatives will lead to a situation where the more powerful players in health service politics (doctors, managers) will come to view nurses and nursing more positively, basically because nurses themselves have a positive view of themselves. Roberts quotes Torres[26]: 'the freedom to develop nursing's own destiny can only come from nursing's own initiative; it will not be freely granted by other groups'.

Nurses, like individuals in all oppressed groups, need to engage in self-empowerment. If this could then be amalgamated with a sense of pride and confidence that what they do is effective and of benefit to society (supported obviously by evidence of their efficacy), the influence that nurses exercise on healthcare and the policy that underpins it will surely come to reflect the proportion of the health services workforce which nurses constitute.

An alternative to learnt helplessness

Martin Seligman,[27] who originally studied the detrimental effects of learnt helplessness, has in the last decade studied learnt optimism. If we can learn to be helpless, we can also learn to be optimistic. By understanding our individual strengths we can learn to be positive, have realistic goals, make plans to achieve them, and be ready to share them when the opportunity arises. Understanding our strengths and how we make good things happen in our lives, we can use this information to find solutions and buffer us when things do not go as well as we planned.

Another important mechanism for staying positive is to be realistic — a key concept related to reactance theory.[28] Those who succeed with it gain a sense of wellbeing from the perception that they can make a difference, not that they necessarily have already — at least not yet. Thinking through what we would like to change and being realistic about whether it is possible to do so, given our sphere of influence, is a basic tenet of being a change agent.

As well as being realistic it is helpful to have a support network. Unfortunately, those who have researched this field[29,30] have found that professionals such as nurses are actually quite bad at asking for and/or accepting help and support from others. Instead, they have a tendency to see themselves as strong, and being seen to be so by others. It is therefore important to develop supports. Some supports may be informal, such as debriefing with colleagues, whereas others can be of a more formal nature, such as critical companions[31] or clinical supervision.[32] Many health services are recognising the importance of providing staff with opportunities to reflect upon their practice and develop systems of peer support.

Solution-focused approaches

Another recent positive innovation for solving problems in nursing has been the advent of a solution-focused approach to nursing.[28] This approach also comes out of the positive psychology movement, especially solution-focused counselling. It can be applied to nursing as both an approach to working with clients and an approach to working with each other to find innovative solutions to workplace issues.[33] In contrast to the problem (or blame)-oriented approach so prevalent in our health services, the solution-focused approach focuses on the future – what's working, progress, influence, collaboration, simplicity and action – rather than the past – what's wrong, blame, control, deficits, complications and definitions.[34] The solution-focused approach assumes that nothing happens by chance. When something bad happens, something makes it happen. However, the same is true when things go well; something makes the good things happen. What we need to do is to explore what makes the good things happen and do more of this, and find out what makes the bad things happen and stop doing that. In this way we take a more positive view of ourselves and others and we build on the strengths that we already possess.[35]

LEADERSHIP AND NURSING'S FUTURE

In all likelihood, the future contribution of the nursing profession will be measured in terms of its ability to influence the delivery of evidence-based, cost-effective care in multidisciplinary, multiagency environments. Success in this will depend on the nursing profession's ability to produce transformational leaders capable of effecting necessary change.

Transformational leadership means changing the realities of our environment to conform more closely to our values and beliefs. Covey[36] identifies the goal of transformational leadership as being to 'transform' people and organisations in a literal sense – to change them in mind and heart; to enlarge vision, insight and understanding; to clarify purposes; to make behaviour congruent with beliefs, principles and values; and to bring about changes that are permanent, self-perpetuating and momentum building. In his book *Creating Culture Change: The Key to Successful Total Quality Management*, Phillip Atkinson differentiates between 'transformational' and 'transactional' leaders.[37] He identifies transformational leaders as independent, visionary and inspirational, driven by long-term goals, visions and objectives. They also possess a clear vision of what they wish to achieve, expecting high standards from others and being little concerned with detail. They are the change makers who provide a mission for others to follow. On the other hand, transactional leaders are good at achieving short-term results, typically by promoting teamwork and working in a practical manner. However, transformational leaders will often provide the frame of reference and strategic boundaries within which transactions can be conducted. Transformational leaders create new initiatives and stimulate action and loyalty, whereas transactional managers are better at administering systems and making things happen on a daily basis, and have an important role in sustaining change once it has been introduced. Both types of leadership are important and, while they develop different approaches, successful exponents of both types give direction and motivation, and reward and recognise success. They also develop and meet the needs of staff. Indeed, the personal styles that managers adopt are important – research has shown that the leadership style and use of emotional intelligence have a measurable impact on work atmosphere and enhancement of team performance.[38]

Davidson and Peck suggest[39] that the key characteristic of good leaders is the ability to tune their responses to the context in which they are working. They assert that what we ideally need are leaders who possess both skill sets, and that one solution may be the acquisition of a repertoire of leadership skills. They propose that leaders should aim to develop skills from a broad range of dimensions which are summarised as:

- intellectual – the theories and concepts available to individuals to inform their personal and intellectual responses
- psychological – the understandings and insights that individuals have of their behaviours and relationships with others
- performative – the range of behaviours individuals can enact in the leadership role.

Davidson and Peck also suggest mechanisms through which this repertoire can be exercised. In summary, these are the abilities to identify and exercise aspects of self and leadership behaviours which have been learnt through experience, whilst being sensitive to the needs and responses of self and others. The underlying assumption of this model is that the effectiveness of individuals as leaders is determined by the range of dimensions available to them and the ability to exercise the appropriate related mechanisms.

To date, nursing has produced many highly skilled transactional managers, but leaders in possession of transformational skills are still less common in the profession. However, strategies to address this have been developed and the Clinical Leadership Programme in Australia is one of these. This program utilises several approaches to develop transformational leadership skills in clinical leaders; central to this is Kouzes and Posner's[40] exemplary leadership behaviours. Evaluation and research to date indicate that transformational leaders in healthcare enhance practice and the patient experience (see http://www.clinicalleadership.com/ for further information). They may also be pivotal to the implementation of evidence-based practice. Kitson et al.[41] highlight that not only is it important for there to be strong evidence to support the change being advocated (along with an environment supportive of that change), but also facilitation of the change by leaders is vital. It seems that high-quality facilitation skills may well be vital to high-quality leadership.

LEADERSHIP AND CHANGE MANAGEMENT

We noted at the outset of this chapter that change is faster and more complex than ever before. It is an inevitable phenomenon and a characteristic of every human condition today, and whether or not we want to accept change we must learn to manage or at least cope with it.[42] The need for change emerges when, as a result of pressure from either intrinsic or extrinsic sources, the balance of a system is disturbed.[43] Although change can create anxiety, successful change thrives alongside risk and uncertainty and this can lead to real opportunities for creating a better way forward – innovation.[44]

It is therefore important to understand change processes, and have insight into why things happen in order to offset feelings of uncertainty and anxiety. Crookes and Froggatt[45] provide useful insights into making a difference in practice. An experienced change manager will encourage participation to engender ownership of change among staff, but having insight into the change process could allow others also to identify how they can play a more active part in the change process. It is interesting to consider how people affected by change react. Rogers and Shoemaker[46] categorise these responses along a continuum: innovators, early adopters, early majority, late majority and laggards; it is interesting to reflect on our personal experiences of change and consider where on the continuum we might find ourselves. For most of us, change management skills are acquired over time through active participation; it is unlikely that we would be successful in managing change if our first exposure was in the leader role. It is surely no accident that people who succeed in effecting lasting change are those who have been in situations where successful change has previously taken place.

The *Oxford Dictionary*[47] defines change as 'the act or an instance of becoming different'. This broad definition includes both planned and unplanned change. Unplanned change, referred to by Lippitt[48] as change by the transmission of culture, is a reaction to an internal or external stimulus that affects the balance of the system. Change by transmission is evolutionary in nature, frequently occurring without reference to design or intention,[48] and is therefore gradual, often piecemeal, and unlikely to meet the demands of a dynamic organisation. Such change would typically occur under the management of a transactional leader.

Planned change, like unplanned change, will also be a reaction to internal or external factors but there is a concerted and organised effort to move the system, the organisation or the individual in a new direction. This conscious effort to bring about change has been referred to as change by transformation,[49] the objective of which is to restructure social patterns. The reforms in health services being undertaken in many countries are examples of radical attempts to restructure social patterns; they emanate from central government and have major implications for the whole population, not just healthcare professionals.

Innovation, or transformational change, is a dynamic process that takes place over a period of time during which planned change may be redefined and modified. The processes of planned change have been explored by several authors who have variously described the stages of change as they see them.[3,41,50,51] These are invariably little more than elaborations on the three stages of the change process first described by Lewin.[43]

Lewin's theory of change

Lewin[43] asserted that the three stages in the process of effecting permanent change are unfreezing, moving and refreezing. Unfreezing refers to the preparatory stages prior to the implementation of an initiative, and takes the form of eliciting that there is a need for change, identifying resistance to change and identifying strategies for overcoming resistance to it. Lippitt et al.[3] subcategorised Lewin's unfreezing concept into the development of a need for change and the establishment of the change relationship. To Meleis and Burton[50] (who call this the 'pre-innovation stage'), it is essential that the innovator not only identifies what is to be changed and why, but also clearly defines the setting in which the change is to take place.

Moving begins when the participants have identified or accepted the need for change, and potential solutions are identified and appropriate changes are made. By taking time and effort to provide an appropriate milieu for change to take place, the chance of successful change is increased. Before embarking on any innovation, it is wise to establish that the intended change has relative advantage over existing ways of doing things and to ascertain whether or not the philosophy and values of the change are in conflict with those of the participants. The complexity, trialability and communicability of the innovation should also be considered. That is, is the change easy for the user to understand? is a trial period possible? and how visible will improvements be? In other words, there should be a good reason for change, and those affected by it need to see that it is a change worth making. The reason(s) should be made clear to all staff, and opportunities for them to discuss the change and contribute ideas on how this could best happen are crucial.

Refreezing occurs when the newly acquired behaviour is integrated into participants' existing behaviour. It is during this period that consequences are realised and evaluated. During this stage resources and facilitation should be provided to help integrate the innovative role into the existing structure. If the new way of doing things does not take the place of previous behaviours it will be only a matter of time before people revert to the old ways of doing things. Meleis and Burton[50] considered this stage to be under way when the innovation becomes part of the language of the organisation and an integral part of the role behaviour of its personnel. In other words, the success of an innovation is manifested in its adoption. Allan and Kraft[52] contend that, if continued use of the change in the absence of the change agent does not occur, this may be because the participants do not own the change, possibly because they were not instrumental in the change, and so their values and beliefs have not been altered.

Other implications of change

Another implication of change, whether successful or failed, is the psychological effect on individuals. Change affects everyone. Knight,[53] in a study of nursing lecturers' responses to organisational change, identified that participants experienced feelings of anger, loss of control and lack of optimism. They also described feeling alienated and voiced their fear that they would no longer be of use to the organisation. An awareness of our own possible reactions to change will help the identification strategies for moving through the change process and emerging with positive self-esteem.

While Lewin's theory of change is overarching in scope, it does little to explain the emotions related to change other than motivations to adopt or reject it. When situations change and previous understanding does not enable decisions to be made, we are likely to experience a sense of loss.[54] Marris[55] contends that the fundamental crisis of bereavement is not due to the loss of others but due to loss of some aspect of self. Mead and Bryar[56] concur that the grieving process could apply in many contexts that would not normally be thought of as bereavement and they contend that, when we lose objects or even an activity, we lose a part of ourselves. The same could be said of a job, or a work role within it.

Esty[54] identifies four kinds of loss experienced by employees in the wake of organisational change: (1) loss of the familiar; (2) loss of security; (3) loss of control; and (4) loss of optimism. All of these things, Esty[54] maintains, contribute to our occupational identity, which in turn is a major contributor to our perception of self. Perlman and Takacs[57] expanded on the acclaimed work *On Death and Dying* by Elisabeth Kubler-Ross[58] to describe employees' grief responses to change. The 10 steps described by Perlman and Takacs[57] (equilibrium, denial, anger, bargaining, chaos, depression, resignation, openness, readiness and re-emergence) detail the emotional responses of individuals confronted with change. Schoolfield and Orduna[59] identified that the process of unfreezing requires changing the values, attitudes and customs of individuals. During this stage, you can expect to encounter some or all of the Perlman and Takacs phases.[57]

Changes for the profession as a whole

Whilst this chapter has discussed change at an individual level, some systematic processes that are being used in nursing bring about change that not only provides for more efficient organisations but also provides better patient outcomes and more satisfied working environments for staff. Probably the most comprehensive approach to this sort of change, which incorporates most of what we have stated thus far about change in bureaucratic environments, is practice development.

Practice development, according to McCormack et al.,[60] is:

a continuing process of improvement towards increased effectiveness in person-centred care, through the enabling of nurses and healthcare teams to transform the culture and context of care. It is enabled and supported by facilitators committed to a systematic, rigorous and continuous process of emancipatory change (p 256).

We believe the single most important element in the definition is also the underlying philosophy: person-centredness. Person-centredness is acknowledging the personhood, or shared humanity, of all people. This is the starting point and shared value of practice development and its guiding principle.

In relation to person-centredness, values are worked out explicitly with all people involved in practice development. Practice development provides many ways of doing this but when done well it breaks down the barriers between 'them' and 'us' and helps people see each other as more similar than different.

It also gives the work a compass bearing so that each solution and action can be evaluated in the light of shared values that are lived – that is, there are good values–practice interaction and good values congruence.

Practice development is also about evolving cultures of innovation through facilitation in order to bring about emancipatory change – change that frees people to work in ways that support dignity for themselves and others. It is practical in that it works with the people and the context at all levels of healthcare. It is very much about personal leadership but not just at the level of people with recognised leadership roles: everyone is seen as a leader of something and someone and everyone can work in ways that facilitate person-centred change, even if they do not have the formal role of facilitator. Most importantly, practice development incorporates the views and knowledge of service users and involves them in the process.

In these ways practice development builds on the strengths already existing in organisations and further builds the social and intellectual capital so that worker agency, rather than worker resistance, is developed. The collective (including clients) is seen as a rich resource of innovative ideas and, through various processes, solutions to problems are generated by the collective wisdom of the group.

There are lots of ways of doing this and the strength of practice development is that, in solution generation, as in all other activities, no one process is prescribed. The key is that whatever process we use, person-centred emancipatory change is the goal. It is our underlying shared humanity that counts.

Practice development as a program of practice change is being undertaken more and more in health services in Australia, New Zealand, the UK and continental Europe. It is beyond the scope of this chapter to detail practice development principles and processes. Manley et al.[61] provide a comprehensive overview of the approach.

CONCLUSION

Change is something that has been with us forever. In fact, that is perhaps the only thing that will never change. In this chapter we have attempted to explain and illustrate why bureaucracies operate the way they do, and present ideas on how nurses may make a difference in these environments. Working through the exercises and undertaking the recommended reading will help to reinforce what we hope is, after the negativity of the earlier part of the chapter, a constructive and optimistic message for the future.

CASE STUDY 7.1

Charles has begun working on a new ward. The staff say they are involved in practice development and are working to develop a person-centred culture.

REFLECTIVE QUESTIONS

- What do you understand by the term 'practice development'?
- What would a person-centred culture mean for both staff and patients?

EXERCISE 7.1

Review the characteristics of transactional and transformational leaders (see Case study 7.2). Next, compare these characteristics with four people you know: one in a senior management position, one in middle management, one an experienced registered nurse and, finally, yourself.

1. Do any of these people demonstrate the characteristics of either of these types of leader?
2. Which type do you most easily fit into, and which would you most like to be?
3. As a registered nurse, do you believe that you have a choice about whether or not you occupy a leadership position?
4. Think now about how you might best go about becoming the leader you would like to be and make a plan to help you get there. Ask colleagues and managers to help you do this.

CASE STUDY 7.2

Elise works in a unit where the staff seem to be innovative and creative and work together to find solutions to shared problems. They say that part of the reason they work so well together is because of the support they receive from their manager. They describe her as being a transformational leader.

REFLECTIVE QUESTIONS

- What is transformational leadership and how does it differ from transactional leadership?
- What does the literature say about the strengths of a transformational leadership style?
- What does the literature say about the strengths of a transactional leadership style?

CASE STUDY 7.3

Declan works in a busy surgical ward. He has been asked to join a group of staff who are working together to improve staff access to learning opportunities and staff development. He has been told the group uses a solution-focused approach.

REFLECTIVE QUESTIONS

- How does a solution-focused approach differ from a problem-based approach to change?
- As a group using a solution-focused approach, what would you explore together in order to find a solution to the problem?

EXERCISE 7.2

Reflect on a change you have been involved in, or affected by, and then try to answer the following questions:

1. Was the change planned or unplanned? Was an established model of change used?
2. Can you identify the actions taken to unfreeze, move and refreeze the behaviour of individuals involved?
3. Was the change process, in this instance, successful or not? How could it have been more successful?
4. Did oppressed group behaviour play any role in events?

   Consider the points put forward about oppressed group behaviour, preferably in light of the recommended reading. What do you think you might do to ensure that you do not suffer from horizontal violence, as well as avoiding treating others in this way?

RECOMMENDED READING

Clinical Leadership Programme in Australia. Online. Available: http://www.clinicalleadership.com/ 16 June 2007.

Covey SR. The 7 habits of highly effective people. 2nd ed. London: Simon & Schuster; 2004.

Crookes PA, Davies S, editors. Research into practice: essential skills for reading and applying research in nursing and health care. 2nd ed. London: Harcourt Brace; 2004.

Kouzes J, Posner B. The leadership challenge: how to get extraordinary things done in organisations. 3rd ed. San Francisco: Jossey-Bass; 2003.

Manley K, McCormack B, Wilson V, editors. International practice development in nursing and healthcare. Oxford: Blackwell; 2008.

REFERENCES

1. Handy C. Understanding organisations. 4th ed. London: Penguin; 1993.
2. Pugh DS, Hickson DJ. Writers on organisations. 5th ed. Thousand Oaks, California: Sage; 1997.
3. Lippitt R, Watson J, Wesley B. The dynamics of planned changes. New York: Harcourt; 1958.
4. Carr A. Critical theory and the psychodynamics of change. Journal of Organisational Change Management 2000;13:289–99.
5. Handy C. Gods of management. 3rd ed. London: Century Business; 1991.
6. Hodson R. Dignity at work. Cambridge: Cambridge University Press; 2001.
7. Walsh K, Kowanko I. Nurses' and patients' perceptions of dignity. International Journal of Nursing Practice 2002;8:143–51.
8. Marx K. Economic and philosophic manuscripts of 1844. New York: International Publishers; 1964.
9. Lawless J, Moss C. Exploring the value of dignity in the work-life of nurses. Contemporary Nurse 2007;24:225–36.
10. Joyce JT, Crookes PA. Developing a tool to measure 'magnetism' in Australian nursing environments. Australian Journal of Advanced Nursing 2007;25:17–23.
11. Seligman M. Authentic happiness: using the new positive psychology to realize your potential for lasting fulfillment. New York: Free Press; 2002.
12. Anderson KN. Mosby's medical, nursing and allied health dictionary. 5th ed. St Louis, Missouri: Mosby Year Book; 1998.
13. Darbyshire P. Thinly disguised contempt. Nursing Times 1988;84:42–4.
14. Green GJ. Relationships between role models and role perceptions of new graduate nurses. Nursing Research 1988;37:245–8.
15. Corwin RG, Taves MJ. Some concomitants of bureaucratic and professional conceptions of the nurse role. Nursing Research 1962;11:223–7.
16. Melia K. Learning and working: the occupational socialisation of nurses. London: Tavistock Publications; 1987.
17. Roberts SJ. Oppressed group behaviour: implications for nursing. Advances in Nursing Sciences 1983;5:21–30.
18. Roberts S, Demarco R, Griffen M. The effect of oppressed group behaviours on the culture of the nursing workplace: a review of the evidence and interventions for change. Journal of Nursing Management 2009;17:288–93.
19. Cleland V. Sex discrimination: nursing's most pervasive problem. American Journal of Nursing 1971;71:1542–7.
20. Freire P. The pedagogy of the oppressed. New York: Herder & Herder; 1971.
21. Carmichael S, Hamilton C. Black power. New York: Random House; 1967.
22. Fanon F. The wretched of the earth. New York: Grove Press; 1963.
23. Farrell GA. Aggression in clinical settings: nurses' views. Journal of Advanced Nursing 1997;25:501–8.
24. Duffy E. Horizontal violence: a conundrum for nursing. Collegian 1995;2: 5–17.
25. Hutchinson M, Vickers M, Wilkes L, et al. A topology of bullying behaviours. The experiences of Australian nurses. Journal of Clinical Nursing 2010;19: 2319–28.

26. Torres G. The nursing education administrator: accountable, vulnerable and oppressed. Advances in Nursing Science 1981;3:1–16.

27. Seligman MEP. Learned optimism. New York: Pocket Books; 1998.

28. Brehm JW. A theory of psychological reactance. New York: Academic Press; 1966.

29. Crookes PA. Personal bereavement in registered general nurses. PhD thesis. University of Hull, UK, 1996.

30. Crawley P. Once a nurse always a nurse—unless you are a patient! International Journal for the Advancement of Counselling 1984;7:261–5.

31. Titchen A. Critical companionship: part 1. Nursing Standard 2003;18:33–40.

32 Walsh K, Nicholson J, Keough C, et al. The development of a group model of clinical supervision to meet the needs of a community mental health nursing team. International Journal of Nursing Practice 2003;9:33–9.

33. Walsh K, Moss C, FitzGerald M. Solution focused approaches and their relevance to practice development. Practice Development in Health Care 2006;5: 145–55

34. Jackson P, McKergow M. Harry Enfield, Hamlet and the solutions focus. Organisations and People 2001;8:26–31.

35. McAllister M, editor. Solution focused nursing: rethinking practice. Houndmills: Palgrave McMillian; 2007.

36. Covey SR. Principle centred leadership. London: Simon & Schuster; 1992.

37. Atkinson PE. Creating culture change: the key to successful total quality management. Bedford, UK: IFS Publications; 1990.

38. Goleman, D. Leadership that gets results. Harvard Business Review 2000; Mar–Apr:78–90.

39. Davidson D, Peck E. Organisational development and the 'repertoire' of healthcare leaders. In: Peck E, editor. Organisational development in healthcare: approaches, innovations, achievements. Oxford: Radcliffe; 2004.

40. Kouzes J, Posner B. The leadership challenge: how to get extraordinary things done in organisations. San Francisco: Jossey-Bass; 1995.

41. Kitson A, Harvey G, McCormack B. Enabling the implementation of evidence-based practice: a conceptual framework. Quality in Health Care 1998;7: 149–58.

42. Zukowski B. Managing change before it manages you. Medsurg 1995;4: 325–33.

43. Lewin K. Field theory in social science. London: Routledge & Kegan Paul; 1951.

44. Poggenpoel M. Managing change. Nursing RSA Verpleging 1992;7:28–31.

45. Crookes PA, Froggatt T. Techniques and strategies for translating research findings into health care practices. In: Crookes PA, Davies S, editors. Research into practice: essential skills for reading and applying research in nursing and health care. 2nd ed. London: Harcourt Brace; 2004.

46. Rogers EM, Shoemaker FF. Communication of innovations: a cross-cultural approach. New York: Free Press; 1971.

47. The Concise Oxford dictionary. 10th revised edition. Oxford: OUP; 1999.

48. Lippitt R. Visualizing change: model building and the change process. Fairfax, VA: NTL Learning Resources Corporation; 1973.

49. Field PA. Implementing change in nurse education. Nurse Education Today 1988;9:290–9.

50. Meleis AI, Burton PS. Innovative educational changes. International Journal of Nursing Studies 1981;18:33–9.

51. Crookes PA, Davies S, editors. Research into practice: essential skills for reading and applying research in nursing and health care. 2nd ed. London: Harcourt Brace; 2004.

52. Allan RF, Kraft C. The organisational unconscious. Harlow, UK: Prentice Hall; 1982.

53. Knight S. A study of the 'lived' experience of change during a period of curriculum and organisational change in a department of nurse education. Journal of Advanced Nursing 1998;27:1287–95.

54. Esty K. The management of change. Employee Assistance Quarterly 1987;2: 90–7.

55. Marris P. Loss and change. London: Routledge & Kegan Paul; 1985.

56. Mead D, Bryar R. An analysis of the changes involved in the introduction of the nursing process and primary nursing using a framework of loss and attachment. Journal of Clinical Nursing 1992;1:95–9.

57. Perlman D, Takacs GT. The 10 stages of change. Nursing Management 1990;16: 820–4.

58. Kubler-Ross E. On death and dying. New York: Macmillan; 1969.

59. Schoolfield M, Orduna A. Understanding staff nurses' responses to change: utilization of a grief-change framework to facilitate innovation. Clinical Nurse Specialist 1994;8:57–62.

60. McCormack B, Manley K, Titchen A, et al. Towards practice development: a vision in reality or a reality without vision. Journal of Nursing Management 1999;7:255–64.

61. Manley K, McCormack B, Wilson V, editors. International practice development in nursing and healthcare. Oxford: Blackwell; 2008.

CHAPTER 8

Caring for self: the role of collaboration, healthy lifestyle and balance

Judy Lumby

LEARNING OBJECTIVES

When you have completed this chapter you will be able to:

- be critically aware of the parameters of remaining healthy inside and outside the workplace
- explore the ways in which values and lifestyle affect health and wellbeing
- build a knowledge of stress, its manifestations and its effects
- understand how to recognise and manage increased dis/stress in self and others
- ensure that a life balance is maintained so that health is central personally and professionally.

Keywords: caring, coping, allostatic load, healthy lifestyle, teamwork

---

INTRODUCTION

Nursing is a role similar to medicine, which demands much of an individual both personally and professionally. My own experience is that the two aspects of one's life, work/recreation or professional/personal, become inextricably linked when undertaking the work known as nursing. To nurse is to become involved. After all, unless another or others are involved then the act is not nursing. Central to being a nurse is being involved with another, either caring for that person or assisting that individual in his or her own care. This can take many forms: chance conversations about health issues; provisional diagnosis of an illness or disease; managing symptoms such as pain or breathlessness; counselling; advising on choices in treatments such as chemotherapy, dialysis or asthma medication; dressing or draining a wound; or assisting someone to die peacefully in the way the individual desires. All these acts, and many more, are a normal part of everyday nursing and all involve interacting with another person or persons.

Over the last two decades technology has made what was already a demanding job even more demanding, not only in terms of skills development but also in terms of managing time and priorities. While the introduction of new technology is usually made by doctors, nurses are the ones expected to manage and manipulate it, thus adding to their workload of caring. It is interesting to note that, of all industries, healthcare is one where the introduction of technology has not meant the loss of staff but the addition of staff, and even specialist staff, to drive the technology. Unlike many industries, most new healthcare technology has not meant simplification of skills or roles but the extension and even sophistication of roles. In many areas, such as intensive care with technology like ventilators and monitors, central lines and renal dialysis, it has also meant the opening up of new wards or units and the education of specialist nurses and doctors to work in the new areas. In most cases the technology is linked to the patient but, because of the safety aspects of technological intervention, it is vital that the nurse keeps an ever-watchful eye on the machinery as well as its impact on the patient.[1] Nurses now have to divide their time between caring for the patient and caring for the technology. But who cares for the nurse?

In 1996 a report on workforce in NSW Australia mirrored the reduction in retention and recruitment of nurses across the Western world with an ageing workforce compounding the problem.[2] In 2008, however, this appeared to have been reversed. The Australian Institute of Health and Welfare's labour force audit revealed that the total number of registered and enrolled nurses was 312,736, an increase of 10.6% since 2004. The number of full-time equivalent nurses per 100,000 population thus increased by 15.2% between 2004 and 2008. The workforce itself continued to age, with the proportion of nurses aged 50 years or over increasing from 18.9% to 34.4%. And despite efforts to reverse a gender imbalance, the profession continued to be predominantly female.[3]

The challenging nature of our contemporary healthcare systems contributes to the current dilemma of how we retain highly skilled younger nurses in our health workforce, given changing social norms and values. After all, nurses were once expected – and even drilled – to care for others, to the neglect of self. Such values were deeply embedded in nursing's, and indeed women's, history. Nursing is a profession founded in the convent and the army, institutions in which women were expected to be selfless, obedient and silent. Cultural shifts, including the education of women, over the past few decades have questioned the belief that selfless dedication leads to healthy and caring individuals.[4] Quite the opposite can occur, with individuals feeling resentful, angry and unfulfilled if their needs are unmet.

Present-day knowledge about self-development shows that, in order to empower and support another, it is important to be aware of who you are and what drives you forward. Caring for others to avoid confronting yourself is not only dangerous; it is unhealthy for those you care for. Often the carer comes from a position of victim or martyr, two very damaging positions for any individual, as well as for those with whom they work. And nurses, like doctors, rely on working with many colleagues and sharing the care of individuals. For this to happen in a way that is in the best interests of the patient we need to explore our personal values and share these with our professional colleagues so that we can work more effectively.

PERSONAL AND SHARED VALUES

The term 'values' means different things to different people. It can refer to our social and cultural principles, goals or standards; it may mean the value we place on another person, or the quality of something in terms of its worth, or the extent to which something is desirable or worthy of esteem.[5] Inherent in any discussion on values is the subject of ethics, which is a system of moral values, values about what it means to be a good person whose actions are based on a moral code of behaviour. There are at least six moral principles in most professional codes of ethics for health professionals. These are autonomy, beneficence, fidelity, justice, non-malificence and veracity. It is incumbent on graduates entering the workforce to analyse their specific profession's code of ethics to ensure that their personal values are not in conflict with such a code. This ensures an integrity of the personal and professional conduct which patients deserve from everyone they come into contact with. In addition, it has been shown that individuals gain a sense of worth and connectedness if the values they hold personally are given expression through their professional practices. This requires us to ensure a balance between our personal and professional lives.

It has become increasingly clear to those who work in systems such as healthcare that the key to good outcomes is effective teamwork, which requires shared values. While our education and healthcare systems educate and employ individual practitioners such as nurses, doctors or therapists, ultimately our diverse skills are complementary. Our boundaries of practice are not nearly as distinct as we would like to believe, and in many cases our work overlaps and interlinks. Nurses in one context may do what doctors do in another, and vice versa. For example, in isolated areas nurses often work alone with no professional support apart from someone at the end of a telephone line (assuming they have a telephone line). Nurses in these contexts triage, diagnose, treat and manage care in the way that a general practitioner in the city might. And, in the city, general practitioners may dress wounds and give injections which in a hospital would be the work of a nurse. One solution to 'turf battles' of practice is to use models of care that place the patient, rather than any one practitioner, at the centre of care. This focuses the mind on the core of healthcare practice – the patient – and away from vested interests. One such model of care is that used by nurse practitioners working in many primary healthcare contexts, either alone or in collaboration with other health professionals.

On 1 November 2010 there was a move towards acknowledging and valuing the role of nurse practitioners in our workforce through groundbreaking changes to Medicare legislation.[6] From this date, approved nurse practitioners and midwives working collaboratively with doctors but in private practice have access to a provider number, thus enabling their patients access to a Medicare rebate for specific itemised services. Nurse practitioners working in the public healthcare system in some states and territories also have access to a pharmaceutical benefits prescriber number which enables them to prescribe medications for their patients through this scheme.

While these changes have taken two decades to achieve, against much criticism from national medical bodies, they represent one more step towards the roles of nurses and midwives being validated as making a difference in people's lives. In turn this validates the lives of those nurses and midwives who are dedicated to improving access to quality care. And in this way their sense of worth and connectedness are reinforced, thus leading to emotional wellbeing for the practitioner.

Collaborative multidisciplinary models of practice that fully involve the patient have been shown to be highly satisfactory and empowering for both providers and patients.[7] It could be said that practitioners who are unwilling to work in a team that involves the patient may be violating the ethical principles inherent in any professional code of conduct. Nevertheless, true collaboration in healthcare remains difficult to put into practice for reasons that are mainly to do with enforcing power and control rather than best patient care.

To work in a team so that care is not fragmented, individual practitioners need to take time out to consider their values individually and share them in a way that underpins the paradigm of care in which they work. This is rarely done, resulting in severe conflict in some cases because individual practitioners may have different values concerning whom to treat, with what and for how long. While ultimately there may be one decision maker, it is worthwhile for the whole team to take time to discuss the patient's wishes, needs and cultural beliefs and to include the patient in the team discussion. In many cases the nurse is often privy to information never shared with the doctor/s. This is not necessarily because the doctor is not a good listener but because the doctor may not be available, whereas the nurse cares for the patient for long periods of time, often in quite an intimate way. And, alternatively, the doctor may have very well-thought-out arguments for why a treatment should be considered. Unless there is a space for such conversations to happen before the event, decisions will always be made from only one perspective, with critical implications for healthy workplaces.

Toni Sullivan[8] comments on the way in which collaboration requires individuals to change or even reaffirm their values if they are to work in new ways with others. Collaboration itself can change individuals in many ways because of the experience of being forced to consider others and their ways of thinking and working. For many, the fact that others may have different values and ways of working is extremely confronting, requiring much reflection on personal values as well as a willingness to balance personal values with shared values when working in a team.

THE PERSONAL IN THE PROFESSIONAL – A MATTER OF BALANCE

In a role that demands so much, personally and professionally, what can a nurse do to maintain a sense of equilibrium, of balance, so that work remains satisfying, indeed rewarding? The mass of material on a healthy, balanced life and health-related issues is complex in terms of what to believe and what to ignore. There are journals, tabloid newspapers, magazines and talk-back shows bombarding us with information about diet, exercise, relationships, cosmetic surgery, alternative therapies and drugs. How does one individual make sense of such a mountain of material? This chapter does not intend to address such debates because of lack of space and because there is so much good research devoted to this area which individuals can access. A reliable way of gaining the most up-to-date data is to download the weekly health report material from the ABC website (www.abc.net.au/health/). Perhaps the most interesting thing to note in all the debate about health, however, is the way in which we have focused on our bodies over the last three decades to the point of obsession, perhaps neglecting other components of wellbeing.

Since the early 1980s particularly, there has been an emphasis on, even a fanaticism over, health and fitness. Health and wellbeing have become big business. And indeed the reality is that, as a population, chronic diseases such as type 2 diabetes are more prevalent as obesity figures increase. Exercise is now one of our largest industries as joggers pound the streets with the latest equipment, expensive personal trainers become increasingly popular, and gymnasiums promise weight loss, weight gain, weight redistribution and happier, more successful lives, all for an annual fee. Pharmaceutical companies bombard us with new and better vitamin/mineral compounds in which the secret to longevity is supposedly contained. Food is dissected to within an inch of its organic components, categorised and labelled accordingly. We can buy it fat-free, chemical-free, preservative-free, sugar-free, calorie-free and taste-free.

The recent demand for perfect health (and the perfect body) – as opposed to 'being healthy' – has created whole new job categories. Fitness trainers, lifestyle managers, beauty therapists and psychic gurus have capitalised on and helped to manufacture our obsession with our bodies. In the USA this has reached manic proportions, with the restructuring, reorganising and reorientation of people now a huge industry. Bodies are manufactured, manipulated and managed. The ultimate medical manipulation of our bodies is, of course, plastic surgery. Advertising constantly bombards us with messages concerning our ability to reinvent our own bodies through diet, exercise and surgery. As a cultural medium, our bodies are also regulated by norms perpetuated through these media images. The advertising associated with the commodification of our wellbeing has had both positive and negative impact. While providing a vector for the dissemination of information, it has also increased the anxiety and confusion we have about avoiding illness (and perhaps even death) and having the perfect life and body.

Accordingly, the general public has become much more likely to seek alternatives to those offered by conventional medicine. One of the most significant consequences of the contemporary focus on physical, mental and emotional wellbeing, and the growing disillusionment with the conventional system, has been the increasing rejection of conventional medicine and medical practices in favour of what are termed 'alternative' therapies.[9] These so-called alternatives are in fact traditional therapies, ousted when modern medicine gained its scientific foothold in the mid-1800s. One study of parents with children being treated for cancer showed that about 50% had also sought alternative therapy.[10]

Treatments that are becoming increasingly popular include acupuncture, homeopathy, iridology, hypnotherapy, naturopathy, aromatherapy and herbs. These have been incorporated into many people's lives for some time now as daily routines.[7] For patients who are accessing both conventional and alternative medicine, the cost of healthcare is doubled and, nationally, this increases the overall amount spent on health and illness.[10]

Recognition of traditional Chinese medicine has recently translated into registration of practitioners and into universities offering undergraduate and postgraduate degrees. Patients with illnesses such as autoimmune disorders, irritable bowel syndrome, cancer, arthritis, infertility and even asthma are the most likely to consult such practitioners because they are often unable to gain relief through conventional medicine. There are also those who attend traditional therapists as a preventive measure and those who simply want to optimise their feeling of wellbeing, of being supremely healthy.

WHAT IS HEALTH AND WHAT IS ILLNESS?

The concepts of health and illness are, of course, not immutable but are constructed culturally and historically. In turn, these constructs structure the way health and illness care are delivered and, therefore, received. For example, whereas most Western countries have traditionally focused their notions of healthcare around illness, specifically acute illnesses, other cultures focus on staying healthy and preventing illness. As a result, the way a society funds its healthcare usually reflects its perceptions of health and illness.

Health is currently defined by the World Health Organization Constitution as being a 'state of complete physical, mental and social well being and not merely the absence of disease or infirmity'.[11] This general definition of health reflects current popular notions of health in the West, although this rarely translates into a different funding regime. As advances in science have enabled mass immunity from certain infectious diseases, at the same time as nutrition and sanitation have improved, people in developed economies have broadened their views of illness and health. They are now able to envisage a life longer and healthier than that of their mothers and fathers (unless they are Indigenous Australians) and, as a result, they can rethink the very notion of what constitutes a healthy life. It is a conception of health that moves beyond the mere absence of disease. As a result, the late 20th century witnessed a new focus on mental/emotional health. Indeed, psychological wellbeing is now considered an essential part of being healthy, although it does not yet receive the same attention or the funding it requires.

A 60-year-old Australian woman, recently discharged from a private hospital after a prolonged illness, spoke to me about what health means to her. Her comments sum up the contemporary, popular, Western understanding of health prevalent in Australia today:

> I don't see that [health] as purely a medical thing. To me, being healthy is how I'm perceiving life, how I'm relating to people, how I'm coping with day-to-day things. And I guess there are more things that influence that than the physical condition of your body.

The World Health Organization's Global Strategy of Health for All by the Year 2000[12] states:

All people in all countries should have at least such a level of health that they are capable of working productively and of participating actively in the social life in which they live.

DEVELOPING A HEALTHY LIFESTYLE

So how can we work productively every day, yet maintain our health and wellbeing so that we have a well-balanced life?

There is an increasing interest in the notion of coping, in individual coping mechanisms, in why stress in one individual may not be perceived as stress by another, and why things such as cancer survival are not necessarily scientifically determined. This research into coping has important outcomes for individuals and organisations attempting to ensure safe, healthy and productive working days and workplaces. It also answers some important questions. Does a heavy workload increase your stress? Do those who work longer hours feel more stressed, and are they more unhealthy, than those who work shorter hours? What are the major stressors for employees?

Interestingly, the most recent research has confirmed that it is certainly not as simple as hours of work; it's more about control, specifically control over work. What Professor Syme from the University of Berkeley, California, calls 'cell mastery' involves 'control over destiny; the ability at work to decide how and at what pace we get the job done, and how to be able to traverse life's difficulties and solve everyday problems so they don't overwhelm us'.[13]

Recently the *British Medical Journal* reported the findings of a Harvard study of 21,000 female nurses which showed that having a high-stress job in which one has little job control or support is as damaging to the health as smoking, alcohol or lack of exercise.[14] And those with poor health outcomes in this study continued to deteriorate over a 4-year period. The measures of health utilised in this Harvard study were physical functioning, limitations due to physical and emotional problems, pain, vitality, social functioning and mental health. Such outcomes have been replicated in a yet to be completed longitudinal study of women's health which is monitoring 42,000 Australian women over 20 years.[15] The healthiest women are those who are self-employed or in family businesses; that is, they feel more in control of their lives. However, a more recent study cautioned about the limitations of occupational health research that does not take into account the broader social environment of workers.[16] When such factors were taken into consideration in Canada's National Population Health Survey, the individual's position at work played a limited role in health and wellbeing when the structures of daily life and the agent's personality were accounted for. Indeed, it was shown that compared with occupational structures, the structures of daily life play a far more important role in psychological distress.

Of course, aspects of work that may have negative effects on an individual's health include lack of control, such as not being able to be one's own boss, have flexible hours or determine ways of undertaking tasks, and lack of support.[16] This knowledge leads to new ways of understanding what interventions are required in terms of making workplaces more satisfactory for workers. Rather than merely reducing hours of work, interventions should enable individuals to feel more in control of their environment at work. Flexible rostering for nurses would be one way of enabling individuals to regain a sense of control over when they work, and if the rostering was done by team negotiation it would add to such control. Control over the practice environment; clinical autonomy; good nurse–physician relationships; clinically competent peers; supportive supervisors; adequate staffing; support for education; and concern for the patients are all characteristics of what have been identified as 'magnet hospitals'[17] – those hospitals that attract and retain staff.

Dr Bruce McEwen, from the Rockefeller University in New York, has made meaning of his neuroendocrinology research into stress by applying it to social policies. According to McEwen, when we are under stress our hormonal response attempts to enable us to re-establish homeostasis through allostasis, which means 'achieving stasis through change'.[18] In this way we survive our minute-to-minute challenges through what is a perfectly healthy response. Thus, while stress is a challenge to the body biologically because it is reliant on the adrenal glands producing catecholamines and cortisol, it is also a means of achieving resilience as individuals in our daily lives. In turn, however, as with most biological mechanisms, balance is crucial. A healthy response can become unhealthy if the body is unable to turn off hormonal responses once the acute stress has passed. This results in a continual stream of hormones being poured into the bloodstream, which can be quite damaging. Inefficient operation of hormonal response is referred to as our 'allostatic load', that is, the load from the stress mediators on our body. This may be protective or it may be damaging, depending on our biological response as well as our environment. Both play a part in our allostatic load.

The two forms of stress discussed here are acute and chronic stress. It is chronic stress that is particularly damaging because of the continual outpouring of the stress hormones, causing damage to organs and tissues. And chronic stress is usually not caused by a sudden incidental event, but by longer-term ongoing events such as a personal or professional environment that is full of conflict, or one in which individuals perceive themselves to be out of control. In such cases hormonal levels are continually high, which over time results in a stress-related disorder such as posttraumatic or dramatic disorder, a disorder in which an individual's body has been sensitised to overreact to things that would not normally be disturbing to others.

McEwen has also identified certain lifestyle choices as responses to stress – for example, overeating, poor dietary choices and lack of exercise – but the problem is that these all synergise with the effects of increased hormonal levels to speed up bodily changes such as increased weight and its side effects. Genetic influences may also add to an individual's allostatic load – for example, familial hypertension and type 2 diabetes, both of which add to biological stress. According to McEwen, cited in Swan,[19] there is also some evidence that certain physical characteristics, such as excess abdominal fat, are indicators of high allostatic load. These characteristics are found mainly in populations that have poorer environments and reduced personal resources, both economically and psychologically. The individuals in such environments have raised hormonal levels due to chronic stress.

One of the alternative techniques which has been proven to reduce stress and thus improve cardiac risk factors in patients with coronary heart disease is transcendental meditation (TM). In a randomised trial reported in the *Journal of the American Medical Association*, one arm of the study offered participants a 16-week trial of TM while the other study arm offered health education. At the end of the trial those in the TM arm had significantly reduced blood pressure as well as improved levels of fasting blood glucose and insulin levels and more stable functioning of the autonomic nervous system, which is significant in controlling stress responses.[20] Another study involving TM was that carried out by Castillo-Richmond and colleagues from the Center for Natural Medicine and Prevention in Iowa. This study investigated the effects of stress reduction on carotid atherosclerosis in hypertensive African Americans using TM as the method of reducing stress.[21] The TM group in the study showed a significant decrease in the intima media thickness of the carotid artery following the adoption of two sessions of 20 minutes of TM in their daily life. Carotid intima media thickness is a significant predictor of coronary heart disease: an increase in thickness predicts an increased risk.

WHAT MAKES US HEALTHY WORKERS?

We certainly know that socioeconomic status has an impact on the risk of disease, with those in lower socioeconomic groups having a higher incidence of disease.[22] Whether this is to do with nutrition or lack of control, or with a factor yet to be uncovered, we can only work with the evidence we have so far. Similarly, the 2006 Gallup World Poll 20, which studies income health and wellbeing around the world, showed that life satisfaction was strongly related to per capita national income.[22] Although not the same as disease, satisfaction with life is a major influence on the quality of day-to-day living and perhaps on an individual's health and wellbeing.

An important factor in lowering people's risk of death is social networks. Having strong social networks and friendships and being involved in social activities are all variables that make a difference in terms of feeling better and living longer with a healthier mental state.[23]

The plethora of research on health is consistent in stating that exercise and diet are major variables. While writings on both these factors form anthologies in their own right, and there are conflicting opinions about both diet and exercise, there is also some unequivocal evidence that we need to heed. The first is that the body does need some activity to keep it able to function. Staying in bed and immobile is not good for circulation, respiration or flexibility.[24] Contradictions enter the debate when it comes to how much and what kind of exercise is ideal, and at what time in life.

Trends in exercise each decade are clear evidence of the lack of any one body of research that points the way. Professor Stuart Biddle, head of sports psychology at Loughborough University, UK, has shown that the increased self-esteem and reduced anxiety observed in those who exercise are due to the biochemical changes that take place as we exercise.[25] This may be a key factor in why exercise has such a positive impact on our health and why some individuals become obsessed with exercise.

The intense high-impact aerobic classes of the 1980s have been gradually replaced by the resistance and strength classes, individual workouts and yoga of our contemporary society. These include boxing, resistance cycling, defencercise and pump classes, moving away from pounding the streets as many of us did during the jogging craze. Indeed, such pounding has been criticised for causing joint and skeletal damage which rarely manifests as pain and impaired mobility until later in life. The two exercises that have remained consistently popular over the years are walking and swimming. These have been identified as the two ideal forms of exercise for the majority of the population who are able to undertake them as activities. And to gain the most benefit they should be undertaken regularly, three times per week.

For postmenopausal women, walking is preferable because of the positive impact of weight bearing on preventing severe osteoporosis. A study into physical activity in postmenopausal women[26] showed that, in those women who engaged in vigorous activity four times per week compared with women who didn't engage in such activity, there was a 43% reduced risk of dying. The risk reduction was also there for women who engaged in moderate activity only once a week. They still had a 24% reduced risk of dying compared with those women who undertook no activity at all. As far as osteoporosis is concerned, genetic predisposition is still a major factor, as are smoking and inadequate calcium intake.

Exercise has also been shown to lower the risk of developing breast cancer. In a 14-year study of 25,000 women aged 20–54 years, those who exercised had a lower risk of developing breast cancer, with the greatest reduction in those women who were leaner than average and exercised at least 4 hours per week.[27]

In terms of adequate nutrition, while the literature is massive and often conflicting, several key factors are central. These are that adequate amounts of protein, carbohydrates and fats, fluids and vitamins and minerals are essential to a healthy daily diet. The conflict in the evidence comes in terms of amounts and types of each, with some diets even dictating the time of day each should be consumed. The National Health and Medical Research Council published *Dietary Guidelines for Older Australians* in which it was claimed that 'fifty per cent of deaths of Australians aged 65–69 are diet-related'.[28] It has also been shown that bad diets appear to be related to loneliness, grief and depression.[19]

THE CULTURE OF THE CONTEMPORARY WORKPLACE

So does following a healthy lifestyle and ensuring that your life is balanced mitigate against the impact of an unhealthy workplace? In answering this we need to narrow the workplace down to the healthcare workplace, which is somewhat different to many other workplaces. Deidre Wicks, a researcher from Newcastle University, has undertaken one of the most indepth and contemporary exposés of the healthcare workplace in terms of nurses and doctors.[29] Her study not only provides insight into the conflict inherent within professional boundaries, but also erects signposts for new graduates entering the workplace.

As Wicks comments, 'Power is ever-present within health settings. It is evident in the way people walk, the way they communicate, in who gets recognised as having a presence and who gets ignored' (p 91).[29] Wicks observed in the 5 months she was in the workplace that it was rare for doctors and cleaners to interact, and this was also the case for doctors and very junior nurses. She also noted that at times both doctors and nurses exhibited behaviours of ownership of the ward and, ipso facto, of the patients.

The exercise of power within the hierarchy of medicine over nurses and even patients surprised Wicks in that it had 'survived the reforms of the "new managerialism" in health care settings' (p 98).[29]

The fact that public healthcare in particular is dominated by the technologically driven medical specialties marginalises the discourses and therefore practices of those wishing to work in a more contemporary framework of healing. Wicks notes that nurses facilitate this marginalisation through their apparent willingness to pick up the invisible caring components of patient care while the doctors continue their visible curing component. This division has implications not only for healthcare policies but, I would argue, for healthy workplaces in which the most effective care can be delivered by a functioning, multidisciplinary team. The research previously outlined in this chapter has emphasised the importance of control over one's role and of support in the workplace. Wicks' study reveals clearly that this is not currently so, and the present difficulty in recruiting and retaining nurses may be a clear indicator of a culture that is outmoded and even disabling for many working in it.

Several studies[30,31] of graduate nurses have revealed similar issues facing new graduates in their first and ongoing years in practice. These centre around the ability to preserve their moral integrity, as the workplace values and their personal values are often incongruent. Living up to their individual perceptions of the nursing role was often in conflict with the role dictated by management and the socialisation of the workplace. The consequences of such a mismatch can cause moral distress, leading to self-blame and self-criticism, as individuals questioned their professional abilities.

To avoid such distress, which can lead to the loss of competent, caring nurses, those entering the workplace need to articulate their practice clearly and to be open and assertive in their dialogue with their fellow practitioners. But it is also up to the healthcare team to engage and support new graduates since they are the future workforce. While Wicks' solution of nurses and doctors undertaking undergraduate degrees together may not be feasible in the short term, her goal is still possible in the workplace. This is to move towards integrating the best of modern medicine with a perspective that emphasises 'holism, illness prevention and the relationships between health, illness, individual life history and social structure' (p 181).[29]

Understanding the workplace and its culture is essential for anyone entering the workforce since it assists the initial assimilation of a new graduate. Entering a new work environment is difficult for even a skilled individual who has been in the workforce before but is now entering a new workplace environment.

Healthcare is a multifaceted system in terms of the contexts, the geographical sites, the personnel and the levels of care. Compounding this is the public/private and the federal/state divides. Contexts include acute hospitals, community centres, nursing homes, rehabilitation centres and people's homes. Geographical sites include city and country and the areas in between. Personnel include nurses, doctors, therapists, technicians, cleaners, dieticians, pharmacists and social workers.

With such complexity in the contexts in which care takes place it is extremely difficult to identify a single culture, as may be possible in a simpler system. Instead we have multiple cultures requiring newcomers to adjust as they move across various areas within the system.

It is little wonder, therefore, that the healthcare system is a difficult culture to traverse for the 'new kid on the block'. More recent changes brought about by the managerialism that has invaded the public sector have created an environment in which the naive tend to struggle. This is mainly to do with the efficiency imperatives that demand productivity gains in the system. And in healthcare, where people rather than, say, whitegoods are involved, the main strategies used to make gains have been to reduce staff, increase workload and increase turnover of patients. Given that we have an increasingly elderly and drug-dependent patient population and more sophisticated technology and pharmacology, we now have an industry in which staff are working harder with fewer resources at a time when patients are more highly dependent and yet are discharged to recover at home.

It is important to note that being in control at work is only one part of the very complex equation that makes up the profile of being healthy, an equation that is in its infancy in terms of being solved. After all, as Michael Marmot,[32] Professor of Epidemiology and Public Health at University College, London, points out, the fact that those in control at work may also be on a higher salary and more educated in nutrition must be factored into the equation. Such individuals are more likely to eat fresh fruit and vegetables, which contain antioxidants and vitamins thought to be protective against certain cancers and other illnesses.

CONCLUSION

The workplace into which new nursing graduates journey is vastly different from the one in which many of us worked several decades ago. The contemporary emphasis on fiscal restraint, organisational restructuring and measurable outcomes rarely takes account of the cost of caring work mainly undertaken by nurses. A Canadian nurse, Brenda Sabo,[33] investigated the consequences of caring work in her doctoral program and discovered that many nurses who care for patients experiencing trauma, pain and suffering themselves suffer from compassion fatigue. Certain qualities, however, appear to offer protection against compassion fatigue. These are resilience, hardiness and social support – qualities that may take time to develop. It is up to each one of us in the nursing profession to support our neophyte nurses in every possible way, not only assisting them in their daily caring work but also ensuring that they are able to pursue healthy, well-balanced lives.

CASE STUDY 8.1

As a first-year graduate registered nurse, you are working in an orthopaedic ward mainly with elderly patients who have undergone surgery. You observe one of the senior registered nurses consistently handling the patients in what you consider to be a rough manner when he is assisting them to get out of bed.

REFLECTIVE QUESTIONS

- What steps would you take in this circumstance?
- Who would you speak to in order to address this?
- If you were unable to do anything about the behaviour what would you do?

CASE STUDY 8.2

You are asked to work in cardiac rehabilitation following graduate studies in the area. The model of care in the unit is collaborative, involving a physiotherapist, psychologist, social worker, doctors and yourself as the specialist nurse. In the case conferences you notice that that your opinion is consistently ignored despite your expertise in the area. In addition you are never asked for your ideas when difficult situations are encountered.

REFLECTIVE QUESTIONS

- What steps could you take to change this?
- Explore the way an effective collaborative model involving practitioners from several disciplines could work most effectively.
- Who should be at the centre of a collaborative model of care? Why?

CASE STUDY 8.3

In your second year as a registered nurse you are asked to mentor a new graduate who is very uncertain and obviously unsure of many procedures and practices. You have a heavy caseload and at the time you are also studying part-time so you feel slightly stressed.

REFLECTIVE QUESTIONS

- Think back to how you felt when you first graduated and began working as a registered nurse. List the feelings and concerns you remember having.
- What helped you most to overcome your concerns?
- Was there a staff member who helped you during that first year? If so, think about what this person did which helped you most and explore what you might do to assist this new graduate while ensuring you remain healthy and safe.

EXERCISE 8.1

Reflect on your own lifestyle and diarise a normal week's activities, including your nutritional intake and exercise. Answer the following questions once you have completed your diary:

1. Do you have a balance of work, play and rest?
2. Is your diet balanced in terms of essential nutrients, ensuring it is low in fat and high in complex carbohydrates? Do you have at least three servings of fruit and vegetables per day?
3. Do you walk wherever possible?
4. Do you feel rested when you wake from your sleep?

EXERCISE 8.2

---

1. Examine your workplace. What is the culture like in terms of enabling effective teamwork, rewarding commitment and initiative and allowing open consultation?
2. What do you contribute to the workplace to enable better teamwork, open consultation and positive reinforcement of colleagues?
3. What three initiatives do you intend to undertake to ensure a more effective work environment?

RECOMMENDED READING

Lumby J. Who cares? The changing health care system. Sydney: Allen & Unwin; 2001.

Peterson A, Lupton D. The new public health: a new morality? In: The new public health: health and self in the age of risk. Sydney: Allen & Unwin; 1996. p. 1–27.

Sullivan TJ. Collaboration, a health care imperative: reflection on values. In: Sullivan TJ, editor. Collaboration: a health care imperative. New York: McGraw-Hill; 1998. p. 622.

Swan N. Good stress and bad stress. Radio National's 'The Health Report', Monday 13 April 1998. Online. Available: http://www.abc.net.au/rn/talks/8.30/helthrpt/stories/s10743.htm

Turkel M, Ray M. Creating a caring practice environment through self-renewal. Nursing Administration Quarterly 2004;29:249–54.

REFERENCES

1. Lumby J. Who cares? The changing health care system. Sydney: Allen & Unwin; 2001. p. 36–53.
2. NSW Health Department. Nursing recruitment and retention taskforce, final report. NSW Health Department: NSW; 1996.
3. Australian Institute of Health and Welfare bulletin no. 81. 13 October 2010. AIHW cat. no. AUS 130.
4. Lumby J. Who cares? The changing health care system. Sydney: Allen & Unwin; 2001. p. 19–35.
5. Sullivan TJ. Collaboration, a health care imperative: reflection on values. In: Sullivan TJ, editor. Collaboration: a health care imperative. New York: McGraw-Hill; 1998. p. 621–4.
6. Health Legislation Amendment (Midwives and Nurse Practitioners) Act. Federal Government Department of Health & Ageing. Canberra. March. 2010.
7. Rose J, Glass N. Community mental health nurses speak out: the critical relationship between emotional wellbeing and satisfying professional practice. Collegian 2006;13:27–32.
8. Sullivan TJ. Collaboration, a health care imperative. New York: McGraw-Hill; 1998. p. 622.

9. Phelan A. Culture, cure: orthodoxy embraces alternative medicine. Health for Life 1. Sydney Morning Herald. 21 October 1997. p. H1–H4.

10. Sawyer MG, Gannow A, Toogood IR, et al. The use of alternative therapies by children with cancer. Medical Journal of Australia 1994;160:320–2.

11. Editorial. Health and Development Aug 1998;181:2.

12. Peterson A, Lupton D. The new public health: a new morality? In: The new public health: health and self in the age of risk. Sydney: Allen & Unwin; 1996. p. 1–2.

13. Swan N. Mastering the control factor, part 4. Radio National's 'The Health Report', Monday 30 November 1998. Online. Available: http://www.abc.net.au/rn/talks/8.30/helthrpt/stories/s17549.htm

14. Stock S. Sick of work? Your job could be killing you. Weekend Australian 2000;Jun 3–4:3.

15. Lee C, Dobson AJ, Brown WJ, et al. Cohort profile: the Australian longitudinal study on women's health. International Journal of Epidemiology 2005;34:987–91.

16. Marchand A, Demers A, Durand P. Do occupation and work conditions really matter? A longitudinal analysis of psychological distress experiences among Canadian workers. Sociology of Health & Illness 2005;27:602–27.

17. Aiken LH. Superior outcomes for magnet hospitals: the evidence base. In: McClure ML, Hinshaw AS, editors. Magnet hospitals revisited: attraction and retention of professional nurses. Washington DC: American Nurses Publishing; 2002.

18. McEwen BS. Protective and damaging effects of stress mediators. New England Journal of Medicine 1998;338:171–9.

19. Swan N. Good stress and bad stress. Radio National's 'The Health Report', Monday 13 April 1998. Online. Available: http://www.abc.net.au/rn/talks/8.30/helthrpt/stories/s10743.htm

20. Paul-Labrador M. Transcendental meditation may improve cardiac risk factors in patients with coronary heart disease. JAMA 2006;June 12.

21. Castillo-Richmond A, Schneider RH, Alexander CN, et al. Effects of stress reduction on carotid atherosclerosis in hypertensive African Americans. Stroke 2000;31:568–73.

22. Deaton A. Income, health and wellbeing around the world: evidence from the Gallup world poll. Journal Economic Perspectives 2008;22:53–72.

23. Swan N. Mastering the control factor, part 2. Radio National's 'The Health Report', Monday 6 November 1998. Online. Available: http://www.abc.net.au/rn/talks/8.30/helthrpt/stories/s17092.htm

24. Allen C, Glasziou P, Del Mar C. Bed-rest: a potentially harmful treatment needing more careful evaluation. Lancet 1999;354:1229–33.

25. Clark A. Exercise your style. Good medicine. Sydney: Network Distribution; 20 April 1987.

26. Kushi LH, Fee R, Anderson K, et al. Physical activity and mortality in postmenopausal women. Journal of the American Medical Association 1997;227:1287–92.

27. Thune I, Brenn T, Lund E, et al. Physical activity and the risk of breast cancer. New England Journal of Medicine 1997;336:1269–75.

28. Reiner V. Senior death by diet avoidable. Health, The Weekend Australian 2000;Feb 19–20:7.

29. Wicks D. Nurses and doctors at work: rethinking professional boundaries. Sydney: Allen & Unwin; 1999.

30. Kelly B. Preserving moral integrity: a follow up study with new graduate nurses. Journal of Advanced Nursing 1998;28(5):1134–45.

31. Kelly B. Hospital nursing: It's a battle! A follow up study of English graduate nurses. Journal of Advanced Nursing.1996;24:1063–9.

32. Marmot M. Inequalities in death specific explanations of general pattern. Lancet. 1984;323:1003–6.

33. Sabo BM. Compassion fatigue and nursing work: can we accurately capture the consequences of caring work? International Journal of Nursing Practice 2006;12: 136–42.

CHAPTER 9

Managing approaches to nursing care delivery

Patricia M Davidson and Bronwyn Everett

LEARNING OBJECTIVES

When you have completed this chapter you will be able to:

- identify the importance of tailoring models of nursing care delivery to meet the needs of patients and their families
- recognise key roles and responsibilities for nurses in delivering patient care
- describe strategies for managing nursing workload and time management practices
- consider the role of the registered nurse in an environment of varying skill mix and diverse scopes of practice
- discuss the overarching professional, legal and regulatory frameworks that can influence delivery of nursing care.

Keywords: models of nursing care, mentorship, time management, lifelong learning, setting priorities

---

INTRODUCTION

Contemporary healthcare systems are characterised by their complexity and also the pressures they experience due to increased demand, technological complexity and fiscal constraints. Nursing is a dynamic profession, delivered in a wide variety of settings and in a range of models and regulatory frameworks.[1] The role, scope and function of nursing practice are driven by the social, political and economic contexts in which the care is delivered.[2,3] For example, in countries such as the USA there is a greater emphasis on independent nursing practice, whereas in other countries (such as Australia) there is less of an emphasis on these roles because of opposition in introducing these roles. It is only in recent years in Australia that the nurse practitioner role has been included in healthcare delivery models.[4] Encouraging a range of policy changes has enabled the enactment of the nurse practitioner role.[5] In recent times funding and policy changes have seen the rapid development of the nursing role in Australian general practice.[6] This represents an exciting time for the nursing role in primary care.

In spite of the diverse range and scope of practice, nursing is focused on facilitating wellness and caring for the vulnerable and infirm in the primary, secondary and tertiary care sectors. Nursing practice is constantly evolving and, despite the explosion of new technology and labour-saving devices, nurses have never before been required to deliver high-quality patient care within a context of organisational pressures for efficiencies. Despite these challenges there is an increasing recognition of the importance of nursing in influencing patient outcomes, and the importance of monitoring and evaluating workforce characteristics, particularly the numbers and ratios of registered nurses to other health workers.[7]

Considerable advances and changes in healthcare have occurred since World War II. Escalating technological solutions for healthcare, beginning in the 1960–70s, have driven the development of nursing specialties. An example is the coronary care unit,[8] where changes in care patterns have evolved in line with diagnostic and therapeutic advances, leading to a diversification of nursing roles and the subsequent restructuring of inpatient cardiac services. Primary angioplasty and other innovative procedures mean that lengths of stay in hospital are shorter, leaving less time for secondary prevention.[9] This has placed an increasing importance on transitional care and models that interface with community-based care.[10] In many settings, technological innovation and telemedicine have facilitated the reach of the nursing role to populations with limited access.[11] However, population ageing, the increasing burden of chronic conditions and increasing fiscal constraints are now leading nurses and other health professionals to search for alternative strategies that lie beyond technology for more inclusive and humanistic models of patient care delivery. In particular the importance of prevention, risk management and patient self-management is an increasing focus of nursing care.[9]

In this chapter we look at models of nursing care, the key roles and responsibilities of nurses, managing workload and time management, setting priorities and planning in clinical practice, mentorship and preceptorship, and measuring the outcomes of nursing care. The discussion relates particularly to moving from senior undergraduate student to newly registered nurse and the skills required in making this transition.

MODELS OF NURSING CARE

Nursing is a diverse and multifaceted profession, and nursing care is delivered across a range of settings and contexts from primary prevention to palliative care. Nursing care can be independent in nature, such as nurse–practitioner-based models, or dependent, based on delegation, such as in intensive care; other models include substitution, such as with physician assistants, and enhancement, such as in nurse-coordinated models of care.[12,13] A comprehensive understanding of the nature of nursing practice requires careful consideration and examination of the dynamic processes that have an impact on the nursing profession, including regulatory and legal frameworks. Models are conceptual tools or devices that can be used to understand and place complex phenomena in perspective. A model is a standard or an example for imitation or comparison, combining concepts, beliefs and intents that are related in some way.[2] This organisation of concepts, together with a philosophy of care, allows nurses to plan, deliver and evaluate nurse care in a systematic manner based on theoretical propositions.[14] Nursing care is both independent and interdependent practice initiated on the basis of nursing assessment and actions within an interdisciplinary setting. Therefore as you develop into the registered nurse role it is important that you also engage in a process of self-reflection to identify the attitudes, values and beliefs you bring to this encounter.

Novel models of care are usually developed in response to perceived deficits in existing care delivery. An example is the care of patients with chronic heart failure (CHF). This condition is an intricate constellation of pathophysiological processes that results in a syndrome eventuating from inadequate cardiac output and neurohormonal activation.[15] CHF has a significant chronic physical and psychosocial impact on the individual and is responsible for substantial family and societal burden. The unpredictable illness trajectory of CHF and subsequent life-threatening complications dictate ongoing management and frequent hospitalisation. Readmission rates of up to 30% have been shown in both Australian and international contexts, with up to 50% of these readmissions attributable to failure to comply with prescribed treatment regimens rather than treatment failure.[16] The need for support in self-management and coordination of care has implications for models of nursing care, discharge planning and community follow-up.[17]

The burden of CHF has led to the development of innovative pharmacological and non-pharmacological interventions. Innovative care models have been developed and continue to be developed. Many of these have been collaboratively developed by nurses, focusing on nurse-directed interventions. Many of these approaches to nursing care are based on strategies that promote self-management and treatment adherence.[18]

Changes in the contemporary management of CHF reflect the evolution of nursing care delivery in response to changes in practice patterns, patient needs and demographic profiles, and importantly demonstrate that the profession of nursing is required to be flexible and dynamic in achieving improved health outcomes for patients in a diversity of care settings.[19] Further, models of nursing care in chronic conditions, such as chronic obstructive pulmonary disease and diabetes, place an emphasis on continuity of care rather than a perception of acute and chronic care as distinct and isolated care providers. Many of the current healthcare reforms internationally seek to build a bridge between these distinct care models.[20]

Contemporary models of nursing practice need to be appropriate to the needs of individual patients as well as local policy and funding models. As a consequence these approaches need to be:

- dynamic – responsive to a changing and diverse environment, subject to social, political, economic and cultural change

- eclectic – looking to other disciplines and philosophies to combine factors to improve and complement nursing practice
- responsive – to the needs of health consumers and fiscal priorities
- multidisciplinary – involving consultation with all healthcare professionals and healthcare providers
- interdisciplinary – where the combination of a range of disciplines is greater than the single application of an intervention of a singular profession.

A range of models of nursing care have developed since the Nightingale apprenticeship style of task allocation based on seniority and experience. Common models of care include team nursing, patient allocation and primary nursing, which all provide a more holistic and patient-centred approach to individual patient care; primary nursing ensures nurse responsibility and accountability beyond the individual shift timeframe. Some health systems have the registered nurse as the coordinator of care, while second-line nurses (e.g. enrolled nurses, nursing assistants), nursing students or unregistered healthcare workers assist in direct and non-direct patient care activities. Since the introduction of tertiary-based education in Australia, direct hospital-based nursing care has been provided primarily by registered nurses with some support from enrolled nurses. Primarily related to the nursing workforce shortage, this composition has changed in recent times and there is increasingly a diversification in skill mix in the clinical setting. This requires the registered nurse to function in a more problem-solving, communication and delegation role. Therefore, when planning nursing care the registered nurse has to consider:

- constructing interventions using a framework of evidence and/or theoretical propositions
- planning of care delivery informed by assessment of patient, health provider and health system needs
- evaluating health-related outcomes and intervention outcomes
- consulting with all stakeholders in a participative context
- promoting the safety and wellbeing of nurses
- incorporating a multidisciplinary approach where applicable
- configuring healthcare resources to promote accessibility and optimal utilisation
- promoting equity of access for all members of society
- negotiating interventions that are culturally sensitive and appropriate.

Underpinning nursing models is consideration of the processes of clinical decision making, organising care delivery and planning care outcomes. An important part of developing effective models of nursing care is ensuring that there is assessment of outcomes on an organisation, provider and consumer basis. With the increasing view that multidisciplinary collaboration is important for continuity of care, an emphasis on a specific nursing care plan is increasingly considered 'nurse-centric' and isolated from the team approach to patient care. One solution offered as a ward-based method of managing patients in the acute hospital setting is the model of case management.[21] Case management plans provide guidelines for time-based critical incidents during a patient's hospital stay, including the appropriate length of stay and recommendations for evidence-based treatment. As well, the plans offer collaborative interdisciplinary management strategies for all health professionals providing direct patient care, by standardising appropriate use of resources, promoting collaborative team practice, coordinating continuity of care during the patient's admission period and improving patient and clinician satisfaction.[22,23]

A critical or clinical pathway is a patient management tool which is a summary and a component of the case management plan.[24] The critical path is an interdisciplinary plan of care which provides guidelines on the day-to-day management for a patient type or diagnosis related group. This approach provides recommendations for interventions and investigations and allows monitoring of resources.[25] A common criticism of clinical pathways is that they are appropriate to acute procedurally based care but are challenging in chronic and aged care because of multiple comorbid conditions. Numerous clinical paths for specific patient types are in evidence in the literature, and many hospitals in Australia and overseas continue to develop their own pathways for patient care using their local multidisciplinary clinical experts. In some practice areas, case managers (often registered nurses) are used to coordinate and monitor patient care activities according to the critical path. In spite of the challenges and criticisms of clinical pathways, the empirical and systematic process of mapping patient care, ensuring accountability and measurement of outcomes often drives organisational efficiencies and improves quality of care. Other models of care include the use of liaison nurses and other consultancy models.[26]

Regardless of the model of care, it is important that the interventions implemented are socially, economically and politically relevant to the local context and treatment patterns. An example of this is cancer care. Increasing consumer advocacy, treatment innovations and improving patient outcomes in cancer care have led to the restructuring of models of nursing care where there is an increasing emphasis on self-management, care continuity and the recognition of social and psychological issues that have an impact on health outcomes.[27]

KEY ROLES AND RESPONSIBILITIES OF NURSES

The Australian Nursing and Midwifery Council (ANMC) has developed a set of competencies for registered nurses and midwives, nurse practitioners and enrolled nurses. These are useful documents, and other useful resources include the Code of Professional Conduct for Nurses in Australia and the Code of Ethics for Nurses in Australia, which you can access from the ANMC website (www.anmc.org.au). Key competencies for registered nurses involve integrating activities of clinical practice, coordinating care, counselling, health teaching, client advocacy, clinical teaching, supervising, working in a team, mentoring, monitoring patient outcomes and researching. The proportion of each of these activities performed on a daily basis varies with context, experience and employment position, but it is evident that the role of a registered nurse is always varied, complex and challenging. Although job titles vary between career structures for each state and territory of Australia, registered nurses in the hospital setting engage in activities ranging from ward-based direct patient care (clinical nurse), autonomous clinical practice (nurse practitioner), clinical education and support (educator), unit or ward management (manager), hospital-wide clinical consultation in a specialty field (clinician) to management of a clinical division, stream or functional area within or across an area health service (senior nurse manager). Nurses in the community setting have equally varied activities, often liaising and collaborating with a range of allied health disciplines and managing clients requiring chronic disease and/or health promotion management.[25]

For the newly registered nurse, certain skills have been identified as requiring additional support to improve clinical performance, specifically medication adminis-tration, time management and issues of patient comfort and safety.[28,29] As these issues form part of the everyday work of registered nurses, it is vital that beginning practi-tioners recognise their personal limitations and seek to improve their performance with experience, reflection and support from colleagues. As newly registered nurses are propelled into the busy and often challenging culture of clinical practice, it is important that they look after their physical and mental health and also take the time to reflect and process events.

WORKLOAD AND TIME MANAGEMENT

Determining the metrics of nursing workload and allocation is a fraught and highly political process.[30] Lower numbers of registered nurses and high workloads have been linked to adverse patient outcomes.[31] Funding of the acute healthcare sector is based on funding models which may include case-mix information and other funding models.[32] The increasing pressure for financial efficiencies presents significant chal-lenges to the practice of nursing and in recent times there has been a change in the skill mix of nurses, particularly in the acute hospital setting. The strong relationship between nursing care and patient outcomes compels nurses to define, describe, measure and cost the nature of their work and contribution to the healthcare experience.[33]

Measuring nursing activities according to physical needs or the dependency of patients alone can fail to include the assessment and clinical decision-making aspects that lead to the subsequent nursing activity and also the coordination and management of the healthcare team. There is also evidence of poor reliability for a number of common workload measurement methods when compared with observations of actual nursing care.[34] When developing nursing workload measures tension exists between caring for the patient as an individual and the categorising of patients via mainly physical tasks into dependency (workload) levels. These measures also do not accommodate unanticipated events and the complex psychological and social aspects of nursing care. In spite of these challenges it is important that nurses work towards developing effective and efficient workload systems, and this is clearly a fertile area for future research.[35]

A number of limitations have been identified when considering the measurement of workload. In particular, the assumption that nursing is a linear activity is incorrect. Nurses commonly perform a number of activities simultaneously and also provide a critical role in the coordination of care. Until recent times research into the ways in which hospitals work and function has been greatly neglected. One key area of deficit in this knowledge base is the lack of data on the contribution of nursing to patient outcomes as well as measurement of nursing workload. Applying systems developed in non–health–related industries can be challenging due to the unique and dynamic nature of the hospital environment. Monitoring workloads using information systems in conjunction with quality improvement activities may enable the three core ele-ments of quality, skill mix and cost of nursing care to be managed more effectively, and certainly nurses should look to technology and health informatics as enabling features of practice.[36,37]

In recent times the skill mix of staff involved in patient care has been broadened, with increasing numbers of nurse practitioners in extended/advanced nursing practice roles, higher numbers of enrolled nurses (division 2) and assistants in nursing who are unlicensed assistive personnel. Many critical care areas that have been traditionally staffed by registered nurse are now challenged to reconfigure models of nursing care to accommodate this diverse skill mix. An additional challenge facing many clinical areas is the ageing of the nursing workforce and the increasing need to accommodate work practices to accommodate these factors.[3,38]

From a beginning practitioner's perspective, managing your workload can be an onerous task, particularly in the early period following registration. Determining priorities and communicating your decisions to patients and your staff colleagues is important, rather than being isolationist in style. Being able to verbalise your rationale for decisions will benefit both you and your team. Never be afraid to seek clarification or question clinical treatment plans, and always consider a second opinion if you are not sure about your clinical decision. In addition be aware of personality issues and your own (mis)perceptions. Sometimes an off-hand remark by a senior member of staff may be related to that individual's own pressure and not to your performance. Developing the capacity to perceive, assess and manage the emotions of both yourself and others is useful. The dynamic nature of clinical environments means that your activities and priorities will need to be adaptive and flexible. The next section discusses these issues further.

SETTING PRIORITIES AND PLANNING IN CLINICAL PRACTICE

Effective time management involves prioritising tasks, and this can be a daunting prospect for the novice practitioner dealing with competing demands in a complex environment. Determining priorities should be based on astute clinical assessment of the patient group. It is important to perform this at the beginning of each shift to provide a baseline of patients' clinical progress. This assessment should include a rapid head-to-toe assessment and notation of patients' diagnoses and clinical progress. Continued assessment and subsequent care will be contingent on patient clinical need. Taking time to plan for your shift can increase your efficiency compared with leaping into your work in a reactive way. For example, taking time to assess patency of intravenous lines and chest drains can avoid more dramatic consequences later in the shift. In essence you need to develop your own risk management plan for your shift. Develop your own system to prioritise your work plan, whether it be a notebook with a checklist or a system as you write your report. Remember that you are part of a team; in spite of your commitment to collegial behaviour, sometimes this may not be evident. For example, a medical practitioner may order a new medication halfway through your shift and neglect to tell you. Regardless of this omission, you as the registered nurse are responsible. Therefore, try to make a point to check with medical staff on changes in care plans, and check at medication times for changes in orders.

To be an effective practitioner it is imperative that you spend some introspective time identifying and evaluating your work style. Are you a person who can deal with multiple and competing tasks simultaneously? Or an individual who needs to identify individual discrete tasks? Recognition of your individual work style is an important strategy in the management of your workload. Identifying time-wasting aspects of your work day is an important component in improving your efficiency. Do you make multiple trips to the treatment room for items? Can you take your time and visualise your equipment needs for clinical activities? Do you attempt to document events in the patient's day directly into the progress notes as they occur? Or do you carry around bits of paper and document events retrospectively at the end of your shift? Observe effective practitioners around you and copy their work styles. Focus on working as a team rather than as an individual and loose collective of discrete practitioners. Attempt to set goals and priorities for your working day and plan accordingly. At the end of each day identify the barriers and facilitators to achieving these and modify your work style accordingly. Seek feedback and mentorship from senior colleagues whom you trust. In addition, take the time to look up quickly information related to the pathophysiology and pharmacology of the patients you are caring for. This clinical reflection is not only an important aspect of professional growth but will also rapidly escalate your clinical knowledge and competence.

Many newly graduated nurses need to overcome possible coercion and power relationships that dictate the cultural priorities of showering and bed-making over time taken to assess patients and plan their care for the shift. Despite their best intentions, many new graduates take on existing practices in clinical areas because of power relationships and the potency of the socialisation process. It is important to evaluate all practices critically and strive to ensure that your nursing care meets patient needs rather than individual staff or organisational demands.[39,40]

It is impossible to plan nursing care appropriately without an accurate understanding of patients' diagnoses and management plans, as well as their individual needs for assistance.[41] It is important to ask questions and look up any unfamiliar diagnoses or related issues. It is fair and reasonable that you demand this time as a beginning-level practitioner. Work more effectively, rather than longer hours. Refusing meal breaks can have countereffects. Accept help readily and in turn offer help and assistance to your colleagues.

A recent review of the Australian healthcare system identified a need for better coordination of care and the need to monitor patient outcomes.[17,42] It is essential that these important factors are heeded in order to provide a safe, quality healthcare system. At every level of the organisation, from direct patient caregivers to the director of nursing, there should be identification of your core business as patient care, with a readiness to recognise current practice limitations and seek consultation and assistance for continuously improving clinical practice.

Clinical learning as a lifelong process

As students approach the end of their undergraduate degree and begin their career as a registered nurse, there is often a notion that the learning experience is over. However, this is only a brief interlude in the process of being a lifelong learner.[43] Much of what you will learn about nursing is experiential in the workplace; this learning will differ from your university studies as it is applied and immediate. The qualities of a lifelong learner include an inquiring mind, a positive self-concept, the ability to establish goals and information literacy. These qualities involve taking in and synthesising information and cues from a variety of sources, including online resources. The internet provides immeasurable opportunities for acquiring information, as well as self-development.

As you enter the workplace, it is important to have a realistic expectation of your abilities, knowledge and limitations. Perhaps the most important lesson for the new graduate is that, despite the fact you are employed as a registered nurse, no one expects you to know everything and therefore you should not expect this of yourself. Become comfortable with asking questions and seeking advice. Embrace all opportunities for learning, including attending multidisciplinary events, such as medical grand rounds.

As part of being a nurse professional, there is an expectation that you will strive for self-improvement and enrichment of your nursing knowledge and skills over time and be accountable in your clinical practice and professional development. A considerable amount of information and resources will be supplied in new graduate and preceptorship programs.[44] Yet, as part of professional behaviour, a significant onus remains on the individual to seek out information and knowledge. This is an important behaviour to nurture not only to increase your competency and proficiency as a nurse clinician, but also to enrich your personal and professional growth.

Therefore, in your beginning years of practice you should take the time to stop and reflect on your day's work and seek clarification of incidents and processes from a senior staff member, your supervisor or mentor. A personal journal is an excellent way to monitor your own progress. It is important not to allow fear and doubt to plague your performance and undermine your confidence. If you feel that your work is dragging you down and you are lacking confidence, seek help from a senior nurse, such as the new graduate program coordinator, earlier rather than later. Like most challenges in life, ignoring these feelings will not make them go away; likely they will only get worse and encroach on other dimensions of your life. Also, remember this is not the first or the last time your senior nurse colleagues will hear this story. It is likely what you are feeling has been experienced by many before you, even by themselves, and will be in the future.

MENTORSHIP AND PRECEPTORSHIP

As well as enhancing their beginning skills through lifelong learning and reflective practice, recent graduates need to engage with effective clinical and professional mentors through their workplace or the various professional colleges or clinical societies; for example:

- Australian College of Critical Care Nurses: http://www.acccn.com.au
- Australian College of Midwives: http://www.midwives.org.au
- Australasian College of Cardiovascular Nurses: http://www.acnc.net.au
- Australian Nurse Practitioner Association: http://www.nursepractitioners.org.au
- Australian Practice Nurses Association http://www.apna.asn.au
- Australian and New Zealand College of Mental Health Nurses: http://www.acmhn.org
- The College of Nursing: http://www.nursing.edu.au
- Royal College of Nursing, Australia: http://www.rcna.org.au
- Sigma Theta Tau International: http://www.nursingsociety.org

The internet provides an excellent medium for obtaining current information. Many professional organisations have chat rooms and you can subscribe to email updates.

The 'reality shock' experienced by new graduates is well recognised.[45] Models of professional learning support have been incorporated in many institutions to ease this transition process. Professional learning support can be derived in a variety of ways, in both formal and informal contexts. The efficacy of a preceptor–preceptee relationship is largely determined by the calibre and commitment of both parties, enthusiasm, personality, and in particular the motivation of the preceptor in that role. In the clinical setting, conflicting rosters can be a major barrier to communication between the preceptor and preceptee. The role of the preceptor is often envisaged as more of a 'how to' or 'where to find' person. The preceptor generally provides collegial support rather than intense clinical supervision and career direction. In many instances, the new practitioner looks beyond the often prescriptive relationship of preceptorship towards a professional mentor.

As with your university clinical placement, in your role as a registered nurse you will be exposed to a variety of role models, some good, some bad. Reflecting on how people around you manage situations and people can assist you in developing your own practice and management style. Many experienced nurses can identify with a particular mentor who has shaped his or her clinical practice development.[46] Heller[47] defines the characteristics of a good mentor as an individual who:

- possesses high integrity, honesty and credibility
- insists on the highest standards
- sets an inspirational example
- insists on getting things done
- demonstrates the ability to envisage the future
- shows deep concern for the other's performance.[48]

In many instances you will find your mentor will stay with you in your professional journey. In essence, your mentor should be the person you look at and say, 'that's the type of nurse I want to be'. Importantly, the mentoring relationship will also be a partnership based on collaboration and the development of trust, loyalty and mutual respect. Morton-Cooper and Palmer[49] stress the importance of reciprocity and collaboration in a mentoring relationship and identify the following strategies in attracting a mentor:

- having a positive attitude to work and career
- standing out in the crowd
- being willing to take risks
- having commitment to your own development
- being receptive to coaching, advice and support
- showing initiative and motivation
- having positive self-esteem
- demonstrating loyalty to individuals and the organisation.

Not all mentoring relationships are successful, and it is important to recognise early relationships that are disabling and do not promote individual growth (e.g. elitism and mutual seclusion); these can cause the mentee to withdraw from other relationships and become excessively dependent on the mentor.[49] In addition to seeking out a mentor for yourself, you also need to consider how to develop these attributes in yourself as part of your ongoing contribution to the profession of nursing and your personal development. We can guarantee that the years will fly by, and soon you will find yourself in charge of a shift and responsible for the transitional development of newly registered nurses and supervision of enrolled nurses and assistants in nursing.

TAKING CARE OF YOURSELF AND YOUR COLLEAGUES

Stress in the workplace can be distressing for nurses. In order to be an effective role model to our patients and colleagues it is important that we pay attention to the messages we preach and look after our own body and mind. This means taking time to exercise, relax, eat and sleep well, together with ensuring we work in a safe environment. Cognisance of these factors, and looking after ourselves and each other, are important strategies in addressing the nursing shortage[50] and minimising the threat of horizontal violence.[51] In order to ensure that nursing is a dynamic and driving force in health, we need to project within and externally to our profession an image of coherence and solidarity.

MEASURING OUTCOMES OF NURSING CARE

The measurement of nursing interventions and patient outcomes is more relevant than ever; the recent drive for an evidence-based approach to clinical management, and the increased emphasis on nursing as a profession, require a patient-centred focus with an emphasis on improving health outcomes.[52,53] However, it is interesting to note that outcome evaluation was first advocated for nursing as early as the 1860s by Florence Nightingale.[54] Although evaluating care has been integral to nursing practice, contemporary trends in management and evaluation create new dilemmas in the selection of methodological approaches and choice of patient and organisational outcomes.[55] It is often difficult to separate nursing from the inputs of other professional groups, as well as incorporating patients' perspectives. As a result there is an increasing focus on nurse-sensitive patient outcome indicators and how these contribute to the quality of care.[56]

Measurements assessing both process and outcome measures of nursing care are imperative for the development of nursing practice and justification for the nursing role in an interdisciplinary milieu. The impact of nursing can be evaluated in terms of costs, length of stay, clinical outcomes, and patient and carer satisfaction, although it may be difficult within highly technological environments to measure the separate value of nursing care, particularly using biomedical and economic measures. Thus mixed-method approaches, using both quantitative and qualitative dimensions, may be useful in determining outcomes.[57]

A mission to ensure the delivery of safe, effective, quality clinical care based on evidence is mandatory in the contemporary clinical environment. Many organisations now focus attention on clinical governance as a means of achieving this aim. Clinical governance is defined as a framework through which health organisations are held accountable for continuously improving the quality of their services and safeguarding high standards of clinical care by creating an environment in which clinical excellence will prosper. Clinical governance refers both to the context and outcomes of clinical activities and, importantly, the involvement of all clinical staff in the monitoring and evaluation process. The necessary framework in which to implement a model of clinical governance comprises three main elements[58]:

1. structures to allow monitoring and evaluation
2. clear documentation of care processes based on evidence
3. organisational support for a culture of evaluation and quality practice.

In such frameworks nursing is considered to be a pivotal element in not only directly facilitating patient care, but also coordinating and monitoring care processes.[59] The importance of interprofessional collaboration and the important role of nurses in directing and coordinating care have led to an increased emphasis on the nursing role.[60] Nurses need to evaluate care, measure patient outcomes and review their practice within a framework of evidence-based practice.[61]

CONCLUSION

Nursing is a complex and multifaceted profession playing a critical role in primary, secondary and tertiary care. High-quality nursing care is dependent on fostering a collegial profession based on caring and mentoring of its members as well as an evidence-based approach to providing care. Professional development should be directed to the continual improvement and evaluation of effective clinical practice models, as well as the growth of the nurse as an individual, not only professionally but personally.

Contemporary clinical practice presents challenges for both recently graduated and experienced nurses in delivering appropriate nursing care in accordance with the best available evidence. This mandate requires the development of flexible, dynamic and eclectic models of care that ensure cost-effective, optimal health-related outcomes for patients. Important in the planning of these services is the implementation of strategies to optimise equity of access for all members of society. Recent graduates need to enhance their beginning skills in lifelong learning and reflective practice, as well as engaging with effective clinical and professional mentors. Additional support for professional growth can be gained through the professional colleges and clinical societies. Taking the time to plan for your professional development and seeking mentorship and support are critical in the period following graduation.

CASE STUDY 9.1

Amy began the second day of her new graduate rotation on an evening shift in the medical ward. Amy had been allocated six patients, all with complex needs and management plans. She was also responsible for supervising an enrolled nurse, who was taking care of patients in adjoining rooms. One of Amy's patients, Mr Joseph Blythe in room 4 bed 2, had end-stage renal failure and diabetes and was in a semiconscious state. He was not taking oral fluids and the medical team had decided to commence nasogastric feeds for nutritional support. Approaching Joseph was daunting for Amy. Even though she had dealt with seriously ill people before, this situation presented Amy with new challenges as the registered nurse responsible and accountable for the care of Joseph.

On returning to the bedside, Joseph's wife Joan looked up at Amy with teary eyes and asked why the nasogastric tube was needed. Amy explained that this was the fourth time her husband had been in hospital in the last 6 months and each time he had become weaker and frailer. For the last month he had not been out of the house and needed the community nurse to shower him. Joan was finding it hard to cope and Joseph's confusion and aggression were highly distressing. She also struggled with his incontinence at night. Amy explained to Joan that the nasogastric tube was necessary for nourishment but Joan was adamant she did not want any further invasive procedures for her husband. She said that Joseph had often said he didn't want to be kept alive if could not take care of himself.

REFLECTIVE QUESTIONS

- Describe the rationale for the decision to insert the nasogastric tube. On what evidence was the decision based?
- What other sources of information need to be considered in this case?
- What are the rights of the patient and his family?
- What is the regulatory and legal framework in this scenario?

CASE STUDY 9.2

Amy paged the resident medical officer who was equally adamant the nasogastric tube had to be inserted. Amy could feel the tears brimming in her own eyes, and her head was fogged with the conflict and the confronting nature of this scene and troubled by the thought of the 4 p.m. medication round and glucometer readings, as well as the needs of her other patients.

REFLECTIVE QUESTIONS

- What would you do in this situation? Why?
- Can you identify the resource people who may be available to give you support and direction?

CASE STUDY 9.3

Tim is feeling tired and exhausted. The first month of his clinical rotation has been a whirlwind. He is feeling frustrated that he can't get on top of his work in spite of skipping lunch and staying late.

REFLECTIVE QUESTIONS

- What strategies would you give Tim regarding time management?
- In planning for your day in the clinical setting, what are the important priorities?

RECOMMENDED READING

Chaboyer W, Najman J, Dunn S. Cohesion among nurses: an end to horizontal violence in Australian hospitals. Journal of Advanced Nursing 2010;35:525–35.

Davidson PM, Halcomb E, Hickman L, et al. Beyond the rhetoric: what do we mean by a model of care? Australian Journal of Advanced Nursing 2006;23:47–55.

Duffield C, Diers D, O'Brien-Pallas L, et al. Nursing staffing, nursing workload, the work environment and patient outcomes. Applied Nursing Research 2010; doi:10.1016/j.apnr.2009.12.004.

Lucero RJ, Lake ET, Aiken LH. Nursing care quality and adverse events in US hospitals. Journal of Clinical Nursing 2010;19:2185–95.

Sochalski J, Jaarsma T, Krumholz HM, et al. What works in chronic care management: the case of heart failure. Health Affairs 2009;28:179.

REFERENCES

1. Bartz CC. International Council of Nurses and person-centered care. International Journal of Integrated Care 2010:10.
2. Davidson P, Halcomb E, Hickman L, et al. Beyond the rhetoric: what do we mean by a 'Model of Care'? Australian Journal of Advanced Nursing 2006;23:47.
3. Duffield C, Roche M, Diers D, et al. Staffing, skill mix and the model of care. Journal of Clinical Nursing 2010;19:2242–51.
4. Middleton S, Gardner G, Gardner A, et al. The first Australian nurse practitioner census: a protocol to guide standardized collection of information about an emergent professional group. International Journal of Nursing Practice 2010;16: 517–24.
5. Considine J, Fielding K. Sustainable workforce reform: case study of Victorian nurse practitioner roles. Australian Health Review 2010;34:297–303.
6. Halcomb EJ, Davidson PM, Brown N. Uptake of Medicare chronic disease items in Australia by general practice nurses and Aboriginal health workers. Collegian: Journal of the Royal College of Nursing Australia 2010;17:57–61.
7. Chan TC, Killeen JP, Vilke GM, et al. Effect of mandated nurse–patient ratios on patient wait time and care time in the emergency department. Academic Emergency Medicine 2010;17:545–52.
8. Thompson P. Acute coronary syndromes: coronary care unit admission and care. Coronary Care Manual 2010:467.
9. Rolley JX, Davidson PM, Salamonson Y, et al. Review of nursing care for patients undergoing percutaneous coronary intervention: a patient journey approach. Journal of Clinical Nursing 2009;18:2394–405.
10. Naylor MD, Brooten DA, Campbell RL, et al. Transitional care of older adults hospitalized with heart failure: a randomized, controlled trial. Journal of the American Geriatrics Society 2004;52:675–84.
11. Rabinowitz T, Murphy KM, Amour JL, et al. Benefits of a telepsychiatry consultation service for rural nursing home residents. Telemedicine and e-Health 2010;16:34–40.
12. Shigaki CL, Moore C, Wakefield B, et al. Nurse partners in chronic illness care: patients' perceptions and their implications for nursing leadership. Nursing Administration Quarterly 2010;34:130.
13. Halcomb EJ. Expansion of nursing role in general practice: studies suggest patients think that nurses can manage simple conditions but have some concerns about knowledge and competence in some areas. Evidence Based Nursing 2011;14:28.
14. Meleis AI. Transitions theory: middle-range and situation-specific theories in nursing research and practice. New York: Springer; 2010.
15. Krum H, Jelinek MV, Stewart S, et al. Guidelines for the prevention, detection and management of people with chronic heart failure in Australia 2006. Medical Journal of Australia 2006;185:549.

16. Muzzarelli S, Leibundgut G, Maeder MT, et al. Predictors of early readmission or death in elderly patients with heart failure. American Heart Journal 2010;160: 308–14.

17. Betihavas V, Newton PJ, Du HY, et al. Australia's health care reform agenda: implications for the nurses' role in chronic heart failure management. Australian Critical Care 2010; doi:10.1016/j.aucc.2010.08.003.

18. Riegel B, Moser DK, Anker SD, et al. State of the science: promoting self-care in persons with heart failure: a scientific statement from the American Heart Association. Circulation 2009;120:1141.

19. Davidson PM, Stewart S. Heart failure nursing in Australia: past, present and future. Australian Critical Care 2009;22:108.

20. Wagner EH, Austin BT, Von Korff M. Organizing care for patients with chronic illness. Milbank Quarterly 1996;74:511–44.

21. Burton CR, Fisher A, Green TL. The organisational context of nursing care in stroke units: a case study approach. International Journal of Nursing Studies 2009;46:86–95.

22. Sochalski J, Jaarsma T, Krumholz HM, et al. What works in chronic care management: the case of heart failure. Health Affairs 2009;28:179.

23. Oeseburg B, Wynia K, Middel B, et al. Effects of case management for frail older people or those with chronic illness: a systematic review. Nursing Research 2009;58:201.

24. Basse L, Jakobsen DH, Billesbølle P, et al. A clinical pathway to accelerate recovery after colonic resection. Annals of Surgery 2000;232:51.

25. Loeb M, Carusone SC, Goeree R, et al. Effect of a clinical pathway to reduce hospitalizations in nursing home residents with pneumonia: a randomized controlled trial. JAMA 2006;295:2503.

26. Wand T. Mental health liaison nursing in the emergency department: on-site expertise and enhanced coordination of care. Australian Journal of Advanced Nursing 2004;22:25–31.

27. Beaver K, Williamson S, Chalmers K. Telephone follow up after treatment for breast cancer: views and experiences of patients and specialist breast care nurses. Journal of Clinical Nursing 2010;19:2916–24.

28. Fero LJ, Witsberger CM, Wesmiller SW, et al. Critical thinking ability of new graduate and experienced nurses. Journal of Advanced Nursing 2009;65: 139–48.

29. Dyess SM, Sherman RO. The first year of practice: new graduate nurses' transition and learning needs. Journal of Continuing Education in Nursing 2009;40:403.

30. Aiken LH, Sloane DM, Cimiotti JP, et al. Implications of the California nurse staffing mandate for other states. Health Services Research 2010;45:904–21.

31. Duffield C, Diers D, O'Brien-Pallas L, et al. Nursing staffing, nursing workload, the work environment and patient outcomes. Applied Nursing Research 2010; doi:10.1016/j.apnr.2009.12.004.

32. Goldfield N. The evolution of diagnosis-related groups (DRGs): from its beginnings in case-mix and resource use theory, to its implementation for payment and now for its current utilization for quality within and outside the hospital. Quality Management in Healthcare 2010;19:3.

33. Lucero RJ, Lake ET, Aiken LH. Nursing care quality and adverse events in US hospitals. Journal of Clinical Nursing 2010;19:2185–95.

34. de Cordova PB, Lucero RJ, Hyun S, et al. Using the Nursing Interventions Classification as a potential measure of nurse workload. Journal of Nursing Care Quality 2010;25:39.

35. Hoi SY, Ismail N, Ong LC, et al. Determining nurse staffing needs: the workload intensity measurement system. Journal of Nursing Management 2010;18: 44–53.

36. Lammintakanen J, Saranto K, Kivinen T. Use of electronic information systems in nursing management. International Journal of Medical Informatics 2010;79: 324–31.

37. Stevenson JE, Nilsson GC, Petersson GI, et al. Nurses' experience of using electronic patient records in everyday practice in acute/inpatient ward settings: a literature review. Health Informatics Journal 2010;16:63.

38. Fairbrother G, Jones A, Rivas K. Changing model of nursing care from individual patient allocation to team nursing in the acute inpatient environment. Contemporary Nurse 2010;35.

39. Rudman A, Gustavsson JP. Early-career burnout among new graduate nurses: a prospective observational study of intra-individual change trajectories. International Journal of Nursing Studies 2011;48:292–306

40. Laschinger H, Grau A, Finegan J, et al. New graduate nurses' experiences of bullying and burnout in hospital settings. Journal of Advanced Nursing 2010;66: 2732–42.

41. Davidson P, Cockburn J, Daly J, et al. Patient-centered needs assessment: rationale for a psychometric measure for assessing needs in heart failure. Journal of Cardiovascular Nursing 2004;19:164.

42. FitzGerald G, Ashby R. National health and hospital network for Australia's future: implications for emergency medicine. Emergency Medicine Australasia 2010;22:384–90.

43. Barnard AG, Nash RE, O'Brien M. Information literacy: developing life long skills through nursing education. Journal of Nursing Education 2010;44: 505–10.

44. DeWolfe JA, Perkin CA, Harrison MB, et al. Strategies to prepare and support preceptors and students for preceptorship: a systematic review. Nurse Educator 2010;35:98.

45. Romyn DM, Linton N, Giblin C, et al. Successful transition of the new graduate nurse. International Journal of Nursing Education Scholarship 2009;6:1802.

46. McCloughen A, O'Brien L, Jackson D. Esteemed connection: creating a mentoring relationship for nurse leadership. Nursing Inquiry 2009;16:326–36.

47. Heller R. Achieving excellence. New York: DK Publishing; 1999.

48. Davidson PM. Becoming a nurse leader. Contexts of Nursing 2009:258.

49. Morton-Cooper A, Palmer A. Mentoring, preceptorship and clinical supervision: a guide to professional roles in clinical practice. Oxford: Wiley-Blackwell; 2000.

50. Twigg D, Duffield C, Thompson P, et al. The impact of nurses on patient morbidity and mortality – the need for a policy change in response to the nursing shortage. Australian Health Review 2010;34:312.

51. Chaboyer W, Najman J, Dunn S. Cohesion among nurses: an end to horizontal violence in Australian hospitals. Journal of Advanced Nursing 2010;35:525–35.
52. Radwin LE, Cabral HJ, Wilkes G. Relationships between patient-centered cancer nursing interventions and desired health outcomes in the context of the health care system. Research in Nursing & Health 2009;32:4–17.
53. Nakrem S, Vinsnes AG, Harkless GE, et al. Nursing sensitive quality indicators for nursing home care: international review of literature, policy and practice. International Journal of Nursing Studies 2009;46:848–57.
54. Munro CL. The 'Lady With the Lamp' illuminates critical care today. American Journal of Critical Care 2010;19:315.
55. Griffiths P. RN + RN = better care? What do we know about the association between the number of nurses and patient outcomes? International Journal of Nursing Studies 2009;46:1289–90.
56. O'Brien-Pallas L, Li XM, Wang S, et al. Evaluation of a patient care delivery model: system outcomes in acute cardiac care. Canadian Journal of Nursing Research 2010;42:98–120.
57. Curry LA, Nembhard IM, Bradley EH. Qualitative and mixed methods provide unique contributions to outcomes research. Circulation 2009;119:1442.
58. McSherry R, Pearce P. Clinical governance. Oxford: Wiley-Blackwell; 2010.
59. Sullivan E, Francis K, Hegney D. Review of small rural health services in Victoria: how does the nursing medical division of labour affect access to emergency care? Journal of Clinical Nursing 2008;17:1543–52.
60. Jennings N, O'Reilly G, Lee G, et al. Evaluating outcomes of the emergency nurse practitioner role in a major urban emergency department, Melbourne, Australia. Journal of Clinical Nursing 2008;17:1044–50.
61. Considine J, McGillivray B. An evidence based practice approach to improving nursing care of acute stroke in an Australian emergency department. Journal of Clinical Nursing 2010;19:138–44.

CHAPTER 10

Dealing with ethical issues in nursing practice

Megan-Jane Johnstone and Elizabeth Crock

LEARNING OBJECTIVES

When you have completed this chapter you will be able to:

- distinguish between an ethical issue, a legal issue and a clinical issue
- understand what might count as a moral reason for taking action in work-related settings
- explore the function of a nursing code of ethics
- understand the application of ethical principles and moral rights to and in nursing practice
- appreciate the role and responsibility of nurses in promoting and protecting the significant moral interests of clients in healthcare contexts.

Keywords: ethics, moral rights, moral duties, moral decision making, nursing codes of ethics

---

INTRODUCTION

Nurses in all areas and levels of practice have to deal with ethical/moral issues every day. Sometimes, the issues encountered are relatively straightforward and easy to deal with. At other times, however, the issues may be extraordinarily complex, perplexing and extremely difficult to resolve. In either case, there is always a risk that an ethical issue may not be handled well and that a good moral outcome is not achieved. Because of this risk (in addition to other considerations such as the demands of ethical professional conduct generally), it is imperative that all nurses – regardless of their years of experience and areas of practice – are well informed about the kinds of ethical issues that may arise in nursing practice. It is also imperative that nurses have the knowledge, skills and aptitude necessary to be able to respond to the issues at hand in an appropriate, ethically warranted and just manner. These imperatives derive from the agreed professional and ethical standards of conduct of the nursing profession in Australia, which make explicit the requirements that all registered nurses must:

- demonstrate satisfactory knowledge of the ethical responsibilities of nurses as morally accountable practitioners
- practise in accordance with the nursing profession's codes of ethics and conduct
- fulfil their ethical responsibilities in all aspects of nursing practice (including identifying and adhering to strategies that promote and protect the rights of individuals/groups, and advocating for individuals/groups when their rights are overlooked and/or compromised).[1]

The ability of nurses to fulfil their ethical responsibilities as morally accountable practitioners, and to respond effectively and appropriately to ethical issues arising in nursing domains, depends on a number of processes, including the ability of nurses:

- to distinguish between ethical, legal and clinical issues
- to discern when it is appropriate and even morally imperative to take action to address an ethical issue encountered in a work-related setting
- to respond decisively and in an informed and morally wise way to the question: 'What should I do?'
- to justify, in moral terms, the stance and action they ultimately take.

Here a number of questions can be raised:

- What is an ethical issue, and how does an ethical issue differ from a legal issue or clinical issue?
- When is it 'right' – and even morally imperative – for nurses to take action in response to an ethical issue they have encountered?
- What (moral) reasons might nurses provide to justify the decisions they make and the actions they ultimately take in response to the ethical issues they encounter?

DISTINGUISHING BETWEEN ETHICAL, LEGAL AND CLINICAL ISSUES

When practising in a professional capacity, nurses will encounter a variety of problems and associated issues (such as those described in the case studies presented in this chapter). And while many of these problems and issues may have an ethical dimension, it is not always the case that they are ethical issues per se, requiring a moral solution. In many instances, the problems at hand are more of a clinical or practical nature, requiring a clinical or practical response. In some instances, the problem may be of a frankly legal nature, for which a legal response is required. Although the ethical, legal and clinical dimensions of nursing practice may, and do, overlap, they are nonetheless grounded in and governed by different concerns. In the interests of promoting accountable and responsible professional nursing practice, care must be taken to distinguish between these dimensions and related concerns.[2] To illustrate this, consider the following three scenarios involving the prescription of analgesia for a client with an end-stage illness.

CASE STUDY 10.1

A nurse discovers that an excessively large intravenous dose of an opiate analgesic has been prescribed by an attending doctor. Based on her knowledge of pain management regimens and a clinical assessment of the client, the nurse is concerned that if the prescribed dosage is administered as ordered, the consequences to the client could be dire (specifically, it could result in the client's premature death). She checks with the prescribing doctor who confirms, with alarm, that he has made 'a terrible mistake' and corrects the error, thanking the nurse for her vigilance. The nurse subsequently administers the revised medication order of analgesia to the client with no ill effects.

CASE STUDY 10.2

A nurse discovers that an excessively large intravenous dose of an opiate analgesic has been prescribed by an attending doctor. Based on her knowledge of pain management regimens and a clinical assessment of the client, the nurse is concerned that if the prescribed dosage is administered as ordered, the consequences to the client could be dire (specifically, it would result in the immediate and premature death of the client). She checks with the prescribing doctor who advises her that the medication order 'is correct' and that the drug is to be given 'as ordered'. He advises the nurse that 'should she fail to administer the drug as ordered, he will regard this as being tantamount to her interfering with his treatment plan for the patient'. He clarifies that the treatment plan has been 'openly discussed with the patient – who initiated discussion about the plan – and totally accords with both the patient's and her family's expressed wishes'. Although perplexed about the drug order, the nurse administers the analgesia without further question.

CASE STUDY 10.3

A nurse discovers that an excessively large intravenous dose of an opiate analgesic has been prescribed by an attending doctor. Based on her knowledge of pain management regimens and a clinical assessment of the client, the nurse is concerned that if the prescribed dosage is administered as ordered, the consequences to the client could be dire (specifically, it would, in all probability, hasten the client's death). She checks with the prescribing doctor who confirms that the medication is to be administered as prescribed and that, even though its administration will probably result in hastening the client's death, this is not the intended outcome. He explains that the dose prescribed is 'in the best interests of the client' and 'necessary to alleviate the patient's pain and suffering'. He further states that the prescription in question is simply 'good medical practice'. The doctor upholds this view despite knowing that the client has requested 'everything possible be done' to prolong her life.

Here we can ask the question: in which of these three scenarios does the medication order constitute an ethical issue, as opposed to, say, a clinical (practical) issue or a legal issue? In order to answer this question it is, of course, necessary to have some understanding of what a moral problem or an ethical issue looks like. In other words, we need some idea of the characteristics of a moral/ethical problem.

The nature of ethical issues

It is generally accepted that something involves a moral problem or an ethical issue where it has as its central concern:

- the promotion and protection of people's genuine wellbeing and welfare (including their interests in not suffering unnecessarily)
- responding justly to the genuine needs and significant moral interests of different people
- determining and justifying what constitutes 'right' and 'wrong' conduct in a given situation.[2]

Justifying a moral decision or action, in turn, involves providing the strongest moral reasons behind it. According to Beauchamp and Childress,[3] 'the reasons that we finally accept express the conditions under which we believe some course of action is morally justified'. Reasons or grounds for justifying our moral decisions and actions are generally thought to derive from three key sources: (1) moral rules, principles and theories; (2) lived experience and individual personal judgments; or (3) a synthesis of both these theoretical and experiential approaches (termed a 'coherentist approach').[3] In the case of nursing, reasons are commonly thought to be provided by appealing to: (1) nursing codes of ethics; (2) ethical principles; (3) moral rights; and (4) nurses' lived experiences.[2]

Given the above, it can be seen that where a client's genuine wellbeing and welfare are at risk, where the significant moral interests of different people (e.g. clients, nurses, doctors) are in competition with each other, and where assistance is required to answer the question 'What should I do?' (that is, what is the morally right thing to do?), a moral problem/ethical issue exists. This is in contradistinction to, say, a legal problem/issue where what is at stake is upholding the principles and standards of law and 'doing that which is required by law'. It is also in contradistinction to a clinical (or technical) problem/issue where what is at stake is upholding agreed clinical principles and standards of practice (e.g. upholding the principles of asepsis and the related standards of aseptic wound care). Some problems/issues may, of course, involve all three of these dimensions – that is, involve a complex of ethical, legal and clinical questions and considerations that, in turn, require a complex response guided by an appeal to the principles and standards pertinent to each of these three dimensions. The outcome of deliberations in these instances will ultimately depend on which of the three domains has the weightier claim.[2]

In all three scenarios above, the consequences to the client of administering the prescribed medication are potentially dire. In the first scenario, however, although the dire consequences stand to be morally and legally significant in that the client's genuine welfare and wellbeing are culpably at risk of being adversely affected, the problem of the incorrect dose of medication being prescribed is not an ethical issue as such. A clue to why this is so can be found in the consideration that remedying the problem requires little more than correcting the prescription error and enabling the prescribing doctor to account for his mistake. The need to correct the medication error is beyond dispute, correcting the medication error does not compromise anybody's significant moral interests, and little, if any, assistance is required in deciding whether it is right, all things considered, to correct the incorrect dose that has been prescribed or to justify the ultimate action that is taken to correct the error. In short, the problem requires a practical/technical solution, not a moral one (i.e. a robust ethical debate about 'What should I do?').

In the case of the second and third scenarios, however, two very different situations are involved. In the second scenario, the consequences of both administering and not administering the prescribed analgesia to the client are morally and legally significant in that they stand to make a material difference to the life and wellbeing of the client. Moreover, the medication order in this case is clearly problematic on legal grounds. Although in accordance with the client's expressed wishes – an important moral consideration – the prescription is highly questionable on legal grounds, not least on account of it involving the illegal act of actively assisting another to die.

The nurse's responsibility to question the medication order is unequivocal: in keeping with the competency standards expected of a registered nurse, the attending nurse in this scenario has a professional and legal responsibility to identify and question any order, decision and intervention that she judges to be questionable and inappropriate. Nonetheless, the case is not clearcut morally, since it begs the question of moral imperatives always to follow the law (we could, for example, imagine that some conscientious health professionals committed to respecting patients' choices might choose not to follow the law, even though the consequences to them personally might be dire).[4] Although having a profound moral dimension, the legal considerations in this instance are arguably weightier in that the primary question that needs to be answered is: What is the legally right thing to do? In order to answer this question an appeal will need to be made to legal (as opposed to ethical) principles and standards.

As in the case of Case study 10.2, the consequences of administering the prescribed analgesia to the client in Case study 10.3 are morally and legally significant in that they too stand to make a material difference to the client's life and wellbeing. However, unlike in the Case study 10.2, the medication order in this case is problematic primarily for moral rather than legal reasons (the order seems, at first glance, to be contrary to the client's expressed wishes – a profound moral consideration). Although the doctor's order, decision and intervention are based on benevolent concerns, he has nonetheless failed to give due consideration to the perspective and expressed wishes of the patient. He has also failed to provide a sound and convincing moral justification for his actions. Despite having a profound legal dimension, the ethical issue in this third scenario is arguably weightier. Resolving the ethical problem(s) discerned requires an appeal to ethical principles and standards of practice, rather than an appeal to legal considerations. Unlike Case study 10.2, the primary question to be answered in this case is: What is the ethically right thing to do? (Being appraised of the clinical facts of the case and the standards of effective pain management also stand to enhance the quality of the ethical decision-making process in this case.)

In sum, the key to identifying an ethical issue/moral problem (as distinct from a legal or clinical issue/problem) lies in recognising that the situation at hand involves a threat to human welfare and wellbeing (including the interests of persons in not suffering unnecessarily), competing and possibly conflicting interests between different people, and the need for assistance in working through what constitutes the 'right' (good) thing to do in the case at hand. Whereas a legal problem/issue is best resolved by appealing to legal principles and standards of conduct, and a clinical problem by appealing to clinical principles and standards of conduct, ethical problems/issues are primarily resolved by appealing to ethical principles and standards of conduct. Upon identifying a given ethical issue, the task remains of deciding how best to respond to it and, more specifically, to justify the responses made. The remainder of this chapter now turns to a consideration of this issue.

TAKING ACTION TO DEAL WITH ETHICAL ISSUES

Are nurses obliged to take action in response to ethical issues encountered during the course of their professional practice? If so, under what conditions might this be so? The short answer to the first question is: yes. Nurses are not only morally obliged to take action in such circumstances, but have a special professional responsibility to do so.

The moral imperative to take action in order to address and remedy a moral problem or ethical issue can derive from a number of sources, including a profound intellectual commitment to upholding given moral standards of conduct and to 'doing one's duty' in the strict moral sense of the term. However, moral imperatives to act can also derive from moral feelings such as pangs of conscience, a passionate sense of justice, an opposition to seeing vulnerable people suffering unnecessarily and an associated altruistic desire to prevent or alleviate that suffering.[2,5] For example, a nurse might feel and state: 'I could not live with myself if I did nothing to help client X. Things were going very badly for him; I just could not stand by and do nothing. I felt I had to intervene to alleviate his suffering. It would have been wrong not to.' Nevertheless, justifying moral decisions and conduct requires more than an appeal to feelings. Nurses also need to be able to articulate good and sufficient reasons to justify their actions, noting here that 'not all reasons are good reasons, and not all good reasons are sufficient for justification'.[3] What kind of reasons, then, are sufficient for justifying our moral decisions and actions? What (moral) reasons might nurses provide to justify the moral decisions they make and the actions they ultimately take?

Reasons or justifications for a nurse's actions can be found by appealing to the following: nursing codes of ethics, ethical principles and moral rights theory. Although there are several other sources that can be appealed to in order to justify moral conduct (see, for example, Johnstone[2]), the sources considered in this chapter are the most common.

Nursing codes of ethics

Nursing codes of ethics are regarded as important guides to ethical professional conduct in nursing. Like other codes of professional ethics, a nursing code of ethics may be described as a (document explicating) conventionalised set of moral rules and/ or expectations devised for the purpose of guiding ethical professional conduct. Although codes of ethics are not fully developed systematic theories of ethics, they nevertheless tend to reflect a rich set of moral values that have been explicated through a process of extensive consultation, debate, refinement, evaluation and review by practitioners over time.[2,6]

Codes can be either prescriptive or aspirational in nature. In the case of prescriptive codes, provisions are 'duty-directed, stating specific duties of members'.[7] In contrast, aspirational codes are 'virtue-directed, stating desirable aims while acknowledging that in some circumstances conduct short of the ideal may be justified'.[7] Either way, codes of ethics have as their principal concern directing:

> what professionals ought and ought not to do, how they ought to comport themselves, what they, or the profession as a whole, ought to aim at.[8]

In Australia, for example, the Code of Ethics for Nurses in Australia[9] and the Code of Conduct for Nurses in Australia[10] both make explicit:

- the ethical standards that Australian nurses are expected to uphold in the interests of promoting and protecting the moral interests and welfare of patients/clients
- the actions that nurses can expect to be taken against them if they breach the agreed standards.

If a nurse breaches the values and standards explicated in the code, this is generally regarded as sufficient grounds for censuring the nurse's conduct such as by formal disciplinary action.[3]

Ethical principlism

Ethical principlism is the view that the best way of dealing with ethical problems is by appealing to sound moral principles.[4] The principles most commonly used are those of autonomy, non-maleficence, beneficence and justice, which are commonly discussed and applied in the healthcare professional and bioethics literature.

AUTONOMY

The principle of autonomy prescribes that people ought to be respected as self-determining choosers and that it is wrong to violate a person's autonomous choices.[11] This is so even if we do not agree with another's choices and regard them as foolish, provided they do not interfere with the significant moral interests of others. Accepting this principle imposes on nurses a moral duty to respect clients' choices regarding recommended medical treatment, nursing and other associated care.[12] Further, this duty is binding even if nurses and other attending healthcare professionals do not agree with the choices that clients may and do make.

NON-MALEFICENCE

The principle of non-maleficence prescribes: 'do no harm'.[11] Accepting this principle imposes on nurses a stringent duty not to injure clients and to avoid causing them to suffer any otherwise avoidable harms. Harm, in this instance, may be broadly taken as involving the invasion, violation, thwarting or setting back of a person's significant welfare interests to the detriment of that person's wellbeing.[13]

BENEFICENCE

The principle of beneficence entails a positive obligation to 'act for the benefit of others' – that is, to promote their welfare and wellbeing.[11] In sum, it prescribes: 'do good'. Beneficent acts can include such virtuous actions as care, compassion, empathy, sympathy, altruism, kindness, mercy, love, friendship and charity – all of which stand to find ready application in nursing and healthcare contexts.

JUSTICE

The principle of justice can be conceptualised in a variety of ways.[2] However, for the purposes of this discussion it is sufficient to conceptualise justice in the following ways: as fairness (an intuitive sense of justice) and as an equal distribution of benefits and burdens (a rational sense of justice). For example, it might be concluded on the basis of both an intuitive and rational appeal to the principle of justice that it is manifestly unfair and disproportionately (unequally) burdensome to withhold care and treatment from a client simply because he is over 65 years of age. In this instance, people over the age of 65 years would be arbitrarily forced to carry a burden of suffering associated with the non-treatment of their medical condition that others under 65 years of age are not forced to bear.

Although ethical principlism is not without its difficulties (e.g. in instances where the respective demands of the different principles conflict, there may be no easy solution), it has increasingly come to replace more classical theoretical approaches to identifying and resolving moral problems in healthcare contexts. Ethical principlism can be especially helpful in providing sound standards against which a nurse's conduct can be measured and judged as 'ethically wrong'. For example, if a nurse's conduct fails to respect a client as an autonomous chooser or results in a client suffering otherwise avoidable moral harm, on the basis of the principles just described, that nurse's conduct could be judged with justification as being in breach of the standards prescribed by the principles in question (e.g. autonomy and non-maleficence) and therefore as 'morally wrong', all things considered.

Moral rights theory

Moral rights theory is also popularly regarded as an important guide to ethical professional conduct. A moral right is a special interest that a person may have and which ought to be protected and upheld for moral reasons. Moral rights claims are generally taken as involving correlative duties on the part of others to respect the claims made.[2] For example, if a client makes a genuine rights claim in a given healthcare context (such as the right to be treated with respect), then a nurse – or any other attending healthcare professional for that matter – has a corresponding moral duty to act in ways that uphold that right – he or she must act respectfully towards that client.

Rights claims can be either positive or negative. Positive rights claims generally entail a correlative duty to act or do something. Negative rights claims, in contrast, generally entail a correlative duty to omit or refrain from something. For example, if a client claims a right to be kept free of harm, this imposes a correlative duty on an attending nurse to omit or refrain from behaving in a harmful way towards that client. Likewise, if a client claims a right to make informed decisions about his or her care and treatment, this imposes on an attending nurse a positive duty to ensure that the client receives sufficient information to enable him or her to make an intelligent and prudent choice about recommended nursing cares and treatment. This may include facilitating consultations with other members of the healthcare team involved in the overall healthcare of the client.

Rights that are commonly claimed in healthcare include the rights to healthcare, informed consent, privacy and confidentiality, being treated with respect and dying with dignity (for an indepth examination of these rights from a nursing perspective, see Johnstone[2]). These rights are also commonly represented in nursing codes of ethics and codes of professional conduct and are often accompanied by explicit statements emphasising that nurses have both a role and a responsibility in promoting and protecting them.

Although moral rights theory is not without its difficulties (e.g. in instances where equally deserving rights claims might conflict, it may not be possible to satisfy all the claims made), it nevertheless has enormous currency in contemporary discussions and debates on ethical issues in healthcare. Furthermore, there is room to suggest that the language of rights has perhaps done more to protect the genuine interests (welfare and wellbeing) of clients in healthcare than any other part of the moral vocabulary at our disposal. An important example of this can be found in the World Health Organization's publication series on health and human rights.[13-16]

Moral rights theory can be especially helpful in providing reliable standards against which a nurse's conduct can be measured and judged as morally right or wrong, all things considered. For example, if a nurse's conduct violates a client's moral rights (that is, a set of special interests which ought to be respected and protected for moral reasons), on the basis of an appeal to moral rights theory, that nurse's conduct could be judged with justification as being unethical ('morally wrong'). In keeping with the agreed nursing standards of ethical professional conduct, the nurse's conduct in this situation would deserve being censured. Conversely, if the nurse's conduct upholds a client's moral rights, his or her conduct could be systematically appraised as being ethical ('morally right') and, thus, meeting the agreed nursing standards of ethical professional conduct.

REVIEW OF CASE SCENARIOS

In light of the discussion so far, it can be seen that all of the case studies presented in this chapter involve ethical issues. Moreover, each of the cases underscores the importance of moral preparedness and the kind of moral capabilities (knowledge, skills and aptitude) that nurses need to develop if they are to be effective in:

- promoting and protecting people's significant moral interests (including their interests in not suffering unnecessarily)
- responding justly to the genuine needs and significant moral interests of different people
- contributing to the positive project of achieving morally just outcomes in morally problematic situations.

The cases also demonstrate how complex and delicate some ethical issues can be and how achieving a morally just outcome can be an extremely difficult task. The question of how best to achieve morally just outcomes in the cases presented is one that you might now like to discuss with others.

CONCLUSION

All nurses in all areas and levels of practice have an obligation to conduct their nursing practice ethically. This includes being morally vigilant with respect to their own nursing practice, and also being alert to the practice of others that may undermine and even violate the significant moral interests of clients. Nurses have a responsibility to ensure that they are educationally prepared to be able to recognise ethical issues in the workplace and to be able to take appropriate action to respond to them. Taking appropriate action need not always involve some grandiose plan, however. Appropriate action may involve little more than behaving well towards clients and co–workers and reminding others of their role and responsibilities (inherent in the profession's agreed ethical standards of conduct) 'to provide just, compassionate, culturally competent, culturally safe and culturally responsive care to the populations they serve'.[9] This, in turn, includes ensuring that people are not disadvantaged or harmed by being treated differently because of their appearance, language, culture, religion, thinking, beliefs, values, perceptions, age (children and the elderly), sex and gender roles, sexual orientation, national or social origin, economic or political status, physical or mental disability, health status (including HIV/AIDS), or other characteristics that may be used by others to nullify or impair the equal enjoyment or exercise of the right to health.[14–18]

CASE STUDY 10.4 THE RIGHT TO REFUSE CARE AND TREATMENT

Ms M is a 29-year-old with advanced cancer. She has decided in consultation with close family members and friends that, despite the severity of her illness and its symptoms, she does not want any treatment. To ensure that her wishes are respected if she loses the capacity to make choices and consent to recommended treatments and care, Ms M has prepared an advance directive. In her advance directive, Ms M has outlined a comprehensive list of medical treatments and nursing cares that she does not want and, if she were competent to decide, would refuse. The healthcare team involved in her care is unanimous that, at the time of preparing her advance directive, Ms M was competent to make decisions and 'knew what she was doing'.

You are a community nurse visiting Ms M at home and notice with concern the progressive deterioration of her condition. She has noticeable difficulty walking and is at risk of falls. You arrange for her to have a personal alarm system in place, but she refuses any additional support services. She also refuses a range of basic nursing interventions that would help to make her more comfortable, including mouth care for a mouth infection, bowel care for constipation and wound care for various superficial cuts and abrasions that she sustained following a recent fall and that have become slightly infected. Workers from other services who come in to assist Ms M are also becoming increasingly concerned about her condition, and report this to your team.

REFLECTIVE QUESTIONS
- What are the key ethical issues raised by this case?
- Should you and the team override or respect Ms M's wishes?
- In either case, what moral reasons would you use to justify your decision?

CASE STUDY 10.5 MANDATORY REPORTING OF KNOWN OR SUSPECTED CHILD ABUSE OR NEGLECT

A newly qualified registered nurse is caring for a young man with a severe infection. Staff are aware that he has a history of injecting drug use, although he seems to be actively trying to address his health problems and has recently made some progress. One afternoon, during visiting hours, the new graduate nurse happened to walk past the young man's room and noticed that he and his wife were both shooting up drugs in the presence of their 4-year-old child. She discusses reporting them to the local child protection authority but the other nursing and medical staff on the ward are strongly against this on the grounds that the client is 'a delightful young man' and 'seems to have been doing so well'. Moreover, they did not want him to lose trust in the healthcare system and disengage from its services.

The new graduate nurse anonymously reports the couple to the local child protection agency, without telling any other hospital staff apart from a social worker. Although knowing that her report would probably make the young man's life harder in the short term, she believes strongly that she has an obligation to protect his child from possible harm. She knows that, as a registered nurse, she is required by law to report suspected cases of child abuse or neglect to a child protection authority, but still wonders if she has done the right thing.

REFLECTIVE QUESTIONS
- Did the new graduate do the 'right thing' in this case?
- Upon what basis have you made your judgment?
- Do you think the graduate nurse's action will achieve a morally desirable outcome in this situation?

CASE STUDY 10.6 RACIAL HARASSMENT OF NURSING STAFF BY PATIENTS

An elderly white Australian man who had been a soldier in World War II is being cared for on a ward where two nurses from Asian backgrounds are employed. Every time one of the Asian nurses comes into his room, the man becomes very agitated and refuses to have them care for him. On one occasion you overhear the man shout at one of the nurses: 'So you're my nurse? Well, I don't want you. Don't come near me. Don't come near me. I only want an Australian nurse to take care of me.' On another occasion, you see the man suddenly tip a hot cup of tea over one of the Asian nurses when her back is turned to him.

The nurses confide in you that they 'do not want to make any trouble' and that because of this they have agreed not to report the incident to the nurse unit manager. They further confide in you that they are very upset about the man's behaviour, that it has made them feel 'very bad', and that it is not the first time that a patient has treated them in this manner. They also tell you that some staff have 'laughed about it' and told them: 'If you can't take it, then go back to where you came from'.

REFLECTIVE QUESTIONS
- What, if any, are the moral issues raised by this case?
- How would you respond to the issues identified?
- What are the moral obligations of co-workers in this case?

RECOMMENDED READING

Forrester K, Griffiths D. Essential law for health professionals. 3rd ed. Sydney: Elsevier Australia; 2009.

Fry S, Johnstone M. Ethics in nursing practice: a guide to ethical decision making. 3rd ed. London: Blackwell Science; 2008.

Fry ST, Veatch R, Taylor C. Case studies in nursing ethics. 4th ed. Sudbury, MA: Jones and Bartlett Learning; 2011.

Johnstone MJ. Bioethics: a nursing perspective. 5th ed. Sydney: Elsevier Australia; 2009.

Nursing Ethics: an International Journal for Health Care Professionals (Sage Publications)

REFERENCES

1. Australian Nursing and Midwifery Council (ANMC). National competency standards for the registered nurse. Canberra: Australian Nursing and Midwifery Council; 2005. Online. Available: http://www.anmac.org.au/professional_standards 23 August 2010.

2. Johnstone MJ. Bioethics: a nursing perspective. 5th ed. Sydney: Elsevier Australia; 2009.

3. Beauchamp TL, Childress JF. Principles of biomedical ethics. 5th ed. New York: Oxford University Press; 2001.

4. Magnusson R. Angels of death: exploring the euthanasia underground. Melbourne: Melbourne University Press; 2002.

5. Johnstone MJ. A reappraisal of everyday nursing ethics: new directions for the 21st century. In: Daly J, Speedy S, Jackson D, editors. Contexts of nursing: an introduction. 3rd ed. Sydney: Elsevier; 2010. p. 145–54.

6. Johnstone MJ. Determining and responding effectively to ethical professional misconduct in nursing. A report to the Nurses Board of Victoria. Melbourne: Nurses Board of Victoria; 1998.

7. Skene L. A legal perspective on codes of ethics. In: Coady M, Bloch S, editors. Codes of ethics and the professions. Melbourne: Melbourne University Press; 1996.

8. Lichtenberg J. What are codes of ethics for? In: Coady M, Bloch S, editors. Codes of ethics and the professions. Melbourne: Melbourne University Press; 1996.

9. Australian Nursing and Midwifery Council (ANMC). Code of ethics for nurses in Australia. Canberra: Australian Nursing and Midwifery Council; 2008 Online. Available: http://www.nrgpn.org.au/index.php?element=ANMC+Code+of+Ethics 23 August 2010

10. Australian Nursing and Midwifery Council (ANMC). Code of conduct for nurses in Australia. Canberra: Australian Nursing and Midwifery Council; 2008. Online. Available: http://www.nrgpn.org.au/index.php?element=ANMC+Code+of+Professional+Conduct 23 August 2010.

11. Beauchamp TL, Childress JF. Principles of biomedical ethics. 6th ed. New York: Oxford University Press; 2009.

12. Case study: competent refusal of nursing care (with commentaries by Dudzinski & Shannon 2006; Tong 2006). Hastings Center Report 2006;36:14–15.

13. Feinberg J. Harm to others: the moral limits of the criminal law. New York: Oxford University Press; 1984.

14. World Health Organization (WHO). 25 questions and answers on health and human rights. Health & Human Rights Publication Series, Issue No. 1. Geneva: WHO Press; 2002.

15. World Health Organization (WHO). WHO's contribution to the world conference against racism, racial discrimination, xenophobia and related intolerance. Health & Human Rights Publication Series, Issue No. 2. Geneva: WHO Press; 2001.

16. World Health Organization (WHO). International migration, health and human rights. Health & Human Rights Publication Series, Issue No. 4. Geneva: WHO Press; 2003.

17. World Health Organization (WHO). Human rights, health and poverty reduction strategies. Health & Human Rights Publication Series, Issue No. 5. Geneva: WHO Press; 2005.

18. United Nations Development Programme (UNDP). Human Development Report 2004: Cultural diversity in today's diverse world. New York: UNDP; 2004.

CHAPTER 11

Communication for effective nursing

Jane Stein-Parbury

LEARNING OBJECTIVES

When you have completed this chapter you will be able to:

- appreciate the importance of nurse–patient communication in establishing therapeutic relationships with patients
- relate the principles of patient-centred communication to therapeutic interactions
- appreciate that communication competence involves both assertive and responsive skills
- understand key factors that affect communication in nursing practice, especially in relation to cultural competence
- differentiate between the intentions of facilitative and authoritative communication.

Keywords: patient-centred communication, therapeutic nurse–patient communication, communication competence, authoritative communication, communication in nursing practice

---

COMMUNICATION IN NURSING PRACTICE

Human communication is a complex process that involves the exchange of ideas, thoughts and feelings, and people communicate continuously through verbal, non-verbal and behavioural means. It is important that nurses appreciate the importance of effective communication in nursing practice, especially in relation to its purpose and function in their interactions with patients.

Effective communication in nursing practice involves an ability to understand patients' personal and idiosyncratic experiences of health and illness, to relay meaningful information to patients that promotes their wellbeing and to provide patients with an opportunity to participate in their care to the extent that they desire. That is, communication with patients is always focused on the patient. This is a feature that distinguishes effective communication with patients from everyday conversational communication in which the needs of both parties are being met. The needs of patients drive nursing communication.

The purpose and function of patient communication in nursing centre on the need to establish therapeutic relationships. An effective therapeutic relationship is characteristically caring, supportive and accepting and offers reassurance to patients that they are safe.[1] These relationships are ones that are helpful in meeting the needs of the patient. Communication in nursing practice serves a vital function in the building of helpful relationships with patients. Taking time to listen to and understand patients' experiences conveys a message that the patient matters as a person. This in turn results in patients feeling cared for and respected – essential aspects of a helping relationship. Such a relationship is one in which the intent of one person is to assist the other by promoting that individual's growth, wellbeing and more functional use of his or her own resources.[2]

It is often assumed that therapeutic relationships need a great deal of time in order to develop in a deep and meaningful way: this is not the case. The relationship can develop with few patient–nurse interactions and in a short period of time.[3] This is because it is the level of vulnerability and dependency of the patient that determines the level of involvement between patient and nurse, not the amount of time spent together.[4-6] The nurse's response to reduce this vulnerability by meeting the patient's needs and providing helpful resources will determine whether an interpersonal connection is established.

Patients do express a desire to connect interpersonally with nurses but they are often reluctant to do so because nurses seem too busy and patients don't want to bother them.[7-9] Patients' experiences with nurses' communication reveals that nurses focus more on tasks than on communicating with them.[9] This suggests that not much has changed since Menzies[10] first described how a task-oriented approach to care functioned to protect nurses from the anxiety they might experience when dealing with patient distress. It seems healthcare institutions still do not have systems and practices that demonstrate the core values of patient-centred care.

This may be due to a lack of recognition that the effort involved in relating to patients goes largely unrecognised in current healthcare.[11] Simply put, establishing and maintaining therapeutic relationships with patients is not seen as work. However, knowledge gained about the patient through interpersonal communication and relationship building is central to nursing work.

Because the interpersonal relational aspects of nursing practice help to construct a professional identity[12] and relational work is grounded in a moral commitment to patients[13] there is good reason to hold the value of therapeutic relationships as beginning nurses struggle to adapt to healthcare systems. The development of these relationships is best promoted through the use of patient-centred communication which is the foundation of patient-centred care.

EXERCISE 11.1 HELPING RELATIONSHIPS IN NURSING

This exercise can be carried out alone or with other people.

Think about the most fulfilling relationship that you have experienced with a patient – one in which you felt you made a difference.

1. What aspects of this relationship made it fulfilling?
2. How did you make a difference?
3. What communication skills did you use?

Now think about the relationship with a patient that was the least fulfilling – one in which you think that you did not help.

4. What were some of the aspects of this relationship?
5. What happened and why?
6. What did you learn from this experience?

Patient-centred communication and care

Patient-centred communication allows patients to have influence over and input into their healthcare.[14] This involves true dialogue and give and take between nurse and patient, in contrast to telling the patient what to do and expecting compliance or obedience. Patient-centred communication is at the heart of patient-centred care, which is a widely used concept in contemporary healthcare.[15]

The essence of patient-centred care is the recognition of patients as unique beings and requires the nurse to listen to and get to know the patient as a person and to work in a collaborative way with the patient.[16] A common misconception is that patient-centred care is simply individualised care. While the concept of being patient-centred does involve care that is unique to the patient, it also includes the promotion of active patient participation[17] and the formation of a therapeutic relationship.[18] Each of these components involves interpersonal communication between nurse and patient. A patient-centred approach to care focuses nurses away from a task orientation and turns their attention to the values and needs of individual patients. Patient-centred care places communicating and relating with patients at the heart of nursing practice.

As you enter into professional nursing practice your biggest challenge in communicating with patients may be working in a system that is not patient-centred.

Consider the following case study.

CASE STUDY 11.1

Maria was almost as frightened as her 17-year-old son, Steve, when she walked into the emergency department (ED) with him. Steve was suffering from delusional thinking, sleep deprivation and extreme anxiety as a result of drugs he had taken at a party. In the car on the way to the hospital Maria promised Steve that she would stay with him at the hospital as Steve was extremely fearful. Because she had called the nurse practitioner in the ED prior to their arrival, Maria was not prepared for the 'red tape' she encountered on arriving in the ED.

When they arrived at the ED the triage nurse informed Maria that she must see the clerk first and instructed her to go through the door to her left. The triage nurse then opened a large automatic door and told Steve to proceed down the hall. A look of panic came over Steve's face and Maria said that she would not leave her son as he was very sick and scared. The triage nurse insisted that paperwork had to be initiated in order to process Steve through the ED, telling Maria that it 'just has to be done'. When Maria insisted on staying with Steve she could see that the nurse was perturbed.

This is a rather extreme example of communication that is systems-focused instead of patient-focused. The triage nurse in this scenario may not have even realised this, as she thought she was offering a service to this mother and son. She may not have intended to focus on the task rather than the patient, but this is exactly what happened.

Had Maria followed the instructions of the nurse, in all likelihood her son would have become more frightened, even panicked. The nurse's action distanced her from Maria by focusing on making the system work rather than considering individual patient needs.

It may be challenging for nurses who are new to healthcare systems to stay focused on the patient, rather than on the requirements of the system, for example to complete tasks at a specified time. In fact the work of the nurse is often carried out in a routine and bureaucratic manner that is at odds with a patient-centred approach.[19]

What difference does a patient-centred approach make for patients? Research demonstrates that when nurses are not rushed and make the time to get to know patients through communicating and relating, patients are more satisfied with their healthcare.[20] Maintaining a calm demeanour communicates to patients that there is time to communicate. When nurses appear rushed patients are reluctant to communicate. In these instances, it is the nurses' needs, not the patients', that are being met.

However, it is not just patient satisfaction that is enhanced with the use of patient-centred communication and care. There is evidence to suggest that it reduces patient vulnerability, and improves illness self-management, treatment adherence and health outcomes.[18,21,22] Being patient-centred when communicating with patients means that the personal experiences of patients, their desires, values and lifestyle are the focus of interpersonal interactions. More importantly, it involves active patient participation in healthcare; solution-focused care is a useful framework to encourage such participation.

EXERCISE 11.2 BECOMING PATIENT-CENTRED

The next time you conduct an initial assessment with a patient, try having the patient take the lead by letting her tell her story before you ask any questions. Don't ask any questions until the patient has finished with the story. Follow the lead of the patient and make sure that you clarify what she says.

1. How long did the assessment take?
2. What kind of information did you gather? Was it different to typical patient assessments that you have conducted in the past? How so?
3. What difference does it make to let the patient take the lead in an interview?

A focus on solutions

One reason why nurses focus on the task rather than engaging with the patient is to protect them from the anxiety that would result in sharing emotional distress. Such protection is needed when the focus is on the problem, that is, the distress. Focusing on problems can lead to feelings of helplessness and hopelessness and nurses may shy away from communicating with patients as a result. It is for this and other reasons that current attention is turning to solution-focused nursing.[23,24]

Solution-focused nursing care enables patients to develop their own resources, builds resilience and promotes wellbeing by focusing on strengths rather than weaknesses. In all likelihood, the healthcare institutions in which you will practise will be dominated by disorder or problem focus. Problem solving in nursing practice has strong cultural roots[23] and focusing on the solutions may cause you to feel like you are swimming upstream.

Training in and use of solution-focused communication have been shown to increase nurses' willingness to engage with patients even when distressed.[25,26] A solution focus involves creative thinking about what patients desire to happen, followed by working through practical ways to make this happen. In this sense solution-focused communication empowers patients and focuses on their strengths rather than their vulnerability.

COMMUNICATION COMPETENCE

By now you will have had some experience communicating with and relating to patients but may not feel competent in doing so. You may feel inadequate and poorly prepared for the challenges of communication. You are not alone. In a study focused on difficult communication,[27] nurses spontaneously revealed that they felt their educational program did not adequately prepare them in relation to communication challenges such as dealing with angry patients.

At this point in your professional life you are probably at the level of advanced beginner in the use of communication skills. That is, you will still be working from rules and general principles such as those reviewed later in this chapter. Through experience in interacting with patients you will have many opportunities to develop into a competent communicator.

Competent communicators are skilled at listening to other people with understanding (i.e. they are responsive) and able to express their own ideas clearly (i.e. they are assertive). Research has demonstrated that nurses are often passive and accommodating of others rather than being assertive.[28] Most likely this is due to their education which focuses on understanding and meeting the needs of patients. In addition, it could be that nurses do not perceive being assertive as compatible with being a caring person. Another study[29] concluded that caring behaviour and assertiveness are not incompatible. For example, when advocating for patients, a caring behaviour, nurses need to be able to articulate their views clearly and assertively.

Communication competence is not an end point but rather a continuous process of reflection and deepening self-awareness. Competent communicators may make mistakes in their interactions with patients, but the difference between them and those nurses who are not competent is that competent communicators recognise errors and contemplate how to address similar situations in the future. Reflecting on experiences with patients is necessary because developing communication skills in nursing involves continuous learning throughout your career.

The importance of clinical context

Different clinical contexts will demand different types of interpersonal skills, and competent communication in one clinical context may not translate to competence in another. For example, patients in emergency departments have heightened needs for information and explanations about what is happening to them, while people in a palliative care unit may have higher needs for comfort and understanding, rather than information. Nurses working in mental health settings need advanced skills in counselling and psychotherapeutic techniques, while nurses in intensive care units are served well if they know how to ask specific closed questions of patients (i.e. questions that require 'yes/no' answers) as communication may be limited to that style of interaction when patients are mechanically ventilated. It is useful to contemplate the specific types of communication that are most frequently called for in your chosen clinical context.

FACTORS THAT HAVE AN IMPACT ON COMMUNICATION EFFECTIVENESS

The most important contribution you can make to the development of professional communication strategies is to improve self-awareness and practise communication approaches that are known to be effective. To improve communication with patients you should consider the following issues: cultural competence/understanding; the importance of positive self-expectations; dealing with emotions; and metacommunication.

Cultural competence

Most people hold preconceptions about others: sometimes these are positive and sometimes they are negative. Many people have beliefs about nurses: who they are, what they do, what they should be like. Nurses are likely to hold preconceptions about some types of patients. Categorising people in this way can lead to the formation of stereotypes in which all members of a particular group are perceived to possess the same personal characteristics. For example, patients may think that all nurses are kind, caring and compassionate.

All too often stereotypes are based on the ethnicity of a particular group of people, assuming that all people of a particular ethnic background share the same values, beliefs and cultural mores. This can be dangerous for effective communication, firstly because there is confusion between ethnicity and culture. More importantly, when acted upon, stereotypes interfere with culturally competent communication and may even be harmful to both the patient and the relationship.

Culturally competent care involves an understanding that people come from diverse backgrounds and may not share the same value and belief systems. It also includes an appreciation of an individual patient's cultural belief systems and values and awareness that there is much diversity within a cultural group.[30] An essential aspect of cultural competence also includes practice that is 'safe' in a cultural sense. The concept of 'cultural safety' has been developed from a nursing perspective because patient safety is always at the forefront of practice.[31] Culturally safe practice includes both sensitivity to patient values and beliefs and an appreciation that social structures, such as healthcare institutions, can be disempowering to certain cultural groups.[32]

Cultural competence essentially relates to the ability to respect other people's way of being and their personal value systems. In this sense cultural competence is embedded in professional codes of conduct. But there is a danger in thinking that it means that all patients are treated the same. For example, when considering what a patient desires in the way of healthcare, nurses might consult with just the patient as a singular identity. This is based on the notion that adults are autonomous individuals who can make decisions on their own behalf. However, there are cultures in which individuality is not stressed and identity is collective; that is, decisions are based on what is best for a community of people as the individual is not the most important social unit. This might be hard for nurses to understand if they have been taught to focus on the individual person.

This 'one size fits all' approach to cultural care can be detrimental to good patient care. Chenoweth et al.[33] discuss the care of a fictitious person in which there was little shared understanding between the nurses and the person being cared for and her family. The reason why this occurred was that nurses made assumptions on the basis of their own values and belief systems, rather than those of the patient. This is the most common error in cultural care: that patients' views and values are shared by nurses.

So how do nurses become more culturally competent? First, it is important that nurses recognise that culture is not the same as ethnicity. Individual families have a culture, as do schools of nursing and healthcare institutions. Culture refers to values, beliefs and ways of behaving that are shared among a group of people.

The first step in becoming culturally competent is for nurses to understand their own values and beliefs, and this is accomplished through the process of reflection. The next step is to listen and learn about patients' values and beliefs by communicating with them and remaining open to views that are different from the nurse's own values. Allowing patients to define who they are and speak for themselves is part of the communication process involved in becoming culturally competent.

Another step is to learn about the social mores, behavioural patterns and beliefs of other cultures. This is especially true when nurses are working with people from cultures other than their own. For example, looking someone in the eye, considered to be a sign of honesty in Anglo culture, is considered rude in some other cultures, especially if there is a social status difference between people. Learning the specifics of certain cultures does carry a risk as this approach can lead to stereotyping of people from a specific culture. There can be as much diversity within a given cultural group as there is between cultural groups.

Culturally competent communication within nursing accommodates diversity while providing equally effective care, regardless of the sex, age, ethnicity, sexual orientation, class or level of education of patients. As nurses you are professionally and ethically obliged to increase your awareness of your own generalised beliefs and prejudices about others. Often the people we hold false beliefs about are those with whom we are not familiar, or those involved in encounters that we remember negatively. Common stereotypes are associated with gender, apparent ethnicity, socioeconomic class and sexual orientation. When, for example, a person says, 'All women …', 'Asian values are …' or 'Gay men always …', that person is stereotyping.

To achieve cultural competence when communicating you need to be aware of your own stereotyping potential and be alert to the possibility that patients may also have unhelpful preconceptions about nurses.

CASE STUDY 11.2

After completing his new graduate program, Mark decided that he would like to work in a remote area of Australia. Shortly after he began working on an acute medical surgical ward at a hospital in the Northern Territory, he came to the realisation that he had little understanding of the cultures of Indigenous Australians. He was aware that his knowledge was limited by stereotypes and prejudices and was careful not to act on this type of information. However, he was having difficulty understanding the sensibilities of the Indigenous Australian patients for whom he cared.

REFLECTIVE QUESTIONS
- What kinds of strategies should Mark undertake in order to become more knowledgeable, understanding and sensitive when caring for patients who are Indigenous Australians?
- Where should Mark go to find the information that he realises he needs?

Expectations of self

Beginning practitioners of nursing often feel inadequate about communicating with patients. If nurses aim to provide holistic care, then it is important to expect to be successful in interactions with others. If you approach another person expecting to fail to get your message across, or not to understand the other person's request, then this is likely to happen. This is an example of a negative self-fulfilling prophecy. Nurses need to develop and maintain positive self-fulfilling prophecies about increasing the likelihood of effective communication. Managing our own professional concerns about 'looking silly' or fearing 'failure' is a good start, together with perseverance and listening carefully to all patients in any situation.

Dealing with emotions

One ongoing challenge for nurses is a commitment to broaden and deepen our communication repertoire. Students enter nursing courses with communicative abilities that are likely to mirror those of the public at large. In his focus on the significance of emotion in human communication, Goleman[34] outlines three prevalent non-productive communication styles: (1) ignoring or trivialising another person's feelings; (2) noticing feelings of distress but aiming to soothe, placate or cover them over; and (3) recognising feelings but putting down or disapproving of the person due to the belief that certain emotions are unacceptable. If these styles of interaction are retained in nursing practice, then some patients will not be treated with the respect and dignity demanded by professional codes of conduct. In other words, such commonplace approaches demean the patient's feelings, constitute a barrier to effective communication and are unprofessional.

As well as stereotyping, ignoring or trivialising feelings and expressing disapproval, there are other messages that nurses may convey that are incongruent with holistic patient care which values people's social, spiritual, cultural and emotional concerns. Such possibilities include the use of clichés, false reassurance and suddenly changing the subject.[35] Clichés punctuate everyday conversation, but statements like 'Keep your chin up' are unhelpful in most health settings. Similarly, ritual statements of reassurance such as 'You'll be OK', regardless of pain or prognosis, also are not helpful or therapeutic. Abruptly changing the subject from a patient-initiated concern to something nurse-centred or technical is frequently experienced by the patient as belittling or dismissive.

Metacommunication

Metacommunication relates to any factors that affect one person's interpretation of another person's communication. The context of the message, as well as verbal and non-verbal actions, impinges on the content and potential meaning in the message and on the listener's understanding of what has been heard.

Effective communicators have qualities in common that distinguish them from less successful communicators. These include a high degree of self-awareness, an appreciation for the views of other people, congruence between what they say and what they do, the use of clear messages and an ability to evaluate the other person's needs and to grasp the main points. These are all essential aspects of a nurse's professional communication responsibilities.

The language spoken, the patient's state of illness/health, expectations, gender and age are factors that affect the sending of messages and their interpretation. Timing is another crucial ingredient. In professional relationships the nurse must assess the patient for readiness to understand information provided or to answer probing questions.[36] Patients who are disoriented, in the recovery room, in pain, have just received a terminal diagnosis or are in an emergency are not candidates for communicating much beyond support and essential information. As nurses often work with patients in these circumstances, the nurse must judge what information has to be conveyed immediately and what should remain for discussion when the patient is in less pain or is more fully alert after surgery or an emergency.

Effective verbal communication involves the nurse ascertaining the patient's concerns; determining the patient's level of interest and ability to understand health information; and using words carefully, appropriately and accurately. Hence, nursing skills include assessment of patient communication capabilities. This is not always documented, but it is important for holistic nursing.

Non-verbal communication is often called body language. Body language relates to the messages that individuals convey by the way their whole body moves, and includes posture, movements, gestures and facial expressions. Assessment of patients' non-verbal communication is often central to recovery. Nurses can observe and recognise patient actions, facial expressions or topic avoidance that indicate they have unspoken health concerns. Patients also assess nurses' non-verbal communications by picking up on incongruities between what the nurse says and how it is being said.

Interpretation of non-verbal communication has the potential to be wrong, so it is essential that nurses reflect on their observations and clarify their concerns with the patient.

CASE STUDY 11.3

In her first year of practice Jenny was having a great deal of difficulty handling her emotions when caring for patients who were dying. She did not feel that she knew how to communicate with them and was afraid of becoming too emotional when interacting with them. She was especially fearful of 'saying the wrong thing' and upsetting patients who were dying.

REFLECTIVE QUESTIONS

- How can Jenny learn more about how to interact with patients who are dying?
- With whom should she talk about this?
- How can she learn not to be so emotional when dealing with clinical situations that are potentially emotionally charged?

THERAPEUTIC NURSE–PATIENT COMMUNICATION

Therapeutic communication is oriented towards the patient and his or her healing needs. John Heron[37] provides a useful schema for understanding therapeutic communication techniques. The schema is based on therapeutic intention and has two major categories, facilitative and authoritative. Facilitative interventions build relationships and encourage patients to express themselves, while authoritative interventions are instrumental, such as offering explanations, advice and information.

Facilitative communication

Facilitative communication is helpful in and of itself, and constitutes the building blocks for a helping relationship between the nurse and the patient. In this type of communication process is as important as content. This means that how you go about speaking and listening is crucial for the patient's recovery and wellbeing. Process relates more closely to non-verbal communication.[35] Some of the main elements of facilitative communication are active listening, sharing observations, questioning (open-ended, closed and focused), clarifying, paraphrasing and the use of silence.

ACTIVE LISTENING

In the everyday world many people only partially listen to others, and they may not notice non-verbal indicators of discomfort, distress or distance. Nurses are therefore professionally obliged to continue to improve both listening and observation capabilities. Within most complex nurse–patient interactions listening is more powerful than speaking, provided it is active listening and the nurse does not interrupt the patient's flow of thought. Active listening requires that the nurse be fully present and attentive to the patient.[36] Listening is characteristically associated with silence, concentration and astute observation, especially of non-verbal communication.[38] The nurse listens not only for facts but also for the attached values, attitudes and feelings. Enhancement of these skills requires ongoing commitment, practice, reflection, perseverance and self-teaching.

One of the most important aspects of listening involves the observation of patient cues, which are indirect messages that express a need, desire or feeling. They often take the form of an implied question, or a hint or suggestion. They are important in relation to communication because patients often convey their concerns indirectly, especially in relation to their emotional needs.[39] The most helpful response to a patient cue is active exploration of what it means and an open invitation for the patient to say more. A study in which cue recognition was explored revealed that nurses responded by distancing over half of the time, acknowledged the cue a quarter of the time and explored the cue 20% of the time.[39] While cues can be explored through direct questioning, it is also helpful to share what you have observed with the patient.

EXERCISE 11.3 LISTENING
_____

Pair up with another student or friend.
1. Person A will tell person B about his or her most memorable recent experience. Person B should try to think about a personal problem, or an assignment coming up, while person A is speaking.
2. Discuss how you felt about both roles and experiences, with person A speaking first.
3. Person A then tells the same story again, taking about the same length of time. This time person B will concentrate as much as possible on person A and on what person A is saying.
4. Share the differences between these two experiences and discuss the relevance this may have when person A is a patient and person B is a nurse.

SHARING OBSERVATIONS

Reflecting back what the nurse observes is a communication response to a patient who has provided information with unclear emotional or social connotations. The nurse first creates a trusting connection with the person that enables that individual to express his or her feelings[36] by making an observational comment such as: 'It seems like you've had a difficult time …'. Such a statement shows an interest in and understanding of the patient's situation. At other times a patient might imply the presence of strong feelings; in this instance the nurse might respond by saying, 'Many people would be angry if that happened to them'. This is not easy and demands that the nurse concentrates on the patient and gains some certainty about the nature of the feeling being conveyed before naming it. The naming of feelings often normalises them – that is, it allows the patient to know that others are also upset by such experiences. The apt and well-timed naming of feelings can create a sense of relief and understanding about what has been bothering the patient.

OPEN-ENDED QUESTIONING

Once rapport with a patient is developed, open questions are the most effective way of gaining information to complete ongoing holistic nursing assessment. Open-ended questions begin with phrases like: 'Can you tell me about …?', 'Would you try to explain …?', 'How do you feel about …?' These questions give patients permission to talk about what is bothering them and to speak of anything that they consider important. A good example of an open-ended question that can be used to start a conversation is: 'Would you like to tell me more about yourself?' Open-ended questions are well suited to exploring emotional cues or unexpressed healing or health concerns.

CLOSED QUESTIONING

A closed question is one that requires a short answer, often just 'yes' or 'no'. This style of asking questions is best suited to situations where you need to gain a simple straightforward answer. For example, asking a patient: 'Are you allergic to any medication?' is an appropriate use of closed questioning. This type of questioning is instrumental and time-saving. If used inappropriately it is likely to bring a conversation to a sudden halt.

FOCUSED QUESTIONING

This type of questioning focuses on a specific topic on which the nurse wants more information. The topic is focused or narrow, but the response is intended to elaborate on something and is therefore longer than one word. Nursing examples of this type of questioning include 'Will you describe the pain to me?' and 'What drew your attention to this problem?'

CLARIFYING

It is important that nurses clarify a patient's vague or implied communication, a cue, as failure to do so may result in lack of important information being conveyed. If a patient speaks of pain, for example, it is essential for nursing assessment purposes that the patient describes the pain location and qualities in detail. When listening to a patient it is important that the nurse clarifies the main points that the patient is trying to convey. To ensure that this is so, the nurse can use questioning to request that the patient expand or explain the message. Alternatively, the nurse can use restatement to clarify meaning. Clarification can also be sought through the use of a statement such as: 'I'm not sure I follow you' or 'That's not clear to me'.[36] Most importantly, it is dangerous to pretend that you understand and not to seek clarification.

PARAPHRASING

Paraphrasing is often used to confirm with patients the meaning of their message, before the exchange goes much further. It involves using your own words to pull together the key points the patient has made. Paraphrasing often begins with something like, 'Tell me if I've got this right' and continues with a short restatement of what you have understood the patient has said. 'Simple, precise, and culturally relevant terms' are used.[35] Paraphrasing is a very important communication technique for use face to face and on the telephone to ensure that you have understood what the person is saying and to give the respondent the opportunity to alter your interpretation if it is not what that person meant.

SILENCE

Many patients feel scared and alone in hospital, as it is an alien environment for them and they inevitably have concerns and worries about their diagnosis, treatment or future health.

When the nurse is attending a patient in hospital, the experience of the patient can suddenly change from boredom, sleep or pain to multiple actions and words. Hence, it is unusual from a patient's perspective to have a nurse just sit with the patient, a nurse who is not carrying out any procedure and who is not giving instructions or asking questions. Silence can emphasise a particular point that either the patient or the nurse has made, or convey its seriousness. Some silences are better left as they begin – without words. If the patient is trying to talk about complex matters and is searching for words, silence on the nurse's part shows respect and the recognition that this is not an everyday conversation topic. Sitting quietly with a patient, even for a brief period, shows concern, caring and empathy. Such a silence is accepting, validating and therapeutic.

CASE STUDY 11.4

Louise has finished her first clinical rotation in surgical nursing in a busy metropolitan hospital; she enjoyed it very much, especially because she was on a unit of mostly female patients. Her second rotation is on a unit where the patients are mainly elderly men. She finds that she is uncomfortable and often embarrassed around these patients; she does not know how to initiate conversations with them. She notices that her male colleagues seem to have no difficulty as they often talk to the men about sport.

REFLECTIVE QUESTIONS

- What can Louise do to become more comfortable and at ease with elderly male patients?
- What communication strategies should she try when initiating conversations with them?

AUTHORITATIVE COMMUNICATION

Much communication between nurses and patients in busy hospital settings is not therapeutic in its own right. Some communication with patients is primarily social rather than facilitative, in that it is spontaneous and not goal-directed. Other communication is instrumental; that is, the communication aims to get something done. Instrumental communication is authoritative in the sense that the nurse takes the lead. In this type of communication the clarity and content of your words are at least as important as the process involved in imparting that information.

Offering accessible and relevant information

It is important not to confuse information provision with effective communication or with knowledge. For most patients, nurses are a valuable source of information. It is important to remember that even as new graduates your knowledge of the body and its workings is greater than that of many patients. The goal is to provide information that will improve patients' ability to understand what is happening or enable them to improve their own self-care activities.

There are a number of ways in which information can be shared with patients and general guidelines ensure that the sharing of information is helpful[36]:

- Share information when the patient has indicated a need for it and is ready to hear the information.
- Find out first what the patient already knows and what he or she wants to know.
- Limit the amount of information at any one time.
- Use language that is appropriate to the patient and tailor to that person, i.e. consider the patient's background and educational level.
- Reinforce spoken information, for example through the use of written material.
- Frequently check if the patient is understanding the information.
- Make sure of your own knowledge base.

Summarising

Summarising is similar to paraphrasing in that it focuses on conversation content, but it occurs near the end of the time that you spend with the patient and aims to summarise the important points you have discussed. Nurses can use summarising as an aid to go over information that has been provided, to show the patient what has been achieved, or to create a break before moving on to the next topic. It is a useful technique as it brings a sense of closure to your interaction, provides the patient with an overview of the issues you have discussed and allows for any last-minute clarification.

EMPATHY

Empathy, the ability to put yourself in the patient's shoes, is an essential aspect to all therapeutic communication and underpins both facilitative and authoritative communication. Egan[40] defines empathy as 'listening carefully to the client and then communicating understanding of what the client is feeling and of the experiences and behaviours underlying those feelings'. Before empathy is possible, you need to put your own interests, concerns and needs aside and concentrate on some as-yet-unknown patient concerns – that is, empathy is altruistic.[34,41] Openness without judgment is the beginning of the possibility of empathy, as any perception of disapproval will encourage patients to hide their worries. Empathy is complex and includes active listening, recognising covert communication, validating feelings and responses, understanding ambiguous cues and validating the 'normality' of strong emotions. There is a twofold process inherent in empathy, involving stepping into another person's emotional shoes, then stepping out of them to use cognitive analytical skills and draw on experience with other patients in similar situations.

CONCLUSION

This chapter aims to increase awareness of communication responsibilities for ethical and holistic nursing practice. The focus of communication in nursing practice is placed in the context of relationship building. The concepts of person-centred care and patient-centred communication are reviewed along with solution-focused communication. Communication competence is discussed in relation to the need for both assertive and responsive communication skills. Precommunication factors such as cultural differences, stereotyping and interpersonal expectations are outlined. A significant part of the discussion focuses on key strategies to improve therapeutic communication, both facilitative and authoritative communication.

RECOMMENDED READING

DeFrino DT. A theory of the relational work of nurses. Research and Theory for Nursing Practice 2009;23:294–311.

Hobbs JL. A dimensional analysis of patient-centered care. Nursing Research 2009;58: 52–62.

Jones A. Admitting hospital patients: a qualitative study of an everyday nursing task. Nursing Inquiry 2007;14:212–23.

Shipley SD. Listening: a concept analysis. Nursing Forum 2010;45:125–34.

Stein-Parbury J. Patient and person: interpersonal skills in nursing. 4th ed. Sydney: Elsevier Australia; 2009.

REFERENCES

1. Mottram A. Therapeuitic relationships in day surgery: a grounded theory study. Journal of Clinical Nursing 2009;18:2830–7.
2. Rogers C. On becoming a person. Boston: Houghton Mifflin; 1961.
3. Shattell M. Nurse–patient interaction: a review of the literature. Journal of Clinical Nursing 2004;13:714–22.
4. Morse JM. Negotiating commitment and involvement in the nurse–patient relationship. Journal of Advanced Nursing 1991;16:455–68.
5. Ramos MC. The nurse–patient relationship: theme and variations. Journal of Advanced Nursing 1992;17:496–506.
6. Graber DR, Mitcham MD. Compassionate clinicians: taking patient care beyond the ordinary. Holistic Nursing Practice 2004;18:87–94.
7. Chang T, Lin Y-P, Change H-J, et al. Cancer patient and staff ratings of caring behaviors. Cancer Nursing 2005;28:331–9.
8. Shattell, M. Nurse bait: strategies hospitalized patients use to entice nurses within the context of the interpersonal relationship. Issues in Mental Health Nursing 2005;26:205–23.
9. McCabe C. Nurse–patient communication: an exploration of patients' experiences. Journal of Clinical Nursing 2004;13:41–9.
10. Menzies I. A case study of the functioning of social systems as a defence against anxiety. Human Relations 1961;13:95–123.
11. DeFrino DT. A theory of the relational work of nurses. Research and Theory for Nursing Practice 2009;23:294–311.
12. Deppoliti D. Exploring how new registered nurses construct professional identity in hospital settings. Journal of Continuing Education in Nursing 2008;39: 255–62.
13. Doane GH, Varcoe C. Relational practice and nursing obligations. Advances in Nursing Science 2007;20:192–205.

14. Epstein RM, Franks P, Fiscella K, et al. Measuring patient-centered communication in patient–physician consultations: theoretical and practical issues. Social Science and Medicine 2005;61:1516–28.

15. McCormack B, McCance TV. Development of a framework for person-centred nursing. Journal of Advanced Nursing 2006;56:472–9.

16. Johnson R. Shifting patterns of practice: nurse practitioners in a managed care environment. Research and Theory for Nursing Practice 2005;19:323–40.

17. Sidani S. Effects of patient-centered care on patient outcomes: an evaluation. Research and Theory for Nursing Practice 2008;22:24–37.

18. Hobbs JL. A dimensional analysis of patient-centered care. Nursing Research 2009;58:52–62.

19. Jones A. Admitting hospital patients: a qualitative study of an everyday nursing task. Nursing Inquiry 2007;14:212–23.

20. Haskard KB, DiMattero MR, Heritage J. Affective and instrumental communication in primary care interactions: predicting the satisfaction of nursing staff and patients. Health Communication 2009;24:21–32.

21. Robinson JH, Callister LC, Berry JA, et al. Patient-centered care and adherence: definitions and applications to improve outcomes. Journal of the American Academy of Nurse Practitioners 2008;20:600–7.

22. Charlton CR, Dearing KS, Berry JA, et al. Nurse practitioners' communication styles and their impact on patient outcomes: an integrated literature review. Journal of the American Academy of Nurse Practitioners 2008;20:382–8.

23. McAllister M. Doing practice differently: solution-focused nursing. Journal of Advanced Nursing 2003;41:528–35.

24. McAllister M. Solution focused nursing: a fitting model for mental health nurses working in a public health paradigm. Contemporary Nurse 2010;34:149–57.

25. Bowles N, Mackintosh C, Torn A. Nurses' communication skills: an evaluation of the impact of solution-focused communication training. Journal of Advanced Nursing 2001;36:347–54.

26. McAllister M, Zimmer-Gembeck M, Moyle W, et al. Working effectively with clients who self-injure using a solution focused approach. Journal of International Emergency Nursing 2008;16:272–9.

27. Sheldon LK, Barrett R, Ellington L. Difficult communication in nursing. Journal of Nursing Scholarship 2006;38:141–7.

28. Timmins F, McCabe C. Nurses' and midwives' assertive behaviour in the workplace. Journal of Advanced Nursing 2005;51:38–45.

29. McCartan PJ, Hargie ODW. Assertiveness and caring: are they compatible? Journal of Clinical Nursing 2004;13:707–13.

30. Schim SM, Doorenbos A, Benkert R, et al. Culturally congruent care: putting the puzzle together. Journal of Transcultural Nursing 2007;18:103–10.

31. Ramsden I. Kawa Whakaruruhau: cultural safety in nursing education in Aotearoa (New Zealand). Nursing Praxis 1993;8:4–10.

32. Richardson S. Aotearoa/NewZealand nursing: from eugenics to cultural safety. Nursing Inquiry 2004;11:35–42.

33. Chenoweth L, Jeon YH, Burke C. Cultural competency and nursing care: an Australian perspective. International Nursing Review 2006;53:34–40.

34. Goleman D. Emotional intelligence. Why it can matter more than IQ. London: Bloomsbury; 1996.

35. Varcarolis E. Communication and the clinical interview. In: Varcarolis E, editor. Foundations of psychiatric mental health nursing. 6th ed. Philadelphia: WB Saunders; 2010.

36. Stein-Parbury J. Patient and person: interpersonal skills in nursing. 4th ed. Sydney: Elsevier Australia; 2009.

37. Heron J. Helping the client. 5th ed. London: Sage; 2001.

38. Shipley SD. Listening: a concept analysis. Nursing Forum 2010;45:125–34.

39. Uitterhoeve R, Bensing J, Dilven E, et al. Nurse—patient communication in cancer care: does responding to patients' cues predict patient satisfaction with communication? Psycho-Oncology 2009;18:1060–8.

40. Egan G. The skilled helper. 9th ed. Pacific Grove, California: Brooks/Cole; 2010.

41. Yegdich T. On the phenomenology of empathy in nursing: empathy or sympathy? Journal of Advanced Nursing 1999;30:83–93.

CHAPTER 12

On gender in nursing: a discussion of issues and directions

Debra Jackson and Jennifer Clauson

LEARNING OBJECTIVES

When you have completed this chapter you will be able to:

- describe occupational segregation and how it affects nursing
- discuss the gendered nature of nursing and its effects on both female and male nurses
- explain the issues that contribute to the hidden advantages of males in career advancement in nursing, and the ways women nurses contribute to these advantages
- discuss the dynamics of the doctor–nurse relationship and its effect on the nursing profession
- detail the role of equal employment opportunity (EEO) in minimising the effects of gender bias in the workplace.

Keywords: gender, nursing, oppression, bias, violence

INTRODUCTION

Nursing has long been considered 'women's work'[1] and a female occupation[2] because of its association with feminine qualities, particularly caring.[3] Many texts discuss the gendered nature of nursing work[4] and the general consensus is that, because of its construction as 'women's work', and its status as a strongly female-dominated profession, nursing has been marginalised and devalued.[5] Indeed, writing in 1997, Gordon and Wimpenny[6] described nursing as 'being a prime example of occupational segregation where women and women's work are less valued'. Occupational segregation can be associated with how professions and occupations are positioned or viewed, and 'occurs when workers of one sex are disproportionately concentrated in a particular sector of the economy or in a particular occupational category'.[7]

There are various consequences of this positioning, including oppression (experienced by female nurses both as nurses and as women) and silencing. Oppression has a number of ramifications.[5,8,9] For example, although nursing is predominantly a profession of women, men hold a disproportionately high number of powerful positions. There is quite a body of literature about this situation, and various arguments are presented that highlight factors contributing to male career advantage in nursing,[4,10–12] an issue we will discuss more fully later in this chapter.

Entrenched oppression can result in difficulties in challenging power inequalities[5] and organisational injustice. Though the sheer size and importance of the nursing workforce mean that nurses have considerable potential political power, the recognised and entrenched oppression of nurses[13] means that nurses do not lobby as effectively as some other, smaller, but more vocal professional groups, One outcome of nursing being an ineffective lobby group is the evidence that registered nurses earn considerably less than other female professionals, due to persistent labour market inequalities in setting comparative wages.[5]

Nurses are exposed to various occupational hazards, including very high levels of violence and assault and aggression,[14–18] and there is evidence that the nursing workplace can be very hostile to nurses generally and women nurses specifically.[4] For example, a study in a UK hospital showed that nurses had the highest exposure to assault and doctors the fewest.[18] Though gender was not addressed as a variable in this particular paper, the fact that nursing is so strongly female-dominated, while medicine is more male-dominated, means that gender is likely a factor. The literature also suggests that nursing is affected by sexual harassment and aggression more than any other occupational group[19] and, furthermore, the majority of harassers are workplace colleagues.[20–22] The vulnerability of nurses to sexual harassment has been seen as a result of the strongly gendered images of nursing[3,4] and the intimate nature of nursing work.[23]

This chapter focuses on the hospital because most nurses work in hospitals, particularly at the beginning of their careers, and explores some of the gender-related issues that have an impact on nursing and nurses. These factors include hospitals as male-dominated institutions; men in nursing; violence and nursing; and the relationship between nurses and medical practitioners. We conclude with a discussion of some ways of minimising gender bias in nursing.

EXERCISE 12.1

Obtain a copy of the Australian Nursing and Midwifery Council's Code of professional conduct for nurses in Australia[24] and Code of ethics for nurses in Australia.[25] What statements included in these documents endeavour to provide a non-discriminatory and inclusive environment for nurses?

HOSPITALS AS MALE-CONTROLLED INSTITUTIONS

Healthcare systems are male-dominated,[10] with hospitals generally run along strongly hierarchical lines. This is because the management structures and systems are historically grounded in institutions of social control such as the church and the army, and traditionally men have held positions of power in these institutions. As well, patriarchal attitudes existing within medicine have influenced hospital environments because, although other institutions (such as government) exercise controlling influences, hospitals are essentially under the control of medicine.[26,27] Medical practitioners from various specialties dominate hospitals and, thus, taken-for-granted hegemonic values and beliefs (those held by powerful groups and cultures) dominate and permeate the hospital as an institution.

The power of men in healthcare is maintained in a number of ways. Nursing and medicine both have a tradition of occupational segregation (nursing being feminine and female-dominated, and medicine being masculine and male-dominated). Though more men are entering nursing, they are disproportionately situated in senior positions with decision-making powers. In medicine, though there are increasing numbers of women doctors in hospitals,[28] the senior medical officers with decision-making powers are most often men.[29,30]

Most of the powerful decision-making forums in hospitals, such as hospital boards, medical committees and institutional ethics committees, are also male-dominated. The power of these forums is reinforced by a patriarchal public service, which controls finance and helps to shape health and financial policy. Although we are focusing on hospitals in this chapter, it is important to consider that similar structures exist within community health settings.

Nurses are the backbone of the hospital system since patients enter hospitals primarily to receive nursing care; otherwise (medical) diagnosis and treatment could occur in the community. Nurses are concentrated at the lower levels of the hierarchical management system within hospitals.[13,31] For example, although nursing has some representation on hospital committees, the level of representation varies according to the power and the prestige of the committee. Nurses generally have considerably less representation on budget-controlling or policy decision-making committees such as area health boards and hospital management boards or committees. However, nurses are generally well represented on working parties, and on (draft) policy-generating or 'doing' committees such as infection control and quality assurance.

MEN IN NURSING

Although nursing continues to be strongly female-dominated, evidence shows that the numbers of men are growing. Indeed, Stott[32] asserts that in Australia the percentage of male nursing students has been steadily increasing. Evans[10] suggests that men have hidden advantages over women when it comes to gaining access to elite specialties and power positions, and that women nurses assist and foster the careers of male nurses, either deliberately or unknowingly. Conventional feminine characteristics such as nurturing, caring, dependence and submission exist, in contrast to masculine traits such as aggression, dominance, autonomy and objectivity. Feminine traits have traditionally been viewed as suited to service and domestic responsibilities. These traits are also advantageous to men in the workplace, where women may be more likely to defer to men.

Women tend to support men in the workforce and at home, and this support often costs women progression in their own careers[4,12,33] or even loss of integrity in the workplace.[34,35] In terms of career advancement, marriage may be advantageous to male nurses but can be disadvantageous to women nurses because of the associated domestic responsibilities.[10,12] This domestic advantage also means men are more likely than women to pursue higher degrees and ongoing education.[10,33] Even the university sector is friendlier to men than women and Gordon and Wimpenny[6] assert that patriarchal structures are entrenched throughout universities and that this may be detrimental to women nurses. Thus a greater proportion of men than women complete higher degrees, which are highly advantageous in the workplace.[36] The repercussion of these and other advantages is the overrepresentation of men in positions of power within nursing.[12] In a very influential and still widely cited work, Evans[10] emphasised:

> the small number of men currently in the profession occupy a privileged position in relation to their women colleagues. This position is established and maintained by patriarchal institutions and the use of strategies by male nurses to separate themselves and their masculine sex role identity from their female colleagues and the feminine image of nursing itself.

However, this position of percieved privilege may be a double-edged sword. There may be an expectation that males naturally progress within the patriarchal and male-dominated healthcare systems into managerial positions. Porter O'Grady[37] suggests that, although males may acquire authority and positional power based on genuine merit, it is often assumed promotions are obtained based on advantage gained through being male. This is disadvantaging to men in these positions.

In the clinical area, men are considered to be attracted to the more 'high-tech', high-status areas of nursing, such as emergency department and critical care areas, and far less represented in slower-stream areas such as aged care. Purnell[38] suggests this is because the 'high-tech' areas are seen as being more 'masculine' specialties. He goes on to suggest that males may feel drawn to these areas to prevent gender-based stigmatisation. Acquisition of skills associated with the highly technical aspects of nursing may also assist in promoting a sense of comfort and mastery in a group that may otherwise feel emasculated.[32] Additionally, uniforms stereotype nurses, and Evans[10] suggests that many male nurses deliberately choose to work in specialties in which non-traditional clothing is permitted, such as mental health (street clothes) and operating theatre (greens).

Despite more men entering nursing,[32] current media images of the nurse as feminine continue to dominate, and may turn men away from nursing. Men who are drawn into female-concentrated professions are often considered by the public as 'less masculine' than those who work in the more traditional male-dominated occupations[11,39,40] and consequently men may reject female-concentrated occupations as potential career choices in order to preserve their masculinity. In the USA, the Oregon Center for Nursing sought to appeal to men by launching the 'Are you man enough to be a nurse?' campaign to project male nurses as strong, self-assured, smart, successful and, overall, masculine. Although aspects of the campaign offended both men and women, it did get the public's attention and assisted in raising the issue of gender-based stereotyping in nursing.[39]

The literature suggests that contemporary nursing education has failed to provide an environment attractive to recruiting and retaining men. In a study by O'Lynn[40,41] of 111 male nurses who had graduated from nursing programs, 10 principal barriers for men in nursing education were identified. These barriers highlighted issues such as: lack of mentorship programs for male students; little acknowledgement of men's contribution to nursing; a lack of support from significant people in their lives for men to become nurses; anxiety about providing intimate body care; and not feeling welcome in the clinical setting as a male student. Stott[32] cited similar themes of male isolation within nursing programs; some issues around the concept of male characteristics were applied to the caring nursing role and concerns about the strongly gendered nature of nursing. Heightened awareness regarding the unique challenges males face within both nursing programs and the nursing workforce is essential in order to understand better the male experience within a feminised nursing world.

EXERCISE 12.2

Look at the governing committees and boards of the institution in which you study or work and analyse the membership based on gender. What is the ratio of male to female members? What professional positions do male and female members hold in the organisation?

NURSING AND VIOLENCE

Like violence against women in wider society, violence against women nurses is a major problem in the nursing workplace.[42-44] Winstanley and Whittington[10] state that nurses are at a higher risk of violence than other healthcare professionals. Trossman[45] suggests that increasing numbers of nursing and other health professionals are suffering the effects of posttraumatic stress disorder as a result of workplace violence.

In a study of Australian nurses ($n = 6326$), Farrell et al.[46] reported that 63.5% of respondents had experienced some form of violence in a 4-week period. Of this sample, 92.8% of respondents were female. These findings are similar to those of Winstanley and Whittington,[18] who found 68% of nursing staff had been verbally abused in a 12-month period.

Although it is known that nurses in areas such as the emergency department and psychiatry are exposed to violence,[16] literature reveals that the general wards are just as hazardous.[42,43] Research by Nabb[15] suggests that managerial decisions related to budget and, in turn, staffing, affect nurses' exposure to occupational violence. Nurses in Nabb's study indicated that they felt more vulnerable to violent outbursts when they were short-staffed with an increased workload. They also felt that myths about nursing and the extension of nurses' roles meant that patients and their visitors had impossibly high expectations of nurses, expectations that could not possibly be met in the current economically stretched healthcare environment. Poor discharge planning and lack of community-based support for families were also identified as factors that created anger in members of the public and caused them to direct acts of violence towards nurses.[15] These findings resonate with similar studies in many countries, demonstrating that violence and aggression towards nurses are common-place.[14,47–50] The NEXT study[16] of nurses across 10 European countries ($n = 13,537$) reported that 22% of respondents were exposed to frequent violent events over a 12-month period, while Solfield and Salmond's[51] study of American nurses found 91% of respondents were verbally abused in a 4-week period.

Not all violence is as overt as actual physical assault, verbal abuse or sexual harass-ment. Nor does all the violence and oppression directed at nurses come from doctors, patients, relatives and hospital visitors. There is ample evidence to suggest that nursing itself perpetuates some forms of harassment and violence within its own ranks.[22,46,47,51,52]

Harassment takes many forms. Bullying is a form of harassment that is increasingly recognised as an occupational issue and has been shown to be a work–based stressor for nurses.[44,53] A large study by Stanley et al.[54] found that 65% of registered nurses reported frequently observing bullying behaviours among co-workers. In Australia, a qualita-tive study of 26 nurses reported accounts of minimisation, trivialisation, denial and sustainment of bullying behaviours, with individual as well as 'cliques' of nurse bullies being protected by senior staff and management.[55] Despite a zero-tolerance approach to bullying in the healthcare sector, management attitudes often serve to enforce the tolerance and acceptance of bullying and aggression in the nursing workforce.

One of the difficulties in addressing bullying as a workplace issue is the problem of definition.[48] Although arriving at a clear, concise definition is problematic, a range of behaviours are considered as comprising bullying. These include excessive abuse or criticism, intimidation, threats, ridicule (especially in front of spectators), making excessive and impossible demands, withholding information, inequitable rostering practices, rumour mongering, blocking opportunities for promotion or training, removing responsibility, public humiliation and misuse of power to incite others to marginalise or exclude the victim.[44,47] It is generally accepted in the literature that bullying involves a series of incidents, not an incident in isolation.[49] Though bullying can occur in a variety of situations and between people of equal rank and status, as well as between people who have power and rank differences, literature suggests that most bullying is carried out by line managers to their subordinate staff,[47,50] and there is evidence to show that workplace bullying and marginalisation can have negative impacts on patient care as well as devastating effects on nurses themselves.[46,50,53,56,57]

If aggression and harassment are taken–for–granted practices in the culture of a ward or unit, the capacity for nurses to advocate and care for themselves and their patients is diminished. Attending to the practice environment and monitoring inter-personal behaviour and professional relationships ought to be a management respon-sibility supported by the willingness of the multidisciplinary team to work together for the benefit of the people who use the service.

EXERCISE 12.3

Obtain a copy of occupational health and safety data for last year from your local hospital's human resources department. Examine the level of violence experienced and reported by nurses. Draw some conclusions from anecdotal evidence and your reading about the level of unreported violence.

NURSES AND DOCTORS: AN INTERDEPENDENT AND PROBLEMATIC RELATIONSHIP

Nurses and doctors work closely together and, in a sense, work to achieve similar goals related to improved outcomes for patients. In most hospital settings, nurses and doctors are engaged in a symbiotic relationship, in that nurses require doctors' orders (for certain treatments and medications) and doctors rely on nursing care for treatment of their patients. Patients are admitted to hospital for nursing care, but under the care of a doctor. There are no other comparable professional situations where two practice disciplines, each strongly gendered, have such close and interdependent relationships. Because of their complexities and uniqueness, the relationships between doctors and nurses are endlessly fascinating for social scientists as well as for nurses and doctors. It is important to try to understand the dynamics of the nurse–doctor relationship, as it has been cited as a longstanding contributing factor to nursing shortages and nurses' role dissatisfaction.[56,57]

Gender has played a crucial role in the relationships between nurses and doctors, and the analogy of the family (the doctor/father/patriarchy and the nurse/mother/ nurturer) has been used to demonstrate these.[58] The inequalities between doctors and nurses in hospital and healthcare settings can be thought to mirror those between men and women in wider society. The relationship has been constructed as a game in some of the literature. The doctor–nurse game[59] was first described by Stein in 1967[60] as a stereotypical pattern of interplay between nurses and doctors, in which nurses offer advice to doctors and show initiative while appearing to be deferential to medical power and control. Disagreements between nurses and physicians were to be avoided at all costs, so the doctor–nurse game meant that nurses would make suggestions and recommendations concerning the diagnosis, care and treatment of patients, but in such a way as to appear that the doctors had in fact been the initiator. In this way nurses could recommend treatments without it being obvious, and doctors could hear recommendations without appearing to ask for them. Thus, out-and-out conflict was avoided. Stein suggested that doctors learned to play the game subsequent to their basic training, while the training of nurses prepared them to play this game,[59] because a fear of autonomous, independent practice was conveyed in strict, highly disciplined nurse training schools.[11] In the past doctors had a teaching role in nurse education and so the primacy of medical knowledge was reinforced in the training schools. Although nursing education has changed considerably since the time of Stein's original paper, fear is still imparted to nursing students through fear of the legal ramifications of acting without the protection of 'doctors' orders', even though nurses can in fact make autonomous decisions in many situations.

Stein et al.[59] also suggest there have been major changes since Stein's first proposition in 1967, though they assert that the game still holds true in 'many settings'. They propose that various social factors have altered the 'game', including a loss of public respect and deference for doctors, a widespread nursing shortage and the rapidly increasing number of women in medicine. They point out that the increasing number of women in medicine means that, although women doctors can play the doctor–nurse game, 'the elements of the game that reflect stereotypical roles of male dominance and female passivity are missing'.[59] They also suggest that, to a far lesser extent, men in nursing have also had an effect on the gendered nature of 'the game'. Sweet and Norman[61] also observe that the doctor–nurse game is seldom seen in current clinical settings, which they suggest may be related to the changing status of women in broader society.

Improved career and educational opportunities for nurses are also considered to be important variables in the relationships between nurses and doctors, as are strong nursing images on popular television dramas. Stein et al.[59] suggest that nursing 'has unilaterally decided to stop playing that game and instead is consciously and actively attempting to change both nursing and how nurses relate to other health professionals', and also discuss the changed goals and motivation of nursing. They identify the changed nature of nurse education as a factor in the changed relationship, although this perception is yet to be supported by research. In discussing university-based education for nurses, these authors observe:

> Hospital-based schools trained students in health care institutions and socialized them to accept physicians' authority, but the academic setting is far different. In academia there is not only an absence of physicians' influence, there is an aversion to it. Instead of being told to defer to physicians, students are told that nurses are equal to other health care providers, in a relationship that is collegial, not subservient, and that nurses are professional and thus obligated to make decisions and take responsibility. Furthermore there is a pervasive attitude within nursing academia that sees physicians as narrowly focused technicians who treat illnesses and are uninterested in the humanistic aspects of health care.[59]

However, there are many other issues that have an impact on nurse–doctor relationships. Power remains a major issue in the relationships between nurses and doctors, particularly women nurses. The potential for this power to be abused is visible in research reports which identify hostility, abuse and sexual harassment directed at nurses by doctors. For example, research findings reported by Solfield and Salmond[51] reported that in a 1-month period a significant number of nurses were verbally assaulted by medical staff.

Further complicating the working relationships between doctors and nurses are issues related to sexual harassment. The literature suggests that nurses experience a relatively high level of harassment, and that much of this harassment is directed at female nurses by male doctors. O'Connell et al.[62] report that 42.8% of nurses in their sample ($n = 209$) indicated they were subject to intimidating acts from hospital medical staff. This is a most unsatisfactory situation, especially when considered in the context of hard work, role confusion and staff shortages. It is clearly intolerable and may well be a contributing factor to high turnover of nursing staff in some areas.

EXERCISE 12.4

Nurses form the largest group of employees in any health service, particularly hospitals. Look at your local hospital's annual report and note the priority given to nursing activities.

THE WAY FORWARD: MINIMISING GENDER BIAS IN NURSING

Given the history of nursing as 'women's work',[1,4] it will likely continue to be affected by occupational segregation. In view of this, some feminists believe that young women should not be encouraged to choose a traditional 'female' profession but be encouraged into non-traditional occupations. However, nursing should be recognised as being work of equal value to other comparable professions.[63] Nursing requires personal investment – intellectual, social and psychological – in the same way that other professions do. A major concern for healthcare managers and, in particular, hospital managers must be the level of workplace bullying, harassment and violence to which nurses are exposed. These are real issues for nurses, their colleagues and the public, and there is an urgent need to ensure strategies are in place to promote workplaces that are safe and free from harassment and bullying.

Institutions have an obligation to provide nurses with a workplace that is as safe as possible. Individual nurses also have a responsibility to exercise their rights to fairness, safety and respect in the workplace by saying 'no' to bullying, and making use of policies designed to maintain a safe and equitable workplace.[44,47,51] Nursing professional organisations have a responsibility to the profession and to the public to uncover gender-related workplace violence, name it and put strategies in place to eliminate it. Changing an established culture in strongly hierarchical organisations such as hospitals is not an easy task. Active leadership for change must be demanded from senior executives and supported by organisational policies and practices benchmarked at a zero-tolerance level.

Creative solutions need to be explored to improve the professionally close yet problematic relationships nursing has with medicine. There are many opportunities for collaboration that could provide more effective and responsive healthcare to people. A theme issue of the *British Medical Journal*[64] briefly described several creative and cost-effective innovations involving increased flexibility between nurses and doctors which aimed to improve patients' experiences. Reports such as this really do provide encouragement and highlight the possibilities if nurses and doctors are prepared to be flexible and open to new ways of care delivery. There is a need to explore further options for collaborative opportunities.[57,58,65]

Feminist philosophy challenges and resists gender-based inequity and so offers opportunities for the nursing workplace, particularly in relation to the misuse of power. It is important that nurses and women get adequate representation throughout health service organisations.[28] There is an awareness in many institutions of the importance of achieving gender equity on decision-making committees of all levels, and in some cases this has become a part of organisational lore. Currently, employing organisations are very aware of gender issues in relation to employment and promotion, including gender-related workplace advantage/disadvantage.

Acknowledgment of women's inherent disadvantage in the workplace is given in the form of policies designed to promote workplace fairness and gender equity. EEO policies are in place in public-sector agencies as well as many private-sector agencies. EEO is practised in a range of ways, and is reflected in staff recruitment and promotion policies. These policies provide recognition that certain groups, including women, may be more likely to be employed in lower-level employment. Most hospitals and healthcare agencies have EEO policies to provide guidance for organisations as well as employees in a range of areas, including composition of interview panels and promotions committees, as well as guidance for the conduct of interviews themselves. For example, EEO policies guide interview panels about the types of questions that can be asked of applicants. Many institutions also have designated EEO advisers who are available to discuss issues of concern. EEO advisers are frequently required to keep statistical information about many issues pertaining to equity.

Pay inequity remains an issue for nurses. In 1996 the Pay Equity Inquiry in New South Wales identified the 'poor bargaining position of women in female-dominated industries and occupations' as a major factor in the gap between women's and men's earnings,[66] and although more than 15 years have elapsed since that observation was made, it remains true. Flexible and family-friendly work policies are also important to assist women in achieving equity in the workplace. Nurses must ensure that they know about and understand these policies so that they can use them to empower themselves to minimise the effects of inherent gender bias.

EXERCISE 12.5

Develop for yourself learning strategies to increase your knowledge about gender relationships in the workplace. Work with your colleagues to identify gender-related harassment and violence, name it and devise strategies to eliminate it.

CONCLUSION

This chapter has explored issues related to the gendered nature of the nursing workplace. We have discussed occupational segregation and its effects on the careers and lives of women nurses, on patient outcomes and on economic implications for the health service. Although there are many problematic areas for nurses in the workplace, notably violence towards nurses, male advantage in nursing and the difficult yet essential relationships between nurses and doctors, there are also many creative possibilities to effect positive change.

CASE STUDY 12.1

James is a slightly built, mature-age nursing student working casually as an undergraduate assistant in nursing in a mental health setting. During a shift, a patient begins to ask personal questions regarding his sexual orientation. When James questions why, the patient replies: 'Nursing is for women! Only queers would want to do women's work! I don't want you looking after me!'

REFLECTIVE QUESTIONS
• What gender-based stereotypes are reflected in this patient's attitude to James?
• What strategies can contemporary nurses employ to shift the perception of nursing as 'women's work'?

CASE STUDY 12.2

Feng is a straight-A student who has recently completed high school. Feng's family has always placed a strong emphasis on education and had been encouraging her to apply for law or medicine. Without telling her family, Feng elects nursing as her first choice. Feng receives a letter of offer from her local university accepting her into the Bachelor of Nursing course. When she tells her family, they become very upset with her, believing nursing is an inferior choice for someone with her grades.

REFLECTIVE QUESTIONS

- What gender-based stereotypes are reflected in Feng's parents' attitude to her decision?
- What evidence could Feng give to her parents to demonstrate the need for smart people in nursing?

CASE STUDY 12.3

During her third-year clinical placement, Sarah is placed on a busy medical surgical ward containing patients with an array of chronic and complex problems. One elderly patient, Mr Julip, has many members of his family visiting. During one busy afternoon shift while Sarah is assisting another very incapacitated patient to the toilet, a male visitor asks Sarah to get Mr Julip an extra pillow. It takes Sarah quite a while to attend to her patient fully, and she doesn't bring the pillow until nearly an hour later. Mr Julip's family member becomes quite irate at the delay, calling her a 'stupid lazy cow', among other gender-specific derogatory terms.

REFLECTIVE QUESTIONS

- What gender-based stereotypes are reflected in this scenario?
- What processes can Sarah undertake to report this experience?
- What actions could an organisation take to reduce gendered abuse against staff?

ACKNOWLEDGMENT

The authors would like to thank and acknowledge Judith Clare for her contribution to this chapter in previous editions of the text.

RECOMMENDED READING

Ferreira M. Nurses' organizational commitment: the discriminating power of gender. Nursing Administration Quarterly. Future Nursing Workforce: Securing Intellectual Capital 2007;31:61–7.

O'Lynn CE. Gender-based barriers for male students in nursing education programs: prevalence and perceived importance. Journal of Nursing Education 2004;43: 229–36.

McMillian J, Morgan S, Ament P. Acceptance of male registered nurses by female registered nurses. Journal of Nursing Scholarship 2006;38:100–6.

Rothstein WG, Hannum S. Profession and gender in relationships between advanced practice nurses and physicians. Journal of Professional Nursing 2007;23:235–40.

Speedy S. The gendered culture of nursing. In: Daly J, Speedy S, Jackson D, editors. Contexts of nursing: an introduction. Sydney: Elsevier; 2010. p. 174–92.

REFERENCES

1. Walker K. Philosophy and nursing? Exploring the truth effects of history, culture and language. In: Daly J, Speedy S, Jackson D, editors. Contexts of nursing: an introduction. Sydney: Elsevier; 2010. p. 65–79.
2. Shea ML. Determined persistence: achieving and sustaining job satisfaction among nurse practitioners. University of Maine, unpublished thesis, 2008.
3. Çelik Y, Çelik SŞ. Sexual harassment against nurses in Turkey. Journal of Nursing Scholarship 2007;39:200–6.
4. Speedy S. The gendered culture of nursing. In: Daly J, Speedy S, Jackson D, editors. Contexts of nursing: an introduction. Sydney: Elsevier; 2010. p. 174–92.
5. Nowak M, Preston A. Can human capital theory explain why nurses are so poorly paid? Australian Economic Papers 2001;40:232–45.
6. Gordon F, Wimpenny P. Sex, gender and research supervision in nursing. Nurse Researcher 1997;4:63–77.
7. Estévez-Abe M. Gendering the varieties of capitalism. A study of occupational segregation by sex in advanced industrial societies. World Politics 2006;59: 142–75.
8. Dendaas N. The scholarship related to nursing work environments: where do we go from here? Advances in Nursing Science 2004;27:12–20.
9. Rose J, Glass N. The importance of emancipatory research to contemporary nursing practice. Contemporary Nurse 2008;29:8–22.
10. Evans J. Men in nursing: issues of gender segregation and hidden advantage. Journal of Advanced Nursing 1997;26:226–31.
11. Lupton B. Explaining men's entry into female-concentrated occupations: issues of masculinity and social class. Gender, Work and Organization 2006;13: 103–28.
12. Tracey C, Nicholl H. The multifaceted influence of gender in career progress in nursing. Journal of Nursing Management 2007;15:677–82.
13. Tracey C. The glass ceiling in Irish healthcare: a nursing perspective. Journal of Health, Organization and Management 2006;20:502–11.
14. Camerino D, Estryn-Behar M, Conway PM, et al. Work-related factors and violence among nursing staff in the European NEXT study: a longitudinal cohort study. International Journal of Nursing Studies 2008;45:35–50.
15. Nabb D. Visitors' violence: the serious effects of aggression on nurses and others. Nursing Standard 2000;14:36–8.
16. Estryn-Behar M, van der Heijden B, Camerino D, et al. Violence risks in nursing – results from the European 'NEXT' study. Occupational Medicine 2008;58: 107–14.
17. Luck L, Jackson D, Usher K. STAMP: components of observable behaviour that indicate potential for patient violence in emergency departments. Journal of Advanced Nursing 2007;59:11–19.
18. Winstanley S, Whittington R. Aggression towards health care staff in a UK general hospital: variations among professions and department. Journal of Clinical Nursing 2004;13:3–10.
19. Chuang S, Lin H. Nurses confronting sexual harassment in the medical environment. Studies in Health Technology Information 2006;122:349–52.

20. Congin J, Fish A. Sexual harassment – a touchy subject for nurses. Journal of Health, Organization and Management 2009;23:442–62.
21. Hader R. Workplace violence survey 2008: Unsettling findings. Nursing Management 2008;39:13–19.
22. Johnson SL, Rea RE. Workplace bullying: concerns for nurse leaders. Journal of Nursing Administration 2009;39:84–90.
23. Bronner G, Pertez C, Ehrenfield M. Sexual harassment of nurses and nursing students. Journal of Advanced Nursing 2003;42:637–44.
24. Australian Nursing and Midwifery Council. Code of professional conduct for nurses in Australia. Canberra: ANMAC; 2008.
25. Australian Nursing and Midwifery Council. Code of ethics for nurses in Australia. Canberra: ANMAC; 2002.
26. McGrath P, Holewa H, McGrath Z. Nursing advocacy in an Australian multi-disciplinary context: findings on medico-centrism. Scandinavian Journal of Caring Sciences 2006;20:394–402.
27. Coombs M, Errser S. Medical hegemony in decision-making – a barrier to inter-disciplinary working in intensive care? Journal of Advanced Nursing 2004;46: 245–52.
28. Phillips SP, Austin EB. The feminization of medicine and population health. JAMA 2009;301:863–4.
29. Gargiulo DA, Hyman NH, Hebert JC. Women in surgery: do we really under-stand the deterrents? Archives of Surgery 2006;141:405–8.
30. Riska E. Towards gender balance: but will women physicians have an impact on medicine? Social Science & Medicine 2001;52:179–87.
31. Salhani D, Coulter I. The politics of interprofessional working and the struggle for professional autonomy in nursing. Social Science & Medicine 2009;68: 1221–8.
32. Stott A. Exploring factors affecting attrition of male students from an under-graduate nursing course: a qualitative study. Nurse Education Today 2007;27: 325–32.
33. Wolfinger NH, Mason MA, Goulden M. Problems in the pipeline: gender, mar-riage, and fertility in the ivory tower. Journal of Higher Education 2008;79: 388–405.
34. Timmons S, Tanner J. Operating theatre nurses: emotional labour and the hostess role. International Journal of Nursing Practice 2005;11:85–91.
35. Riley R, Manias E, Polglase A. Governing the surgical count through commu-nication interactions: implications for patient safety. Quality and Safety in Health Care 2006;15:369–74.
36. Hawes C, Flanagan A. The experience of honours at Flinders University: perspec-tives of students and coordinators. In: Kiley M, Mullins G, editors. Quality in postgraduate research: making ends meet. Proceedings of the 2000 Quality in Postgraduate Research Conference, 13–14 April, Adelaide. University of Adelaide; 2000. p. 237.
37. Porter O'Grady. Reverse discrimination in nursing leadership: hitting the con-crete ceiling. In: O'Lynn CE, Tranbarger RE, editors. Men in nursing history, challenges and opportunities. New York: Springer; 2007. p. 143–51.

38. Purnell JD. Men in nursing: an international perspective. In: O'Lynn CE, Tranbarger RE, editors. Men in nursing history, challenges, and opportunities. New York: Springer: 2007. p. 219–32.

39. Burton DA, Misener TR. Recruitment and retention of men in nursing. In: O'Lynn CE, Tranbarger RE, eds. Men in nursing history, challenges, and opportunities. New York: Springer; 2007. p. 255–69.

40. O'Lynn CE. Gender-based barriers for male student nurses in nursing education programs. In: O'Lynn CE, Tranbarger RE, editors. Men in nursing history, challenges, and opportunities. New York: Spinger; 2007. p. 169–87.

41. O'Lynn CE. Gender-based barriers for male students in nursing education programs: prevalence and perceived importance. Journal of Nursing Education 2004;43:229–36.

42. Chapman R, Styles I, Perry L, et al. Examining the characteristics of workplace violence in one non-tertiary hospital. Journal of Clinical Nursing 2010;19: 479–88.

43. Hahn S, Zeller A, Needham I, et al. Patient and visitor violence in general hospitals: a systematic review of the literature. Aggression and Violent Behaviour 2008;13:431–41.

44. Johnston M, Phanhtharath P, Jackson BS. The bullying aspect of workplace violence in nursing. JONA's Healthcare Law, Ethics, and Regulation 2010;12:36–42.

45. Trossman S. Behaving badly? Joint Commission issues alert aimed at improving workplace culture, patient care. AM Nurse 2008;40:1, 6, 12.

46. Farrell GA, Bobrowski C, Bobrowski P. Scoping workplace aggression in nursing: findings from an Australian study. Journal of Advanced Nursing 2006;55: 778–87.

47. Cleary M, Hunt GE, Horsfall J. Identifying and addressing bullying in nursing. Issues in Mental Health Nursing 2010;31:331–5.

48. Dellasega CA. Bullying among nurses. AJN: The American Journal of Nursing 2009;109:52–8.

49. Vickers MH, Jackson D, Wilkes L. Bullying as circuits of power: an Australian nursing perspective. Administrative Theory & Praxis 2010;32:25–47.

50. Johnson SL. International perspectives on workplace bullying among nurses: a review. International Nursing Review 2009;56:34–40.

51. Sofield L, Salmond SW. Workplace violence: a focus on verbal abuse and intent to leave the organization. Orthopaedic Nursing 2003;22:274–83.

52. Hutchinson M, Vickers MH, Jackson D, et al. Like wolves in a pack: predatory alliances of bullies in nursing. Journal of Management and Organization 2006;12: 235–50.

53. Hughes RG, Clancy CM. Complexity, bullying, and stress: analyzing and mitigating a challenging work environment for nurses. Journal of Nursing Care Quality 2009;24:180–3.

54. Stanley KM, Martin MM, Nemeth LS, et al. Examining lateral violence in the nursing workforce. Issues in Mental Health Nursing 2007;28:1247–65.

55. Hutchinson M, Vickers MH, Jackson D, et al. 'They stand you in a corner; you are not to speak': nurses tell of abusive indoctrination in work teams dominated by bullies. Contemporary Nurse 2006;21:228–38.

56. Rosenstein AH, O'Daniel M. Invited article. Managing disruptive physician behavior: impact on staff relationships and patient care. Neurology 2008;70: 1564–70.

57. Schmalenberg C, Kramer M. Nurse–physician relationships in hospitals: 20 000 nurses tell their story. Critical Care Nurse 2009;29:74–83.

58. Rothstein WG, Hannum S. Profession and gender in relationships between advanced practice nurses and physicians. Journal of Professional Nursing 2007;23:235–40.

59. Stein L, Watts D, Howell T. The doctor–nurse game revisited. Nursing Outlook 1990;38:264–8.

60. Stein L. The doctor-nurse game. Archives of General Psychiatry 1967;16: 699–703.

61. Sweet S, Norman I. The doctor–nurse relationship: a selective literature review. Journal of Advanced Nursing 1995;22:165–70.

62. O'Connell B, Young J, Brooks J, et al. Nurses' perceptions of the nature and frequency of aggression in general ward settings and high dependency areas. Journal of Clinical Nursing 2000;9:602–10.

63. Allan H, Tschudin V, Horton K. The devaluation of nursing: a position statement. Nursing Ethics 2008;15:549–56.

64. British Medical Journal 2000; 320 (7241). Online. Available: http://bmj.com/content/vol320/issue7241.

65. Pullon S. Competence, respect and trust: key features of successful interprofessional nurse–doctor relationships. Journal of Interprofessional Care 2008;22: 133–47

66. Spencer C. The changing roles of women: women on the move. NSW Government: Office of the Director of Equal Opportunity in Public Employment; 1999.

CHAPTER 13

Perspectives on quality in nursing

Rhonda Griffiths and Carol Walker

LEARNING OBJECTIVES

When you have completed this chapter you will be able to:

- describe the key components of a quality improvement program
- identify approaches to measuring quality in health from an individual and system-wide perspective
- describe the activities implemented by nurses to measure and enhance quality and promote professional development
- discuss the importance of consumer perspectives in the measurement and improvement of the quality of nursing care
- reflect on practice and consider examples of initiatives to promote quality and aspects that require attention to quality.

Keywords: performance quality, clinical indicators, consumers, patient safety, clinical governance

---

INTRODUCTION

Leaders of industry realised some time ago that in order to build a successful business, attention needs to be directed to ensuring that products and services are of high quality and appropriate for the market. Organisations have adopted increasingly stringent standards to ensure quality is achieved and maintained through models such as continuous quality improvement and total quality management.

The impetus for quality in business began in earnest in the 1940s and 1950s, with Fiegenhaum, Crosby and Deming being the founding experts. While the early focus was on cost,[1] the definition has now broadened to include compliance with defined specifications or standards, with quality being measured as compliance with these standards.[2] In industry quality is seen as separate from luxury or goodness. The focus of quality is compliance with standards and providing effective goods and services with an emphasis on outcomes. However, these definitions were not always appropriate for service organisations (which includes health) and, in that context, quality was redefined as meeting or exceeding customer expectations.[3]

Health services are committed to providing quality care and the concepts defined by industry have been adapted to measure the performance and outcomes of individuals and organisations. However, quality in healthcare is difficult to define and is, in fact, a multifaceted concept. Different but legitimate perceptions of the critical aspects of quality vary according to various stakeholders such as patients, healthcare workers, healthcare managers, policy makers and governments.[4-6] Nevertheless, attempts have been made to elicit the key dimensions of quality in healthcare and these are seen to include (but are not limited to) safety, effectiveness, appropriateness, consumer participation, access and efficiency.[3] These dimensions are often included in the frameworks and criteria organisations that governments use to measure quality in healthcare.[7]

The dominant quality issue in health is ensuring patient safety. This has become a major concern of governments, healthcare providers and the public in developed countries. Patient safety has emerged as a compelling healthcare issue and an international priority research field.[8,9] New ways of addressing patient safety problems and seeking their solutions have emerged, with the most powerful aspect of the reforms being to shift blame from individuals to systems, and an emphasis on investigating 'how people do things' rather than 'what people do'.[8,10]

The requirement for healthcare providers to demonstrate the quality of services is paramount in the quest for good practice, professional standing, accreditation and, ultimately, funding. Health professionals, government and consumers are working individually and with each other to advance the quality culture in health.

The aim of this chapter is to discuss how quality can be achieved in nursing care. Clinical, organisational and consumer perspectives of quality relating to healthcare in general, and nursing care specifically, will be discussed.

JUDGING QUALITY IN NURSING

The measurement of quality is constructed through the use of standards, criteria and outcome measures. The first documented example of quality assurance in nursing is credited to Florence Nightingale.[11] She identified principles of care, which she developed into the standards she used to measure the structures and processes by which care was provided in military hospitals. Methods of evaluating care have increased in sophistication and precision since that time, and nurses have realised the diversity of ways in which quality of care can be measured and predicted.[12] Each member of the healthcare team has an important role to maintain the momentum by identifying problems and contributing to solutions to establish effective systems and processes.[13] There will always be errors in health, and some will become adverse events. Errors are defined as the failure of a planned action to be completed as intended or the use of an inappropriate plan to achieve an aim.[10] Adverse events are defined as a consequential bad outcome, an injury to the patient, in response to an error that occurs during care.[10] An error does not lead to an adverse event in all cases.

It is the responsibility of all clinicians to be part of a culture that strives to provide quality care; however, clinicians are reluctant to report incidents when they occur[14] and, as a result, the ocurrence of incidents is underreported.[15] Ensuring a safe environment for clinicians and people who use the health system is paramount in the design and planning of health services. Nurses have direct and continuous contact with patients, and therefore they can play a vital role in the development of an organisation that promotes safety. Within that environment nurses must be, and indeed will be, empowered to speak out, prepared to report errors and near misses when they occur, and analyse situations and events to discover why errors occur and to change systems when necessary.

We encourage all nurses, and particularly new graduates, to reflect on their clinical experiences and consider how quality of care is evaluated. Consider also how the results of this evaluation might inform future clinical practice, and how it is documented to inform reviews of the quality of the nursing care that is delivered.

THE HEALTHCARE PERSPECTIVE

Performance management initiatives have been adopted by Western health systems to provide a system-wide approach for ongoing improvement by clinical services and facilities. There are three components to management of performance: (1) guidance by policies; (2) monitoring through data collection of outcomes; and (3) appropriate remedial interventions in response to adverse events.[3,16] Nurses are increasingly being urged to demonstrate the quality of their practice in terms of its effect on consumers,[12,15] and they have responded by taking a proactive role in the development of mechanisms to assure quality.[17]

Criteria and procedures for the accreditation of programs,[18] standards of practice, competencies for practitioners and indicators of outcome have been developed to provide a measure against which the quality of clinical performance by all care providers and outcomes of organisations can be judged. A brief description of the quality measures used is provided below.

The new graduate has a responsibility to identify the accreditation programs, standards of practice, competencies and indicators of outcome that are used in their practice setting. If these tools are not being used the nurse may have a facilitative role in the establishment of these quality measures in a particular practice setting.

Performance standards

Standards are developed for two primary reasons: to protect the public from harm, and to improve the quality of services.[19,20] A standard is defined by Standards Australia as:

> a document, established by consensus and approved by a recognized body, that provides, for common and repeated use, rules, guidelines or characteristics for activities or their results, aimed at the achievement of an optimum degree of order in a given context.[21]

Standards reflect values because they are statements derived from a consensus of professional thinking, and are based on research, expert opinion and observation.[22]

Standards determine what and how performance will be measured,[23] and, when applied to healthcare, standards are directed towards outcome (e.g. the number of deaths due to falls in hospitals), process (e.g. number of completed falls risks assessments) and structure variables (e.g. establishment of a falls coordinator position) to monitor the performance of healthcare facilities and the clinical practice of health professionals.

Standards provide a framework that identifies the boundaries and essential elements for practice, and in doing so links three key professional practice accountabilities: care, quality and competence.[22,24] Standards are key to the success of nursing as healthcare evolves, monitoring the roles and settings of nursing practice and thus providing the link between institutional standards of care, competency-based education programs and quality assurance activities.[12]

In Australia, performance in the health system is measured and reported against three broad domains described by the national health performance framework.[4] Each domain has multiple dimensions that direct development of specific standards that can be implemented at national, state and local levels. The first of the three domains, health status, addresses policy on the general health of Australians, for example, Indigenous mortality rates. Reporting against the outcomes provides data to identify the relative health status of groups or regions, and identifies opportunities for improvement. The second domain, determinants of health, takes into account factors that influence the health status of Australians, for example smoking rates and obesity. The third domain, health system performance, measures variables such as access to and equity of service provision, safety and sustainability; for example, screening rates for breast cancer.

The quality of standards does vary, and criticisms have arisen from a lack of research evidence and poorly defined links between practice and organisational policy evident in standards.[4] Nevertheless, nationally established professional standards are a useful starting point and can provide the benchmark for healthcare organisations with regard to standards of care, competency-based education and quality assurance and improvement. It is important to note that, while clinical practice may differ across settings, the standards continue to serve as a unifying link for nursing practice, regardless of the setting.

Competency standards

Once the performance standard has been established, the level of competence (knowledge, skills and abilities) necessary to achieve the standard can be described. In healthcare, the development of competency standards provides a measure of quality against which practitioners and organisational policy are measured with regard to three key elements: attributes (knowledge, skills, attitudes and abilities), performance and standards.[23] The Australian Nursing and Midwifery Council has developed standards of competence for registered nurses,[24] enrolled nurses,[25] midwives[26] and nurse practitioners.[27] These documents, which are customised for each group, present the core competency standard against which the performance of practitioners is assessed to obtain and retain a licence to practise. A measure of performance and accountability is articulated which can be used to promote and demonstrate best practice, guide occupational classification and restructuring, and as a basis for education and training.

Ensuring competence at the point of entry to the profession and on an ongoing basis benefits the nurse, the profession, the community and employers. Over the past two decades most regulated professions in Australia have developed statements of competence, including the majority of disciplines associated with health. All accredited nursing courses preparing registered and enrolled nurses in Australia are required by the nurse-registering authority, the Nursing and Midwifery Board Australia,[28] to reflect the Australian Nursing and Midwifery Council competency standards.

Competency standards can be used to differentiate between levels of competence and, in doing so, provide an objective measure against which nurses can be judged for recognition of advanced and/or specialist practices, skills or knowledge. They also provide a means of evaluating adverse outcomes by providing a reference point for reviewing the incident.

Indicators as a measure of quality

Evaluating the effect of nursing care on patient outcomes is complex and contentious.[13,29] Measuring the quality of nursing care is difficult, although researchers are developing valid indicators that reliably measure the contribution nursing care makes to patient safety.[9,17,30]

A clinical indicator is simply a measure of the clinical management and/or outcome of care. A well-designed indicator should screen, flag or draw attention to a specific clinical issue. Indicators usually identify the rate of occurrence of an event, and are usually expressed as the percentage of events in a population, for example, rate of caesarean section. They are designed to indicate potential problems that might need addressing, and usually demonstrate statistical outliers or variations within data results rather than provide qualitative information. Nevertheless, indicators are useful as a tool to assist in assessing whether or not a standard in patient care is being met.[19,31]

Clinicians and managers realise that it is important to assess not only how healthcare is delivered, but also to assess changes in clients' condition as a result of these interventions.[22] The potential for those data to inform clinical decision making underpins the increasing interest in valid outcome indicators of care.[30,32] The need for healthcare providers to demonstrate the quality of services is paramount in the quest for good practice, professional standing, accreditation and, ultimately, funding. Facilities have been encouraged to scrutinise the quality of services they provide using clinical indicators and process outcomes as measures of quality. The shift in focus to include outcomes as well as process means that nurses must develop measures and reporting mechanisms that will enable them to demonstrate the benefits of nursing interventions to patients.[33]

Monitoring clinical indicators is considered to have the potential to stimulate a variety of quality activities within healthcare organisations, including changes to procedures and policy.[30] In the case of nursing care, measuring the effect of interventions on patient outcomes is complex and contentious.[29,34,35] Nevertheless, if patient outcomes are to become markers of quality and effectiveness in healthcare, the identification of appropriate clinical outcomes, selection of assessment tools and appropriate processes for documentation and retrieval of data are critical.[36,37]

Much of the early literature that addressed nursing indicators has focused on a simple examination of outcomes that have been proposed to be the result of nursing interventions.[38] More recently factors such as patient characteristics, clinical priorities and models of care that influence how care is provided in addition to patient outcomes are being included.[3] For that reason, when considering how, and indeed which, indicators may be used to measure the outcomes of nursing care, the diversity of factors related to patient care must be considered. The questions being asked, along with the pragmatic constraints of available data and resources, will determine whether structure, process or outcome variables are measured.

It is increasingly acknowledged on an international level that the development and use of clinical indicators can positively influence clinical practice. Since 1989 the Australian Council on Healthcare Standards (ACHS) has liaised with medical colleges, associations and societies to develop clinical indicators, and both hospital-wide and discipline-specific sets of clinical indicators have been developed.[31] Therefore if patient outcomes are to become markers of quality and effectiveness in nursing care, it is critical that as a profession nurses identify appropriate clinical outcomes and use valid and reliable tools and processes for documentation and retrieval of data.[35,37]

Credentialling

Credentialling is the process by which an individual's performance is measured against the relevant practice standards. It is a peer review process which requires an individual nurse to present evidence that he or she has achieved the prescribed level of competence (attitudes, skills and standards) for recognition as a specialist practitioner. The main objective of credentialling practitioners is to ensure high-quality care and provide a process by which:

- the profession can extend expectations of clinical practice
- clinical standards can be scrutinised
- the nursing role in healthcare can be promoted
- nurses can demonstrate their accountability
- professional education can be planned.[39]

Specialty nursing groups around the world are undertaking development of standards, competencies and credentialling procedures, driven by the desire of advanced practitioners to be recognised for the contribution they make to nursing and healthcare. While these activities represent a commitment to promoting quality clinical care and accountability by nurses, there are reservations about:

- the ability of small specialty nursing groups to develop standards
- the diversity, or overlap, of approaches
- methods for monitoring quality of the processes.[39]

Nevertheless, credentialling does provide a process by which specialisation and advanced practice can be recognised and the image of nursing enhanced.

National registration for health professionals was introduced in July 2010 at the direction of the Council of Australian Governments as a safety and quality initiative. While it is not yet determined whether credentialling for advanced practice or to undertake high-risk procedures will be included under the national framework, it is now feasible for specialist organisations to form associations with a central registering body to control and monitor practice.

Evidence-based practice guidelines

McKenna and Hsu[40] suggest that only 10% of all clinical care is based on evidence, and, of that 10%, only about half is based on the best available research. While ensuring that nurses are appropriately credentialled for the roles and functions they undertake is one way to ensure quality care, outcomes will also be enhanced by attention to clinical procedures and processes. The benefits that come from systematically reviewing and rating the evidence for interventions has been recognised and evidence-based practice has gained prominence as a scientific approach to developing clinical policy and guidelines.[6] The emergence, and current prominence, of evidence-based practice has compelled clinicians to reflect on the origins of their practice techniques and procedures. The establishment of the Cochrane Collaboration and the Joanna Briggs Institute has provided a unique opportunity to pursue this ideal with some vigour.

Clinical practice guidelines have been developed to improve the care received by patients by promoting the use of interventions with proven benefits and discouraging ineffective interventions.[41] Clinical guidelines function as education resources for clinicians and consumers by providing evidence for clinical decision making and information about treatment options, services and standards of care.[42,43]

Guidelines are developed from research, expert opinion and clinical experience, often in combination.[44] Research has demonstrated that the development and use of clinical guidelines can change the process of health and improve health outcomes; however, the potential for health gain is dependent on the quality of the evidence and acceptance by clinicians. Development of evidence-based guidelines requires extensive financial and human resources to complete the research process that is required.

While there is evidence about effective ways to encourage clinicians to change practice when appropriate,[33] there continues to be a gap between the evidence and actual clinical care, and researchers, managers and clinicians are turning their attention to identifying the barriers and incentives to change practice.[45,46]

While Pearson et al.[44] caution that evidence-based nursing is not a 'cure-all' for nursing ills, these structures, and the collective energies of clinicians, researchers, educators and managers, can advance clinical practice change in an orderly manner. The development, implementation and evaluation of clinical guidelines have application across a wide range of health services, and are fundamental to narrowing the theory–practice gap and promoting best practice.

ORGANISATIONAL PERSPECTIVES

At a local level organisations are required to provide high-quality health services delivered with efficient use of resources.

Clinical governance, risk management and patient safety

Healthcare organisations have always been responsible for corporate governance, which includes providing strategic direction and ensuring operational, financial and risk management systems are in place to meet required corporate standards.[47] Clinical governance 'is an umbrella term for everything that helps to maintain and improve high standards of patient care'.[48] It draws together a range of quality improvement activities (such as incident monitoring, risk management, clinical audit, morbidity and mortality meetings) in a way that ensures an organisational focus on the development of a culture, systems and processes that promote quality of care as the main focus of the organisation.[3]

The move towards clinical governance has promoted the use of risk management as a patient safety tool.[49] Commitment to risk management has long been a feature of industries such as aviation, shipping and car manufacturing and is defined as 'the culture, processes and structures that are directed towards realizing potential opportunities whilst managing adverse effects'.[50] The Australian risk management standard is a generic guide which articulates a framework of communication and consultation to establish the context and identify, analyse, evaluate and treat risks.[2,50] The framework, with its emphasis on ongoing monitoring and review, is well suited for use in healthcare.

Clinical risk management is the systematic approach to developing strategies that enable healthcare organisations and clinicians to learn from past events in order to minimise future risk. Whilst clinical risk management encompasses some of the topics already discussed in this chapter, such as credentialling, evidence-based practice and clinical guidelines, it has also resulted in increased interest in monitoring adverse events and incorporation of risk management methodology into clinical care.[51,52]

The landmark study, *To Err Is Human: Building a Safer Health System*, quantified the extent of errors and adverse events in hospitals and identified a plan for action to enhance patient safety.[10] As well, inquiries into reported poor care both in the UK and Australia have resulted in governments realising the need for healthcare organisations to focus on clinical as well as corporate governance.[20] In most Australian states incident-reporting systems have been implemented and clinical incidents stratified using a risk assessment matrix to quantify the consequences and likelihood of incidents. This enables a numerical risk rating and the most serious incidents are analysed using root cause analysis methodology, where the aim is to find out what happened, why it happened and how it can be prevented from happening again.[53,54] Nurses need to be vigilant in identifying potential errors and recognising errors when they occur.[55] They need to have the knowledge and skills to participate in incident root cause analysis to identify causes and contributing factors of errors. The roles and responsibilities of nurses place them in a perfect position to recognise and intercept errors.[56]

Benchmarking

Quality is measured against the performance of similar organisations through benchmarking activities and against standards established by external accrediting bodies.

The concept of benchmarking has emerged from the manufacturing sector and is defined as:

> an improvement tool whereby a company measures its performance or process against other companies' best practices, determines how those companies achieved their performance levels, and uses the information to improve its own performance.[7]

Benchmarking is one of the foundations of both total quality management and continuous quality improvement. There are two aspects to a successful benchmarking exercise. The first is to identify other organisations that are good at providing a product and, second, to learn how it can be done.[57] Issues of process in addition to outcome are pivotal to this understanding. Benchmarking should not be randomly conducted with as many agencies as possible, but restricted to comparable agencies. It is important to do this because 'apples need to be compared with apples'. Issues such as size and location of the agency as well as the target population and the types of services delivered must all be considered.

For nursing, benchmarking is aimed at producing clinical guidelines to establish high-quality nursing care.[58,59] Nurses can be instrumental in the determination of the clinical guidelines to be measured, the measuring of these guidelines, the production of data and the implementation of the clinical change required to bring a service into step with best-practice guidelines.

Clinicians and managers recognise the importance of ensuring consistently high-quality care and have become acutely aware of competing priorities in health. Healthcare managers are aware of the hard decisions that must be made around issues such as levels and mix of staff, case mix and priority services.

Benchmarking criteria that have an impact on quality and govern cost-effectiveness include staffing levels, average length of stay, infection rates, mortality rates, readmission rates and staff absenteeism. Although the majority of nurses are removed from decisions regarding the distribution of a health services budget, they can be directly involved in providing the clinical measures necessary to inform managerial decisions about budgetary and quality of clinical care issues.[57,58]

Accreditation of facilities

Accreditation is a mechanism whereby an external body assesses an organisation to determine its performance and compliance with agreed standards. Accreditation procedures measuring the quality of hospital and community-based healthcare are well established in Australia. The aim of accreditation is to ensure and improve quality. Therefore, clinicians should understand the importance of embracing the accreditation process and its relevance to clients and the delivery of nursing care.

Accreditation programs have been specifically designed for hospital and community health services. The ACHS has implemented and monitored an accreditation procedure for Australian hospitals since the 1980s.[20] The program is now also used for community health services and indepth reviews are available for some services, including mental health and drug and alcohol services. The core accreditation program is the Evaluation and Quality Improvement Program, which guides organisations through a 4-year cycle of self-assessment, organisation-wide survey and periodic review to meet ACHS standards.[60] The Quality Improvement Council, previously known as the Community and Health Accreditation and Standards Program, developed national standards (Australian Health and Community Service Standards) using a continuous quality approach to assist organisations with primary healthcare service development.[19] The program operates throughout Australia; however, in Queensland, Western Australia and the Northern Territory, the accrediting organisation for the Quality Improvement Council is the Institute for Healthy Communities.

Generic accreditation programs with application to health facilities include the International Standards Organisation (ISO 9001).[50] The ISO 9001 provides independent accreditation to certify organisations against international standards to ensure they remain competent to perform their functions.

EXERCISE 13.1

- As a student completing your studies in nursing or as a new graduate working in the clinical area, are you aware of when that clinical area was last accredited, by whom, and what recommendations were made by the accrediting body?
- Is the process of accreditation viewed by clinicians as a bureaucratic process or as a method of ensuring quality of the service?

CONSUMER PERSPECTIVES

Donabedian, long considered the authority on quality in healthcare, considered that consumers played a key role in measuring the quality of care.[61] Traditionally the term 'patient' has implied a passive recipient of healthcare. The word 'consumer' is more frequently used today as it implies agency, choice and voice in choosing and using healthcare services.

Consumer feedback

The views of consumers are increasingly regarded as providing important information for service development and quality review. This feedback has traditionally been gained from satisfaction surveys but increasing emphasis is being placed on various forms of consumer participation, as a more effective means of including the consumer perspective in healthcare.[61]

Complaints

Another source of feedback is provided by complaints and complaints management. The Health Care Complaints Commission has been established in Australia and is supported by state governments to monitor service providers and practitioners, record and publish the incidence of complaints, and to investigate and if necessary conduct prosecutions.[62] Heightened concern about consumer issues and rights, and unacceptable levels and rates of adverse events in hospitals, were raised in early, but still influential studies relating to adverse events in hospitals.[63,64] The response to the increased awareness of complaints and complaints handling in health led to the establishment of a healthcare complaints commission in each Australian state and territory.[20] A quality improvement approach promotes the integration of complaints management into other adverse event management, and recognises the systemic analysis of adverse events, including complaints, as important components of quality improvement and risk management.[65] Nurses need to be aware of the need for open communication with patients and carers when things go wrong and the need to promote a culture that ensures adverse events and consumer feedback generate opportunities for learning at both a personal and organisational level.[66]

Consumer satisfaction

Consumer satisfaction surveys have frequently been used by clinicians, facilities and government to provide a quality measure. They have been seen to provide information that can inform policy and service development, assess the effectiveness of policies and programs, provide a means of benchmarking with similar health services and as a means of identifying opportunities for improvement.[67] However, satisfaction surveys per se may not give consumers a voice, as they are often based on nurses' perceptions of what constitutes quality care rather than the consumer perception. Other limitations include the potential for oversimplification of complex problems and wariness about using a unitary measure which attempts to represent the complex nature of satisfaction as a single score.[67] Healthcare is not objective or easily measured and sometimes individuals have inaccurate recall of their experience. Further, healthcare from a consumer perspective is an 'undesirable purchase' and for that reason it is to be expected that consumers may be less satisfied with services received when they are physically and/or psychologically stressed and feeling vulnerable.

Beyond consumer satisfaction surveys – consumer participation

Consumers do need to be heard, and mechanisms should be in place to ensure that their suggestions can be considered for action. Increased consumer participation in healthcare is one of 10 national actions recommended in the final report of the National Expert Advisory Group on Safety and Quality in Australian Health Care.[68]

There are various levels at which consumers can participate in healthcare, ranging from inclusion in decision making about their personal healthcare to being members of peer support groups, consumer representatives on boards and committees and acting as consultants and advocates (using their own experience and knowledge) in service development.[69,70] It is important to note that a context of relationships is seen to be one of the most effective approaches to consumer participation.[71] This is in keeping with the findings of a number of workshops as part of a project to support nurses to involve consumers in their care,[72] which identified communication as one of the greatest barriers to achieving this.

CONCLUSION

The provision of safe, effective and accessible health services is of interest to the nation. Funders and providers of services have recognised the need to demonstrate the quality of care and have adapted the concepts and principles developed by industry to focus on the characteristics of their service that indicate quality. Nurses have also been challenged to demonstrate the quality of their care, approaching the task from clinical, consumer and organisational perspectives.

From the clinical perspective, the quality of nursing care is examined and measured using a combination of standards, credentialling, clinical guidelines and outcomes. Evaluation is an important component of quality activities and nurses are realising the benefits of assessing not only how care is delivered, but also assessing changes in clients' condition as a result of interventions. Nursing-specific outcomes have been developed to provide nurses with a framework for recording the effects of the care they provide. The processes promoted by the evidence-based care movement have provided nurses with a scientific approach to developing clinical policy and guidelines, thereby advancing clinical practice in an orderly manner.

Consumer perspectives of quality have traditionally been measured through consumer satisfaction surveys, although the limitations of satisfaction surveys are now recognised and researchers are working to develop a range of patient-focused standards related to the outcomes of nursing care. The inclusion of consumer representation on boards and committees at both organisational and government level is a further move toward the promotion of the consumer voice.

From the organisational perspective, nurses are using a variety of methods to demonstrate and identify quality. Benchmarking, accreditation of facilities and educational programs, and legislation covering the practice of nurses and midwives are used to monitor standards of education, practice and professional behaviour and to determine performance and compliance with agreed standards.

The future challenge for nurses is to continue to be vigilant in their pursuit to demonstrate quality and diligent in their efforts to develop and implement reliable and valid measures. It is a challenge that clinicians, educators and researchers in nursing must embrace to promote the professionalism of nurses and the clinical value of nursing care. The additional challenge for new graduates is to develop an awareness of quality issues within the clinical setting and become actively involved in the process of measuring and evaluating quality activities. The new graduate also needs to develop an appreciation of how the results of these activities can inform and improve clinical practice, and become involved in the process of translating outcome and research findings into quality client-centred nursing care.

CASE STUDY 13.1

Jane is completing the final rotation of her graduate year in a medical ward at a tertiary referral hospital when she is invited to join the Quality Improvement Committee established by the director of nursing. Jane has been asked to talk to other registered nurses on her ward and compile a list of the quality indicators used in that area to monitor the quality of nursing care.

REFLECTIVE QUESTIONS

- What are the nursing activities where the measurement of: (1) process; (2) outcome; and (3) structure would be appropriate?

  Note: Structure may need to be considered in relation to an overall service rather than a specific nursing activity.

CASE STUDY 13.2

At a recent meeting of the Quality Improvement Committee, the group was addressed by a representative from the hospital's consumer participation network who spoke about the ways consumer feedback can be obtained and information used to improve the quality of care.

REFLECTIVE QUESTIONS

Based on your experiences in clinical areas, how could Jane respond to the following questions?
- How is consumer feedback obtained in clinical settings?
- What are examples of consumer input in the evaluation of quality at a clinical level?

CASE STUDY 13.3

Jane has been asked to review the ward clinical guidelines for removal of sutures, removal of indwelling catheters and administration of intravenous antibiotics.

REFLECTIVE QUESTIONS

• What are the sources of evidence used to develop clinical guidelines?

• Where could a clinician look to locate clinical guidelines that are evidence-based?

RECOMMENDED READING

Australian Commission on Safety and Quality in Healthcare. Developing a safety and quality framework for Australia. Sydney: Australian Commission on Safety and Quality in Healthcare; 2008.

Johnstone MJ, Kanitsaki O. Processes influencing the development of graduate nurse capabilities in clinical risk management: an Australian study. Quality Management in Health Care 2006;15:268–78.

Kohn LT, Corrigan JM, Donaldson MS, editors. To err is human: building a safer health system. Institute of Medicine; Washington DC: National Academy Press; 1999.

NSW Department of Health. The clinician's toolkit for improving patient care. Sydney: NSW Department of Health. www.health.nsw.gov.au 2005.

NSW Health Department. Easy guide to clinical practice improvement. Sydney: NSW Health Department; 2009.

REFERENCES

1. Kelemen M. Managing quality: managerial and critical perspectives. London: Sage Publications; 2003.

2. Standards Australia and Standards New Zealand. AS/NZS ISO 9001:2006 Quality management systems – fundamentals and vocabulary. Sydney: Standards Australia and Standards New Zealand; 2006.

3. Australian Commission on Safety and Quality in Healthcare. Australian safety and quality framework for health care. Sydney: Australian Commission on Safety and Quality in Healthcare; 2010.

4. Australian Commission on Safety and Quality in Healthcare. Windows into safety and quality in health care 2010. Sydney: Australian Commission on Safety and Quality in Healthcare; 2010.

5. Australian Council for Safety and Quality in Health Care and the National Institute of Clinical Studies (ACSQHC). Charting the safety and quality of health care in Australia. Canberra: Australian Council for Safety and Quality in Health Care and the National Institute of Clinical Studies; 2004.

6. Schouten L, Hulscher M, van Everdingen J, et al. Evidence for the impact of quality improvement collaboratives: systematic review. BMJ Online First [serial on the Internet]. 2009: Online. Available: http://www.bmj.com/content/336/7659/1491.full.pdf.

7. Australian Council on Healthcare Standards. The EQUIP guide. Standards and guidelines for the ACHS Evaluation and Quality Improvement Program. 4th ed. Sydney: Australian Council on Healthcare Standards; 2006.

8. Zhan C, Kelley E, Yang HP, et al. Assessing patient safety in the United States: challenges and opportunities. Medical Care 2005;43(Suppl.):142–7.

9. Drosler E, Klazinga N, Romano P, et al. Application of patient safety indicators internationally: a pilot study among seven countries. International Journal of Quality in Health Care 2009;21:272–8.

10. Kohn L, Corrigan J, Donaldson M. To err is human: building a safer health system. Washington DC: Institute of Medicine; 2000.

11. Marek K. Outcome measurement in nursing. Journal of Quality Assurance 1989;4:1–9.

12. Farquhar M, Kurtzman E, Thomas A. What do nurses need to know about the quality enterprise? Journal of Continuing Education in Nursing 2010;41: 246–56.

13. Clancy M, Farquhar M, Sharp B. Patient safety in nursing practice. Journal of Nursing Care Quality 2005;20:193–7.

14. Wakefield JG, Jorm CM. Patient safety – a balanced measurement framework. Australian Health Review 2009;33:382–9.

15. Johnstone MJ, Kanitsaki O. Patient safety and the integration of graduate nurses into effective organizational clinical risk management systems and processes: an Australian study. Quality Management in Health Care 2008;17:162–73.

16. Smith P. Performance management in British health care: will it deliver? Performance Management 2002;May/June:103–15.

17. Montalvo I. The National Database of Nursing Quality IndicatorsTM (NDNQI(r)). Online Journal of Issues in Nursing 2007;12:Manuscript 2.

18. Australian Nursing and Midwifery Council. Standards and criteria for the accreditation of nursing and midwifery courses leading to registration, enrolment, endorsement and authorisation in Australia—with evidence guide. Canberra: Australian Nursing and Midwifery Council; 2009.

19. Quality Improvement Council, ed. Health and community services standards. 6th edn. Melbourne: Quality Improvement Council; 2010.

20. Australian Commission on Safety and Quality in Healthcare. Developing a safety and quality framework for Australia. Sydney: Australian Commission on Safety and Quality in Healthcare; 2008.

21. Australian Commission on Safety and Quality. Discussion Paper. National safety and quality accreditation standards. Sydney: Australian Commission on Safety and Quality; 2006.

22. National Health Information Standards and Statistics Committee (NHISSC). The National Health Performance Framework, 2nd ed. Sydney, Australia: National Health Information Standards and Statistics Committee (NHISSC); 2009.

23. Australian Commission on Safety and Quality. National safety and quality accreditation standards. Sydney: Australian Commission on Safety and Quality; 2006.

24. Australian Nursing and Midwifery Council. National competency standards for registered nurses. Canberra: Australian Nursing and Midwifery Council; 2006.

25. Australian Nursing and Midwifery Council. National competency standards for the enrolled nurse. Canberra: Australian Nursing and Midwifery Council; 2006.

26. Australian Nursing and Midwifery Council. National competency standards for the midwife. Canberra: Australian Nursing and Midwifery Council; 2006.

27. Australian Nursing and Midwifery Council. National competency standards for the nurse practitioner. Canberra: Australian Nursing and Midwifery Council; 2006.

28. Nursing and Midwifery Board of Australia. About the Board. 2010 [cited 2011 10th January]. Online. Available: http://www.nursingmidwiferyboard.gov.au/.

29. Considine J, Botti M. Who, when and where? Identification of patients at risk of an in-hospital adverse event: implications for nursing practice. International Journal of Nursing Practice 2004;10:21–31.

30. Fung C, Lim Y-W, Mattke S, et al. Systematic review: the evidence that publishing patient care performance data improves quality of care. Annals of Internal Medicine 2008; 248:111–23.

31. Australian Council on Health Care Standards. Clinical indicator program information. Sydney: Australian Council on Health Care Standards; 2007.

32. Cranely L, Doran D. Nurse's integration of outcomes assessment data into practice. Outcomes Management 2004;8:13–18.

33. Doran D, Harrison M, Laschinger H, et al. Nurse-sensitive outcomes data collection in acute care and long-term-care settings. Nursing Research 2006;55: S75–81.

34. Mattke S, Needleman J, Buerhus P, et al. Evaluating the role of patient sample definitions for quality indicators sensitive to nurse staffing patterns. Medical Care 2004;42(suppl):11-21–11-33.

35. Albanese MP, Evans DA, Schantz CA, et al. Engaging clinical nurses in quality and performance improvement activities. Nursing Administration Quarterly 2010;34:226–45.

36. Richardson J, McKie J. Increasing the options for reducing adverse events: results from a modified Delphi technique. Australia and New Zealand Health Policy 2008;5:25.

37. Nix M, Coopey M, Clancy C. Quality Tools to improve care and prevent errors. Journal of Nursing Care Quality 2006;21:1–4.

38. Pierce S. Nurse-sensitive health care outcomes in acute care settings: an integrative analysis of the literature. Journal of Nursing Care Quality 1997;11:60–72.

39. Cioffi J, Lichtveld M, Thielen L et al. Credentialling the public health workforce: an idea whose time has come. Journal of Public Health Management Practice 2003;9:451–8.

40. McKenna H, Hsu H. Quality and evidence in nursing. Quality in Health Care 1998;7:179–80.

41. National Health and Medical Research Council. A guide to the development, implementation and evaluation of clinical practice guidelines. Canberra: Commonwealth of Australia; 1998.

42. The Guidelines International Network. The Guidelines International Network. 2010 [cited 2011 10th January]. Online. Available: http://www.gin2010.org/?page_id=33.

43. National Institute of Clinical Studies (NICS). Clinical practice guidelines portal. Australian Government; 2010. Online. Available: http://www.clinicalguidelines. gov.au/.

44. Pearson A, Field J, Jordan Z. Evidence-based clinical practice in nursing and health care. Assimilating research, experience and expertise. Melbourne: Blackwell; 2007.

45. Fong J, Marsh GM, Stokan LA, et al. Hospital quality performance report: an application of composite scoring. American Journal of Medical Quality 2008;23: 287–95.

46. Scott IA, Poole PJ, Jayathissa S. Improving quality and safety of hospital care: a reappraisal and an agenda for clinically relevant reform. Internal Medicine Journal 2008;38:44–55.

47. Callaly T, Arya D, Minas H. Quality, risk management and governance in mental health: an overview. Australasian Psychiatry 2005;13:16–20.

48. Royal College of Nursing. Clinical governance: how nurses get involved. London: RCA Publications; 2000.

49. Hovenga E, Kidd M, Garde S, et al. Resource, quality and safety management. Studies in Health Technologies & Informatics 2010;151:360–84.

50. Standards Australia and Standards New Zealand. Quality Management Systems AS/NZS ISO 9001:2008 Self assessment checklist. Sydney: Standards Australia and Standards New Zealand; 2008.

51. Cranston M. Clinical effectiveness and evidence-based practice. Nursing Standard 2002;16:39–43.

52. NSW Health. Performance management framework. North Sydney: NSW Department of Health; 2009.

53. Middleton S, Chapman B, Griffiths R, et al. Reviewing recommendations of root cause analyses. Australian Health Review 2007;31:288–95.

54. Woloshynowych M, Rogers S, Taylor-Adams S, et al. The investigation and analysis of critical incidents and adverse events in health care. Contract No. 19. London: National Health Service; 2005.

55. Johnstone M-J, Kanitsaki O. Processes influencing the development of graduate nurse capabilities in clinical risk management: an Australian study. Quality Management in Health Care 2006;15:268–78.

56. Hughes R, Clancy C. Nurse's role in patient safety. Journal of Nursing Care Quality 2009;24:1–4.

57. Guven-Uslu P. Benchmarking in health services. Benchmarking: An International Journal 2005;12:293–309.

58. Tran M. Take benchmarking to the next level. Nursing Management 2003;34: 18–23.

59. Wait S, Nolte E. Benchmarking health systems: trends, conceptual issues and future perspectives. Benchmarking: An International Journal 2005;12:436–48.

60. Australian Council on Healthcare Standards. EQuIP5. Sydney: The Australian Council on Healthcare Standards; 2010.

61. Greco M. Raising the bar on consumer feedback – improving health services. Australian Health Consumer 2006;3:11–12.

62. Health Care Complaints Commission. Understanding and managing patient complaints. Sydney: NSW Government; 2008.

63. Wilson R, Runciman W, Gibberd R. The Quality in Australian Health Care Study. Medical Journal of Australia 1995;163:458–71.

64. Leape L, Brennan T, Laird N, et al. The nature of adverse events in hospitalized patients. Results of the Harvard Medical Practice Study II. New England Journal of Medicine 1991;324:377–84.

65. Romios P, Newby L, Wohlers M, et al. Turning wrongs into rights: learning from consumer reported incidents, summary annotated literature review. Canberra: Department of Health and Ageing, Commonwealth of Australia; 2003.

66. Iedema R, Jorm C, Wakefield J, et al. Practising open disclosure: clinical incident communication and systems improvement. Sociology of Health & Illness 2009;31:262–77.

67. Burford B, Bedi A, Morrow G, et al. Collecting patient feedback in different clinical settings: problems and solutions. The Clinical Teacher 2009;6:259–64.

68. National Resource Centre for Consumer Participation in Health. Information series – an introduction to participation in health. Melbourne: La Trobe University; 2004.

69. Gregory J. Conceptualising consumer engagement: a review of the literature. Melbourne: Australian Institute of Health Policy Studies; 2007.

70. National Resource Centre for Consumer Participation in Health. Information Series – An introduction to participation in health. Melbourne: La Trobe University; 2004.

71. Powell R, Powell H, Baker L, et al. Patient partnership in care. A new instrument for measuring patient-professional partnership in the treatment of long term conditions. Journal of Management and Marketing in Healthcare 2009;2: 325–42.

72. Australian Nursing Federation. Project to support nurses to involve consumers in their health care. Melbourne: Australian Nursing Federation; 2001.

CHAPTER 14

Managing emotional reactions in patients, families and colleagues

Paul Morrison and Christine Ashley

LEARNING OBJECTIVES

When you have completed this chapter you will be able to:

- identify causes of emotional stress in nursing
- examine your responses to emotional conflict
- develop a greater level of self-awareness
- explore ways of managing emotional reactions in yourself and others
- take a positive and constructive approach to dealing with conflict.

Keywords: conflict, coping, interpersonal skills, self-awareness, strategies for managing conflict

---

INTRODUCTION

The care context is a microcosm of society. It exposes us to the whole gamut of stresses and strains that unfold during a person's lifetime. But it does so in an intense way and sometimes over a very short and compressed period of time. Whether you work primarily in a hospital or community setting, you will be exposed to a wide range of stressful events that elicit attendant emotional reactions and upset in you and others. You will also have to learn to cope with the routine stresses and strains that affect us all outside work. How you deal with these will have an impact on how you deal with work–related issues. Learning to cope with and respond positively to the emotional side of things will not only help you to function more effectively at work; it will also help you to stay healthy.

STRESS AND YOU

One useful way of considering how much stress you are under is to use the life events scale developed by Holmes and Rahe some years ago.[1] Take a few minutes to rate yourself on the life events scale and calculate your overall score.

EXERCISE 14.1

Mark each item on the list that has occurred in your life during the past 12 months. Then add the points together.

LIFE EVENTS SCALE

Life event	Lifechange unit	Life event	Lifechange unit
Death of spouse	100	Son or daughter leaving home	29
Divorce	73	Trouble with in-laws	29
Marital separation	65	Outstanding personal achievement	28
Imprisonment	63		
Death of close family member	63	Spouse begins or stops work	26
Personal injury or illness	53	Begin or end school	26
Marriage	50	Change in living conditions	25
Dismissal from work	47	Revision of personal habits	24
Marital reconciliation	45	Trouble with boss	23
Retirement	45	Change in work hours or conditions	20
Change in health of family member	44	Change in residence	20
Pregnancy	40	Change in schools	20
Sexual difficulties	39	Change in recreation	19
Gain of new family member	39	Change in church activities	19
Business readjustment	39	Change in social activities	18
Change in financial state	38	Minor mortgage or loan	17
Change in number of arguments with spouse	35	Change in sleeping habits	16
Major mortgage	32	Change in number of family reunions	15
Foreclosure of mortgage on loan	30	Change in eating habits	15
		Vacation	13
Change in responsibilities at work	29	Christmas	12
		Minor violation of the law	11

Reproduced from Holmes TH, Rahe RH. The social readjustment rating scale. *Journal of Psychosomatic Research* 1967; 11: 213–218,[1] with the permission of Elsevier Science.

The life events scale lists 41 positive and negative common occurrences that require adjustment and affect your risk of illness. A score of over 300 in 1 year greatly increases your chance of illness. A score of 150–299 reduces the risk by 30%, and less than 150 indicates a small risk of illness. However, even if you are at great risk due to major changes in your life, you can reduce that risk through the use of effective stress management techniques.

We respond to these sorts of stresses in individual ways as we evaluate the impact they will have on our lives and our capacity to cope effectively with them over time. Not all stress is bad. The normal stress in our lives – called eustress – helps us to perform and achieve things on a daily basis. The process of appraising the tasks facing us and our capacity to deal with these effectively helps to identify support networks and personal resources that may be helpful. These networks, coupled with an optimistic attitude, tend to promote good coping in student nurses.[2]

Consider how you tend to cope with these general stresses. Some coping strategies may create more problems – excessive use of alcohol, food, recreational drugs and tobacco can lead to additional problems in your worklife, and at home with your partner and children. They will also have a negative impact on your identity and general wellbeing. It is important to develop an awareness of the sort of things that you find especially stressful, and learn positive ways of coping with them. Self-awareness is perhaps one of the first steps in this direction. Being aware of the issues and having someone to talk to will help. It is surprising how sitting down to complete a simple scale like the one you have just done can provide helpful feedback that raises awareness and generates personal insight. This is an important step in promoting change and positive coping.

EMOTIONAL REACTIONS IN NURSING PRACTICE

There are many potential sources of emotional reaction at work. We have divided some of these into three major categories but in reality they blend into each other depending on the complexity of the situation. In addition, you will probably be able to generate your own list of emotionally trying situations from your clinical experiences and those of your close colleagues. The examples outlined below should provide a realistic flavour of some of the common issues that elicit strong emotions.

Patients

Patients can be a major source of emotional reactions in you. Consider a few scenarios. A mother and child with a relatively minor complaint have to wait in the accident department for 2 hours because the staff is busy following a major road accident. As you walk by the mother complains in a rude and hostile manner that nobody has examined her child yet and the child may be seriously ill. She describes the nurses as 'arrogant bitches'. On other occasions you may come across people who are drunk or on drugs and demand that you see to their needs now. Some patients may have unrealistic expectations about what you can do and the level of resources at your disposal. They simply assume that you can give them what they want.

In emergency situations such as resuscitation or dealing with major traumas, people's emotions will be working overtime. Verbal assault and occasionally physical assault are almost inevitable in some areas of healthcare, especially in the emergency department. It is wise to prepare for these.[3] It is also vital that, if this happens to you or to a colleague, the incident is reported and dealt with appropriately. This includes you or the colleague who has been exposed to verbal or physical assault being provided with support and care.

CASE STUDY 14.1 DEALING WITH VICTIMS OF CRIME

Jane was a new graduate in her first week on a medical ward. During an evening shift, an elderly man was admitted to the ward from the emergency department suffering from severe head and facial injuries and fractured ribs. The patient had been the victim of a brutal attack during a robbery in his home.

During the attack, the man's wife had been killed. The man was accompanied by a police guard and by members of his family. During the first two shifts that Jane cared for this patient, she was kept very busy dealing with the victim's physical injuries. The family members were cared for by the senior nurses, who organised support and counselling. The man gradually gained consciousness, and it was then that the full horror of the incident became apparent to Jane. She listened to a description of the events leading up to the assault, and she stayed with the patient as he begged to be allowed to die. He didn't want to live without his wife. Jane also found the constant presence of the police officers an intrusion on the nurse–patient relationship.

By the fourth day Jane realised that she was becoming emotionally drained by nursing the patient, dealing with his distress and trying to comfort the family. She broke down on the ward and found it hard to come back to work the next day, thinking that she obviously wasn't cut out for nursing. A senior nurse on the ward recognised that several other nurses were also experiencing similar distress. She organised for a counsellor from a support group for victims of crime to hold a debriefing session for staff. Everyone attended, including several of the police officers.

Jane found great comfort in being able to recognise that the trauma associated with such violence was a normal reaction, and that her response did not indicate weakness on her part. She felt much stronger as a result of the counselling session and returned to caring for the victim with increased empathy and understanding.

There are times when you will come across people from different cultures whose language, value system and beliefs are all different from yours. This can create enormous difficulties in communication and arriving at a mutual understanding of events, needs and expectations. It can be a major source of frustration in you and others. From time to time you may come across the victims of serious crimes such as rape, domestic violence and torture, or people who have attempted suicide or the relatives of those who have committed suicide. All these will elicit strong emotional responses in you as a nurse and as a person.

Families

Dealing with the families of patients can be an additional pressure. One of the most difficult aspects of working with families is breaking bad news about the results of tests or telling family members that their mother or father has just died. You may be torn between the need to inform them and your desire to shield them from the pain that will inevitably follow your disclosure. It is an unsolvable dilemma.

However, we all have to face the inevitability of death in our families. Most family relatives respond with great courage but, sometimes, family members react by blaming you and the hospital and this may be uncomfortable for a while. As you spend time with family members of dying patients you will inevitably get to know them and share some of their grief and the sense of loss they are experiencing.

The parents of very sick and dying children will need a lot of psychological support and help. Watching parents spend time with a dying child (or any member of the family, old or young) can be especially traumatic. If you happen to be a parent too then it is an even more difficult experience. The sense of crushing vulnerability[4] you will experience as a parent and nurse may help you to empathise more fully with the family.

CASE STUDY 14.2 PERSONAL VULNERABILITY

Dave was an inexperienced registered nurse in charge of an accident and emergency admission unit in a country area in Wales. On a very hot July day an 18-month-old child was brought into casualty in a semiconscious state accompanied by his mother. He had been transported directly from the beach by helicopter. On examination, nothing unusual was found but it was clear that the child was very ill – he had developed a grey ashen colour and his breathing was very slow and shallow. He could not be roused.

The child's mother was very distressed and kept asking Dave what was wrong with the child. Like everyone else in the unit, including the doctors, Dave (himself a parent of a small child) had no idea what was wrong, but everyone there was very nervous and very concerned for the child's welfare. He did not know what to say and felt totally inadequate and ill prepared for the role he found himself in.

The mother became increasingly agitated and distressed, demanding that someone 'do something' to help her child. Some time later, a policeman arrived and reported that some people on the beach had seen the child pick up a snake – obviously the snake (an adder) had bitten the child. A quick phone call to the poisons unit in a large metropolitan hospital produced effective treatment principles and the child was then transferred to that hospital where he made a full recovery some days later.

The unusual incident was traumatic for the small unit but no action was taken to debrief the staff or to explore how similar incidents could be managed more effectively in the future. The staff did not talk about it among themselves as it highlighted deficiencies in their performance and knowledge. Dave had nightmares about the incident for months afterwards and found that he had to talk to other nurses outside the unit to help him to put it aside.

Colleagues

This category may seem slightly strange and out of place here for someone working in a 'caring' profession like nursing. However, as you become more experienced you will find, if you have not done so already, that colleagues and other members of the healthcare team can be a major source of conflict in your working life.[5] Sometimes managers, supervisors or colleagues make unfair demands on you: asking you to work unreasonable rosters or ignoring your requests for special shifts, or you may feel unreasonable pressure to come to work when unwell. In the workplace, you may feel that your contribution to discussions relating to patients' issues or ward management are deliberately ignored. In other words, you feel undervalued or 'picked on' in your workplace. 'Horizontal violence' is the term used to describe intergroup conflict of this nature.[6,7]

There may also be times when you come into conflict with colleagues from other disciplines. For example, you may feel that an elderly patient with terminal cancer should be left to die in peace while the surgeon insists on performing another traumatic and expensive operation in the hope that it might prolong the patient's life for another 6 months.

It can be very difficult to challenge another colleague in a situation like this because of the power differences that exist. Nurses often just accept the situation without question and this may be part of the hidden curriculum they have been exposed to as students or new graduates, that is, not to question the doctor or other senior colleagues. However, a clash of values, especially if they occur in a particular workplace setting, needs to be dealt with constructively or people will feel very stressed and disempowered and their effectiveness will deteriorate.

There may be times when a situation at work raises ethical dilemmas for you. You suspect that a colleague (and friend) may be taking medications from the ward and using or selling them. Yet you have no proof. Do you confront your friend and run the risk of ruining the friendship? Or do you report your suspicions to the supervisor? Both options carry the risk that your friend's career may be in jeopardy. Yet you also have a responsibility to the patients whose medication your friend may be stealing by falsifying their medication records. As a registered nurse you must report any incident of this nature. 'Dobbing in' someone who is acting inappropriately or unethically is now a legal responsibility of registered nurses.[8]

CASE STUDY 14.3 WORKPLACE BULLYING

Sue started work in a busy psychiatric ward in a regional hospital. She had gained a year's experience in a large city psychiatric centre after completing her postgraduate studies in mental health nursing. There were several nursing practices in the new workplace that Sue knew were outdated and not evidence-based. She spoke to the nurse manager about these and asked if she could revise them. The manager told her that the current practices worked very well and she saw no reason to revise them.

From then on, the manager often ridiculed Sue in front of her fellow workers and gave her tasks to do with unrealistic timeframes. Sue began to feel intimidated and lost confidence in her ability. When she confided in her fellow workers, she was told, 'If you want a quiet life, keep your head down and do as you're told.' Senior nurses on the ward also constantly made sly comments about her psychiatric training, saying that she thought she 'knew it all' because she had had a university training.

Sue became so depressed about her work situation that she contemplated leaving nursing, until a colleague from her student days advised her of some strategies to use, and told her about the role of antiharassment officers in the workplace. As a result, Sue was able to learn some skills for dealing with conflict in the workplace, and also gained comfort from learning about her legal rights and the steps she could take if the situation became untenable.

Gradually, over a period of time, the other staff members accepted Sue. Later, another new staff member experienced the same difficulties, and Sue was able to assist her by sharing her own experiences.

Personal dilemmas

There may be times when you have to make important decisions that affect your ability to balance a career and personal life successfully. Getting married, deciding to start a family or to return to full-time study, take on a mortgage or work overseas for a few years can interrupt your career, sometimes with negative consequences.

There are no right answers here. Lots of people, in an effort to be supportive, will tell you what to do. This type of advice is rarely helpful. What is very important is for you to explore different perspectives in order to clarify your values and long-term goals. When you are clear about these you will be able to make informed choices that suit you and those closest to you. Important decisions are never easy. Whatever circumstances might emerge, it is important to remember that humans have a great capacity to adapt and find happiness and contentment in life.[9]

STRATEGIES FOR MANAGING CONFLICT CONSTRUCTIVELY

Acknowledge the conflict

The situations described above may all be considered sources of conflict that elicit strong emotional reactions – such as feelings of anxiety, tension, guilt, depression or anger and hostility – for those involved. These occurrences can range from minor discomforts, incidents and misunderstandings to serious crisis situations that can have an impact on a whole ward team and across disciplines. Most importantly, these forms of emotional reactions will often lead to stress, sour relationships and poor work performance.[10] Acknowledging a conflict or situation is important because it will help you to make sensible plans to address the issue and to arrive at a point where you feel a stronger sense of self-control.

EXERCISE 14.2

Take a few moments to think about a situation that elicited strong emotions in you, and complete sections 1–4 below.
1. Describe a situation and identify the people involved.
2. Describe your emotional reaction and label the feelings you experienced during and after the situation. What changes did you notice in your breathing, heart rate and stomach during the event?
3. How did you react to the situation? How did you behave? What did you say and do?
4. How was the situation resolved or managed? Did you react negatively or constructively?

Notice how completing a short exercise like this may elicit again some of the feelings, thoughts and bodily experiences that you felt at the time of the incident. If it has, then it suggests that this incident is a form of 'unfinished business'. You need to work through this, perhaps by talking with a supportive friend, if you are to move forward at work.

Take care of yourself

Unfortunately, many nurses downplay the effects of emotional abuse or violence in the workplace. Exposure to this sort of working environment, in the long term, will have a very negative effect on your performance both at work and at home.[11] If you are a victim of violence or abuse of any sort, the literature is clear in advocating that you will benefit from debriefing and posttrauma counselling.[12] In many cases, the support of peers and workplace colleagues can facilitate a positive outcome in the short term. However, 'spot debriefing' is often not enough, and more formal follow-up should be sought. Unfortunately, in rural or remote areas there is often inadequate support available. It is important, though, if your employer is unable to provide you with follow-up that you seek professional help from your doctor, counsellor or another health professional.

You can also take care of yourself by ensuring that you have a balanced lifestyle. Avoid overworking, overeating and overdrinking and take regular exercise. Make sure that you take all the vacation time that you are entitled to and that you get enough sleep and relaxation. Plan to review your work situation and lifestyle at three or four points in the year. Too many people don't take time out to reflect on how things are and where they are headed. If you find that some people or situations are continually causing you to feel overwhelmed and exhausted, do something about it. Learn how to say no (and mean it) to taking on more than you can reasonably deal with. Where possible, avoid interacting with those people who add to your stress at work. Focus on a small number of priorities – don't try to do everything at once. Work on being happy and take steps that will help with this goal.[13,14]

Know your rights

Employers in Australia are required under occupational health and safety legislation in each state and territory to provide a safe place of work and to provide and maintain a safe system of work.[12] Equal employment and antidiscrimination legislation also protects you from unfair discrimination and certain objectionable conduct. So if you work in a situation which, you believe, leaves you exposed to physical risks or sexual or emotional abuse, you have a right to take this up with your supervisor or employer.

Perhaps you are working in a rural or remote setting on your own at weekends. You are caring for several potentially aggressive patients, and you have limited access to back-up in an emergency. Potentially you consider you are at risk, but you don't want to appear to your colleagues as if you can't cope. Don't assume that, because no one else has done anything about the situation, you should avoid doing anything too. Remember, when you go to work you have a right to feel safe[9] and you also have a responsibility to your patients, your profession, and to yourself and your family. It is vital that you discuss the situation with your supervisor, and try to be constructive in your discussions. Remember that knowing that the law is on your side is, in itself, empowering.

Use interpersonal skills and build rapport with others

How you cope with a given situation will depend very much on how you interact with others in the workplace. In a complex social environment such as a hospital or healthcare centre, working cooperatively and being able to get along with others is vital. Understanding how you interact is important if you are to develop skills to deal with conflict. Learning to enhance your awareness of your interpersonal approach and skills is an on-going process. Try Exercise 14.3 below for yourself. The items are adapted from the Opener Scale.[15]

EXERCISE 14.3 ITEMS FROM THE OPENER SCALE

- People often tell me about themselves
- I like listening to people's stories
- People trust me with their secrets
- I am very accepting of others
- People feel comfortable around me

Consider each of these statements in turn along a continuum from 'very much like me' to 'not at all like me' and ask yourself the following questions:

1. To what extent is this statement a good description of me at work?
2. Are there things I would like to change? If so, why? If not, why not?
3. How does this description of me shape how I relate to others at work?
4. How does this description of me shape how others relate to me at work?
5. Do you see this description of you as a strength or a weakness in your approach to others? If so, why? If not, why not?

Now that you have considered your own strengths and weaknesses more carefully, you can use this information to improve your skills in dealing with conflict. Having the ability to listen and be empathic is important in all aspects of nursing, not least when we are expected to resolve conflict or defuse emotionally charged situations. When attempting to manage a conflict, it is really important to develop a clear understanding of the other people involved and their particular wants and needs. This takes time and patience and very good communication skills. The ability to empathise with the other parties is fundamental. Remember too that people may have very good reasons to be angry, so it is important to explore the situation from different perspectives.[16] Being able to take on board the perspectives of others will help you to acknowledge and accept that some stresses cannot be avoided, mishaps and mistakes are inevitable and learning to forgive is an important skill in successful coping.[17]

Realise your potential as a professional and a person

Part of dealing effectively with challenging situations as a nurse comes about through life's experiences over time and developing personal maturity. Most new graduates are concerned by their lack of experience but, remember, while you may lack extensive clinical expertise, your ability to deal with tricky situations comes about not only through knowledge gained at university and on clinical placements but also through the experiences you have gained throughout your life. Travel, working in other environments and dealing with family crises are important in developing coping skills and shaping you as a person. So when opportunities present themselves, always consider the potential benefits that may result from, for example, an overseas trip or the invitation to be part of the child care centre management committee. These opportunities will increase your self-esteem and self-awareness, and provide you with unexpected extra knowledge and skills.

As you prepare to embark on your career as a nurse, you will be experiencing the relief of having come to the end of several hard years of study. However, don't make the mistake of thinking that your studying days are over! Sociologists tell us that we will be likely to undergo several career changes during our working lives, so it is vital to recognise the importance of continuing professional development as part of your working life. Learning is a lifetime commitment, so seize opportunities as they arise and keep yourself informed and up to date. Look upon the acquisition of knowledge and skills as the key to your success in the future.

Learn to live with pressure

Living with pressure and coping with rapid change is now a routine requirement in most professional careers. Many of us view 'pressure' as a stress that can lead to conflict in our daily lives. Part of learning to cope with pressure at home, at university and at work is to recognise that pressure can also be a stimulus for enhancing our performance – some anxiety helps us to perform better. Too much pressure for lengthy periods of time becomes exhausting and leads to deterioration in performance.

Similarly with change: we all need to accept change as a positive experience rather than something that should be avoided or that can have only negative consequences. Consider the following example: as a cost-cutting exercise, the staffing on your ward has been cut by one registered nurse on the evening shift. At first, you feel overwhelmed at the thought of how you will get through the resulting extra work, and you worry through your days off about returning to the workplace. This is responding negatively to change and pressure. However, when you start to consider what you normally do each shift, you begin to realise that much of the evening work is done simply because that's the way it has always been done rather than being based on best practice. By using your professional judgment and some creative skill you realise that in fact you can work more efficiently and effectively than before, and with fewer staff. Change in this case has had a good outcome, and you have responded to the pressure positively.

Some of us thrive on pressure – we all know the old saying that if you want something done, you go to the busiest person. Yet others aren't able to cope so well. It is important that you know your own capabilities, and don't expose yourself to unnecessary pressure. Don't fall into the 'Messiah trap'[18] and get caught up in the belief that you are 'indispensable' and everyone else's needs must come before your own. Being a Messiah can make you feel indispensable but it can also leave you feeling worthless, unimportant and isolated because your personal needs are being ignored.

EXERCISE 14.4 THE MESSIAH TRAP[18]

Berry describes the 'Messiah trap' as a two-sided lie into which many caring people fall:

Side 1	If I don't do it, it won't get done. (You take responsibility for everything and feel indispensable.)
Side 2	Everyone else's needs take priority over mine. (You believe you are expected to put everyone else first at the expense of caring for yourself.)

Nursing will always involve a certain amount of pressure in any specialty but some clinical settings are recognised as high-stress areas, such as emergency departments and intensive care units. If you know you don't cope well with stressful situations, use this knowledge to guide you as you choose your career path. If you are starting to feel 'burnt out' by your work then recognise this as a sign that you aren't coping well with pressure. Depending on its severity, dealing with burnout may involve debriefing with colleagues, seeking counselling from a professional, having a well-earned holiday or even reviewing your place of work.

Find your niche

Sometimes we find roles and areas for which we are really well suited and sometimes we don't. For example, it was found that those who were more effective helpers in professions like the clergy and teaching were more likely to view the world from a basically person-centred perspective. It may come as no surprise to hear that many people in professions like nursing and social work change their career and enter counselling. Their system of beliefs may be in conflict with the daily practices of their former profession.[19] However, the search may be a long and arduous one and many blind alleys may have to be explored first. Not everyone finds the niche they hope for.

CONCLUSION

In this chapter we have examined a number of areas that have the potential to elicit strong emotional reactions in patients and relatives and in us as professional carers. Emotional stress is a byproduct of nursing work and cannot be avoided. However, it can be managed effectively through the development of self-awareness and good interpersonal skills. These skills are prerequisites for establishing sensible boundaries to protect yourself against the inevitable stresses that will emerge in clinical work. They can help to 'inoculate' you against the negative consequences of emotional stress and to be an assertive professional. Changes in organisational culture and an increasing awareness of employment safety issues will also help to alleviate stress and conflict in the workplace. Work should be challenging but it should also be rewarding and fulfilling.[20] Making sure that you develop positive strategies to deal with emotional reactions in yourself and others will help to ensure that it is.

CASE STUDY 14.4

During her first week on placement on a busy ward environment, Jacinta found that some of her new colleagues continued to refer to her as a student. On the third day she asked a senior registered nurse for advice – whether or not to give a patient PRN Seroquel when the patient reported feeling very agitated. The senior registered nurse said: 'I'm busy, you should know what to do anyway'.

REFLECTION QUESTION
- How would you support Jacinta in this instance?

CASE STUDY 14.5

Six months after graduating and completing a mental health and a surgical placement, Oisin found that the key skills that helped him to cope with the challenges in that time were reflection and journalling of his experiences, feelings and thoughts on a regular basis. Moreover, he found himself rereading old notes and revisiting things that he did not fully understand as a student. Oisin found this very odd; during his undergraduate years he just did not see the point of reflection!

REFLECTION QUESTION

- What questions would you like to ask Oisin?

CASE STUDY 14.6

As part of her graduate program, Jill has just completed a 6-month allocation in a small country hospital, working in various settings, including the emergency department, operating rooms and the general ward. She has been collating various incidents for her professional portfolio and recalls that there have been two episodes where she has witnessed nursing staff bullying other members of the team. Although she hasn't experienced this directly herself, she feels on reflection that she needs to record these events in her portfolio and examine what affirmative action she could have taken.

REFLECTION QUESTIONS

- What steps could Jill take in terms of developing her skills to handle bullying at work?
- How could these events best be recorded in a professional portfolio in order to provide evidence of reflective learning?

RECOMMENDED READING

Albom M. Tuesdays with Morrie. London: Time Warner Books; 2003.

Blumenthal E. Believing in yourself: a practical guide to building self-confidence. Oxford: Oneword; 1997.

Burns GW, editor. Healing with stories: your casebook collection for using therapeutic metaphors. Hoboken, New Jersey: John Wiley; 2007.

Cornelius H, Faire S, Cornelius E. Everyone can win. Responding to conflict constructively. 2nd ed. Sydney: Simon & Schuster; 2006.

Seligman MEP. Learned optimism. Australia: Random House; 1992.

REFERENCES

1. Holmes TH, Rahe RH. The social readjustment rating scale. Journal of Psychosomatic Research 1967;11:213–8.
2. Gibbons C, Dempster M, Moutray M. Stress and eustress in nursing students. Journal of Advanced Nursing 2007;61:282–90.
3. Flores N. Dealing with an angry patient. Nursing 2008 2008;May:30–1.

4. Morrison P. Understanding patients. London: Bailliere Tindall; 1994.
5. Farrell GA. Aggression in clinical settings: nurses' views. Journal of Advanced Nursing 1997;25:501–8.
6. Duffy E. Horizontal violence: a conundrum for nursing. Collegian 1995;2: 12–17.
7. Longo J. Horizontal violence among nursing students. Archives of Psychiatric Nursing 2007;21:177–8.
8. AHPRA 2010 Online. Available: http://www.ahpra.gov.au/Legislation-and-Publications/AHPRA-FAQ-and-Fact-Sheets.aspx. Accessed 20 January 2011.
9. Peterson C. A primer in positive psychology. Oxford: University Press; 2006.
10. Cornelius H, Faire S, Cornelius E. Everyone can win. Responding to conflict constructively. 2nd ed. Sydney: Simon & Schuster; 2006.
11. Fisher J, Bradshaw J, Currie BA, et al. Context of silence: violence and the remote area nurse. Rockhampton, Queensland: Central Queensland University, 1995.
12. Fisher J. Violence against nurses. In: Horsfall J, editor. Violence and nursing. PDS Series No. 8. Canberra: Royal College of Nursing Australia; 1998.
13. Myers D. The pursuit of happiness. New York: Quill; 2002.
14. Fredrickson BL. Positivity. New York: Three Rivers Press; 2009.
15. Jackson J. Violence in the workplace. In: Horsfall J, editor. Violence and nursing. PDS Series No. 8. Canberra: Royal College of Nursing Australia; 1998.
16. Farrell G. Therapeutic response to verbal abuse. Nursing Standard 1992;6:47.
17. Lambert VA, Lambert CE. Nurses' workplace stressors and coping strategies. Indian Journal of Palliative Care 2008;14:38–44.
18. Berry CR. When helping you is hurting me: escaping the Messiah trap. New York: Cross Roads; 2003.
19. Combs AW. What makes a good helper? Person-Centred Review 1986;1: 51–61.
20. Csikszentmihalyi M. Finding flow: the psychology of engagement with everyday life. New York: Basic Books; 1997.

CHAPTER 15

Clinical leadership

Debra Thoms and Christine Duffield

LEARNING OBJECTIVES

When you have finished this chapter you will be able to:

- understand the responsibility everyone has for leadership
- identify how transformational leadership behaviours can be implemented
- identify opportunities to display leadership behaviours
- start building your own leadership capability
- recognise the role that emotional intelligence has in leadership.

Keywords: leadership behaviours, transformational leadership, emotional intelligence, new reg istered nurse, capability

---

INTRODUCTION

Health systems today still have hierarchical structures, and the nursing profession is no exception. Whilst senior managers may be the most visible leaders in the nursing work environment, it is important to note that they are not the only people who can and do display leadership. In this chapter, we show that everyone, including newly registered nurses, has an important part to play in nursing leadership. We also consider some simple strategies you can use to increase your leadership knowledge and skills in the nursing work environment. Good leadership encompasses a range of capabilities such as communication and social awareness – a number of which you may have read about in other chapters. Understanding the links between these various capabilities will assist in identifying how to build your own leadership capability.

THE LEADERSHIP RELATIONSHIP

Health systems are complex organisations and working within them brings many challenges. At times the management and leadership can appear to be rigid and somewhat mechanistic. While this may be how a unit or service may appear, organisations are also capable of adapting and shifting to meet new challenges. There may be opportunities for local solutions to be developed and implemented. Often these may appear to be the informal structures sitting alongside the more formal structures. Within these settings leaders have an important role to play. Leaders create and support the environment that allows the team to find the solutions and put them into action.[1] Within your workplace you may find opportunities to contribute to the development of solutions and their implementation while enhancing your growth as a leader.

Leaders do not exist without followers, and at various times, we can be either the leader or the follower, depending on the circumstances. However, as Kouzes and Posner show in their research, in order for leaders to be followed, they have to create a relationship with other people who are willing to follow them to progress to a desired goal.[2] Whilst at this stage of your career you may find yourself predominantly in the role of follower, there will be opportunities to lead in various activities and functions within your unit. By creating good relationships with team members and your unit manager from the beginning, you may be able or may be asked to take on leadership activities, which will assist you in building your leadership capability. At other times, you may find yourself taking on an informal leadership role with a small group of staff on a particular activity. By increasing your understanding of leadership, you will be better able to take advantage of these opportunities if and when they arise. As you develop these leadership capabilities we would encourage you to review your understanding of transformational leadership and the role of emotional intelligence, which are covered here.

TRANSFORMATIONAL LEADERSHIP

In 1978, James McGregor Burns wrote about the need to bring together conceptually the role of the leader and that of the follower.[3] He defined leadership as 'leaders inducing followers to act for certain goals that represent the values and the motivations – the wants and needs, the aspirations and expectations – of both leaders and followers'.[3] As a newly registered nurse, there will be opportunities for you to facilitate a small group of staff (possibly as part of a team) to achieve common goals, and in this way you will be building your leadership capability. At times, the team may include various levels of staff, such as enrolled nurses and assistants in nursing, who will have different competencies and skills. Your interaction and work with these other staff members will be enhanced if you can successfully engage them in achieving your common goal of good patient care. One way in which this may be done is by recognition of shared values and common purpose, namely to make patient care the best that it can be within the given constraints of practice.

You may have heard the term 'transformational leadership' during your studies, and read about it elsewhere in this book. Once again, it was Burns who first distinguished between transformational and transactional leadership. He defines 'transactional leadership' as 'when one person takes the initiative in making contact with others for the purpose of an exchange of valued things' and that this exchange can be 'economic or political or psychological in nature'.[3] Transactional leadership is found in all organisations and it has an important place in many interactions, such as those requiring adherence to standards or procedures. However, the transactional model tends to be associated with lower levels of staff satisfaction and innovation than the transformational model, and, for this reason, transformational leadership is often emphasised.

Transformational leadership occurs when 'one or more persons engage with others in such a way that leaders and followers raise one another to higher levels of motivation and morality'.[3] In this situation the purpose of both the leader and the follower is shared, and the leader acts to inspire the follower to greater creativity and originality. As mentioned above, researchers have found that nurses who work with transformational leaders tend to report higher levels of satisfaction and lower rates of turnover.[4-6] For these reasons, it is especially important that newly registered nurses aiming to develop their leadership skills pay particular attention to transformational leadership characteristics. Whilst you may find that you work with some nurse leaders who display more transactional leadership behaviours than transformational, this does not necessarily prevent you from endeavouring to work in a more transformational way with other members of staff.

EXERCISE 15.1

Think about leaders and managers you have encountered and the type of leadership they demonstrate. Which did you prefer and why?

BUILDING TRANSFORMATIONAL LEADERSHIP CAPABILITY

A number of writers have identified capabilities for transformational leadership, and it is possible to consider how these can be developed and applied as a newly registered nurse.[4,7-9] This may at times be challenging, particularly early in your first year, when you will be coming to terms with a wide range of issues, and may occasionally find some other staff less supportive than you would desire. Nevertheless, even in such difficult situations, it is still possible to consider the various strategies that transformational leaders use, and to think about these as you grow and develop your overall practice. In the next section, we list some important strategies that transformational leaders employ. We will describe how effective leaders apply these strategies, and put forward some ideas about how you might use these in your practice.

Get to know your people

A key strategy for leaders is to get to know their staff. This involves simple approaches, such as greeting people each day; taking an interest in their lives outside the workplace; listening to ideas and seeking input; and letting them know they make a contribution.[10]

By greeting people each day and taking an interest in them and their lives, you will not only build this capability as a leader for the future, but you will also be creating positive relationships with other staff. Additionally, by listening and asking questions from more experienced staff members, you can build your clinical knowledge and skills. At times, you may not be met with a positive response from some other staff members. However, this should not discourage you. If your inquiries are met with negative feedback from some staff, this may simply alter who you seek advice and information from. By actively asking and questioning, you will grow in knowledge and skill, knowing that you are building your leadership capabilities at the same time.

Help people to learn and develop

People generally like to learn, and as a transformational leader an environment which supports and encourages learning should be developed. Additionally, as a leader it is important to model a desire and willingness to learn and discover. By setting such an example, you will help encourage other staff members to learn.[10]

Naturally, there will be much to learn within your work environment when first starting as a newly registered nurse. However, as you become more comfortable and confident, it is important to look for further opportunities to develop professionally. This may be achieved through attending in-house learning programs or tutorials and seminars. There may also be external conferences and short courses that you may find of benefit. Consider and demonstrate your commitment to your own ongoing professional development by being prepared to contribute your own time and resources to participate. Good leaders seek not only to further their own professional development, but also to motivate and inspire other staff to seek such opportunities. Therefore, when working with other staff members take opportunities at appropriate times to encourage them to participate as well. Nonetheless, it is important to have created a good working relationship with your co-workers (see Get to know your people section, above) before sharing your knowledge or suggesting future opportunities for them.

Give plenty of feedback

People in leadership roles need to provide appropriate feedback to team members in a timely way. It is as important to give positive feedback (for instance, praising a staff member for high-quality work) as it is to give negative feedback (such as advising a staff member to take additional care with tasks). When providing negative feedback, this should be done in private, whereas positive feedback can often be shared more publicly. When giving feedback, it is important to ensure that active listening is used. Active listening incorporates both verbal skills (such as open-ended questions, summaries and clarification) and non-verbal skills (such as open body language) and helps to show that you are paying attention to the other person.[11,12] It is a particularly helpful skill if giving negative feedback.

In the early stages of your career as a newly registered nurse, it is likely that you will not have to give feedback regularly. Rather, it is much more probable that you will be receiving feedback, rather than supplying it. Nonetheless, in some circumstances, newly registered nurses may find themselves in a position where they are expected to provide feedback to team members. The strategies outlined above provide some guidance on effectively giving feedback, but, importantly, can also be used when receiving feedback. For instance, it is relevant for both those giving and receiving feedback to listen actively. The giver of the feedback should ask questions to ensure that the receiver understands the message being given, whilst the receiver should seek clarification to make sure that he or she has accurately grasped the speaker's meaning.

Give responsibility and status

This is achieved by delegation, which helps to support the growth and development of individuals. In delegating, it is important to understand the individual's knowledge of the job, and provide the person with the opportunity to ask questions so that he or she feels comfortable with undertaking these new responsibilities.

Delegation can be one of many challenging areas that you will come across as a newly registered nurse.[13] Initially, you may not find yourself in a position to be delegating but that will change rapidly. Make use of tools such as the decision-making framework from the Australian Nursing and Midwifery Council website (www.nursingmidwiferyboard.gov.au),[14] as this will assist you in understanding how to make a decision to delegate, and what your responsibilities are when delegating to another team member.

It is important that you have a good understanding of the skills and capabilities of those you are working with before you delegate. This may mean that you need to familiarise yourself with the education programs undertaken by enrolled nurses and assistants in nursing, so that you have a sound knowledge of their abilities.[15] Additionally, you should ensure you are familiar with any policies that guide the roles of staff members within your particular organisation. When you have delegated and the staff member has performed well, remember to thank the person and offer positive feedback if possible (see Give plenty of feedback, above).

Give your people rewards

Identify strategies such as credit for good work and development opportunities as ways of rewarding people.[10]

Again, as a newly registered nurse or new member of a team, you may find you have limited opportunity to reward people in comparison to more senior staff. Remember, though, that a positive word or thank you to someone who assists you is a form of reward. Simple expressions of gratitude will encourage people to continue their good work, and improve staff morale. Giving thanks also allows you to practise providing positive feedback in a natural and genuine manner. This is an important skill to have, especially as you develop and move into more formal leadership positions, as providing genuine support and encouragement to staff members will be seen as a positive behaviour which will contribute to your capacity to motivate staff.

Communication of information

There are two important strategies here. The first is developing trust through creating a positive communication atmosphere. The second is inclusive communicating, which involves sharing information with all relevant staff, not just a few. Communicating information as soon as possible through a range of methods such as meetings, newsletters, bulletins and email lists is an important aspect of transformational leadership. Good communicators are skilled not only in delivering information, but also in receiving information, so once again, being a good listener is vital.[10]

Communication is a key capability no matter what role you find yourself undertaking. It is important to develop your skills in this area from the beginning of your career. Be prepared to admit if you do not know something and actively seek assistance from others. Although some staff may respond to your inquiries negatively, do not see this as a reason not to seek advice in the future (see Get to know your people, above). Instead, you may wish to think about different ways of communicating with those whom you find challenging, or perhaps seek advice from other staff members. Succeeding in finding good strategies at this stage will contribute to your career as it develops. Also, be willing to share information that you may have learnt about a patient or the activities of the unit.

EXERCISE 15.2

Think about how you might be able to apply these strategies in your workplace. Consider the barriers and enablers to you applying them and how you might manage the barriers and use the enablers to develop your leadership capabilities further.

EMOTIONAL INTELLIGENCE

Being emotionally intelligent is useful for everyone in day-to-day work and enhances the skills and capabilities of leaders. Emotional intelligence is about managing our feelings in an effective way so that we can work well with people and enhance the ability of people to work together.[16] Emotional intelligence is something that can be learnt and, while it will continue to develop throughout our life, we can assist that growth in understanding and capability.[16] Daniel Goleman outlines the main domains of emotional intelligence, which are as follows.[17,18]

Knowing one's emotions (self-awareness)

The ability to monitor your feelings with insight and understanding is a crucial element of emotional intelligence. Self-aware people have an indepth understanding of their emotions, strengths and limitations, as well as their values and motives. This self-knowledge assists them in making decisions; Goleman suggests that people who have greater certainty about their feelings are better able to steer their lives in the direction they wish.[17]

Self-management (being able to handle feelings appropriately)

Unless we have a good understanding of our feelings, we will not be in a good position to be able to manage them well and in a positive manner. Self-management refers to being in control of your feelings, rather than letting your feelings control you. If we do not manage how we feel, this can have a major impact on others (such as colleagues or patients), and so it is important to be able to recognise and respond to our own positive or negative emotions.[18]

Social awareness (empathy)

Empathic people are able to recognise when others need or want something – they are able to 'put themselves in the other's shoes', and respond accordingly.[17] In terms of leadership, this means taking into account how others feel, and making intelligent decisions that recognise those feelings.[18] Being empathic will help you to respond better to patient needs, but also to manage some of the more challenging behaviours you may experience from other staff.

Relationship management

Relationship management is the final domain of emotional intelligence. In managing relationships, there is a need to manage people's emotions. However, this must be done with authenticity and genuineness. By being aware of their own values, leaders skilled in relationship management are able to articulate a vision, and to share that with others. Additionally, such leaders are skilled at managing conflict and change, and are able to use their capacities to build teams, encourage collaboration and help team members develop their skills.

As a newly registered nurse it is useful to understand these domains, because, as Goleman indicates, the skills and capabilities that contribute to emotional intelligence can be learnt.[17,18] Even when not in a leadership role, emotional intelligence is critically important. You can begin building your emotional intelligence by identifying your capacity in each of the domains, and endeavouring to increase your skills. For example, if you are experiencing negative emotions about your work or an incident in your life, using your emotional intelligence can help you to deal with these feelings in an appropriate way. This is important, as your actions and emotions affect not only yourself; they also have an impact on your co-workers and the patients for whom you may be caring. We believe that, whilst emotional intelligence is particularly important for leadership, it is also important for all staff, and can enhance how the whole team works.

EXERCISE 15.3

Consider each of the domains and think about how well you meet them. Reflect on this and consider how you might develop your capabilities further.

CONCLUSION

It is hoped that through reading this chapter and undertaking the exercises, you will have identified opportunities to develop your leadership capability at this early stage of your career. You should also recognise that, although you may not be in a formal leadership position, you still have an opportunity to display leadership capacity, and this will stand you in good stead as you progress in your nursing career.

CASE STUDY 15.1

Mary has just started work at a small country hospital in the mixed medical and surgical ward. John is the nursing unit manager and has not worked with newly registered nurses before; this is the first time the hospital has employed a new registered nurse. John has a quick chat with Mary after about 4 weeks and does not seem entirely happy with her but Mary is unsure what the issues are.

REFLECTIVE QUESTIONS

- How often should Mary expect to receive feedback from John? What are the important aspects for Mary to develop in her practice as a registered nurse?
- What should Mary do about the 'quick chat' that John has had with her?
- Mary feels that perhaps staff have a limited understanding of her education and clinical experience. What could she do to address their knowledge deficit?

CASE STUDY 15.2

Mark is a newly registered nurse of 4 weeks, working with Susan, an eighth-year registered nurse in charge on night duty and a very experienced enrolled nurse.

REFLECTIVE QUESTIONS

- How will Mark respond if Susan delegates tasks to him that he does not feel able to do?
- The enrolled nurse offers to assist Mark with some activities but Mark is not sure of the scope of practice of the enrolled nurse. What should Mark do?
- Mark notices that some care is not being carried out according to the required standard. What should he do?

CASE STUDY 15.3

Jill is a very experienced clinical nurse educator on a rehabilitation ward. She has been working with Libby, a newly registered nurse, for a few weeks now. Jill believes that Libby is performing at a very high level for a new nurse; in fact, she is more productive than many of the more experienced registered nurses on the ward.

REFLECTIVE QUESTIONS

- How might Jill provide incentives to Libby for her performance?
- Jill asks the nursing unit manager to let Libby lead a team on morning shift to develop her capabilities further. How will Libby respond to the other registered nurses in her team who may be more experienced?
- Libby sometimes finds herself in conflict with one very experienced registered nurse who does seem to recognise Libby's skills. What should she do?

RECOMMENDED READING

Clark CC. Creative nursing leadership and management. Sudbury, MA: Jones & Bartlett Learning; 2009.

Garber PR. Giving and receiving performance feedback. Amherst, MA: HRD Press; 2004.

McBride P, Maitland S. The EI advantage: putting emotional intelligence into practice. Berkshire: McGraw Hill International; 2002.

Moss MT. The emotionally intelligent nurse leader. San Francisco: John Wiley; 2009.

Shaw S. International Council of Nurses: nursing leadership. Oxford: Wiley Blackwell; 2007.

REFERENCES

1. Wheatley M. Finding our way. leadership for an uncertain time. San Francisco: Berrett-Koehler; 2005.
2. Kouzes J, Posner B. The leadership challenge. 3rd ed. San Francisco: Jossey-Bass; 2003.
3. Burns J. Leadership. New York: Harper; 1978, pp. 3, 19, 20.
4. Weberg D. Transformational leadership and staff retention: an evidence review with implications for healthcare systems. Nursing Administration Quarterly 2010; 34:246–58.
5. Gardner BD. Improve RN retention through transformational leadership styles. Nursing Management 2010;41:8–12.
6. Tomey AM. Nursing leadership and management effects work environments. Journal of Nursing Management 2009;17:15–25.
7. Failla KR, Stichler JF. Manager and staff perceptions of the manager's leadership style. Journal of Nursing Administration 2008;38:480–7.
8. Govier I, Nash S. Examining transformational approaches to effective leadership in healthcare settings. Nursing Times 2009;105:24–7.
9. Aarons GA. Transformational and transactional leadership: association with attitudes toward evidence-based practice. Psychiatric Services 2006;57:1162–9.
10. Cottingham C. Transformational leadership: a strategy for nursing. In: Hein E, Nicholson M, editors. Contemporary leadership behavior. Selected readings. 4th ed. Philadelphia: J.B. Lippincott; 1982.
11. Fassaert T, van Dulmen S, Schellevis F, et al. Active listening in medical consultations: development of the Active Listening Observation Scale (ALOS-global). Patient Education and Counseling 2007;68:258–64.
12. Derkx H, Rethans J, Maiburg B, et al. Quality of communication during telephone triage at Dutch out-of-hours centres. Patient Education & Counseling 2009;74:174–8.
13. Bittner NP, Gravlin G. Critical thinking, delegation, and missed care in nursing practice. Journal of Nursing Administration 2009;39:142–6.
14. Australian Nursing and Midwifery Council. A national framework for the development of decision-making tools for nursing and midwifery practice. ACT: ANMC, 2007. Online. Available: http://www.nursingmidwiferyboard.gov.au/Codes-and-Guidelines.aspx

15. Keeney S, Hasson F, McKenna H, et al. Nurses', midwives' and patients' perceptions of trained health care assistants. Journal of Advanced Nursing 2005;50: 345–55.
16. Goleman D. Working with emotional intelligence. New York: Bantam; 1998.
17. Goleman D. Emotional intelligence: why it can matter more than IQ. London: Bloomsbury; 1995.
18. Goleman D, Boyatzis R, McKee A. Primal leadership: learning to lead with emotional intelligence. Boston: Harvard Business School Press; 2002.

Excellence in practice: technology and the registered nurse

Alan Barnard

LEARNING OBJECTIVES

When you have completed this chapter you will be able to:

- discuss the meaning and implications of technology for nursing care
- outline concepts for appropriate use and integration of technology in clinical practice
- discuss strategies for developing technology skills and knowledge
- debate technology in relation to the organisation of nursing and healthcare
- reflect on the relation between technology and person-focused care.

Keywords: technology, knowledge, skills, clinical practice, technique, technological competency

---

INTRODUCTION

Technology is everywhere. We nurses use it to care for people and manage our working day. Nurses talk about technology, develop skills and knowledge to apply technology, praise the qualities of the latest technology development and sometimes blame it for the demise of human contact. In addition, we write about technology, attend courses to learn about new equipment, work within highly organised healthcare systems and live in a world that is organised increasingly in accordance with efficiency and logical order. Healthcare is increasingly technology-dependent and understanding the influence and impact of technology is essential for effective clinical practice.

Technology has often been interpreted as machinery and equipment; however, it is much more than the things we use. Our meaning of technology also needs to include the knowledge and skills used to apply, develop, design and assess objects, and the development of a human, organisational and political system aimed at the maximisation of efficiency. Technology is in fact a complex interrelationship between a range of important elements, including machinery, equipment, tools, utensils, automata, apparatus, structures, people, organisations, science, culture, systems, gender, values and politics. Technology assists with many diagnostic, assessment and treatment responsibilities but at the same time can challenge our moral, cultural and social development. It remains an important component of nursing practice and is valued highly since technology provides us with evidence for patient care, extends communication and treatment options, assists us to organise time-consuming responsibilities and is used as part of a number of hospital and community activities in healthcare.

This chapter explores technology and the beginning registered nurse in acute and hospital-based care with specific reference to skills and knowledge development for patient care delivery. The primary goal is to unite examples of practical issues common to clinical nursing practice with theoretical concepts in order to assist beginning registered nurses to work better with technology. The chapter examines the meaning of technology and the various types of technologies typical of acute care. It also explores issues related to skill and knowledge development with specific emphasis on personal implications of working with the influence of technology.

WHAT IS TECHNOLOGY?

The word 'technology' refers to the practical arts, and the knowledge and/or activity of a group (i.e. technologist). Technology is more than the sum of all the equipment we use in healthcare, the latest piece of machinery or the internet. Technology has associated characteristics that include the development of skills, knowledge and the incorporation of social and cultural values.[1-3] One way to portray this interpretation of technology is as three concentric circles (Fig 16.1). Concentric circles highlight the characteristics of technology that together emphasise a characterology of the phenomenon. The concentric circles focus our attention on not only the things of nursing at the centre, but also their relations with other characteristics such as skills change, knowledge development, gender and cultural differences, competency development and a growing emphasis on efficiency and rationale order (rationale order means the organisation of behaviours, actions and ways of thinking about nursing into preplanned and predictable processes).

Artifacts and resources

The smallest and central concentric circle depicted in Figure 16.1, entitled artifacts and resources, is technology at its most obvious and refers to the integration, use and application of the 'things' of nursing. Rinard[4] noted that in modern nursing three key periods of change have been significantly influenced by technology. The first period was 1950–60 and was characterised by new medical techniques and a

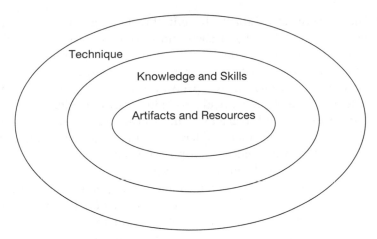

Fig 16.1 A characterology of technology.

significant introduction of pharmaceuticals to care. The second period identified was 1965 80 and was associated with increasing machinery and specialisation; and the third period was from 1980 to 1995, and was associated with increasing technical control, streamlining and prediction of care. Although not noted by Rinard, a fourth period of change has emerged that could be characterised as a period of information access, retrieval and computerisation of care. We each have greater knowledge availability, communicate with more immediacy, and there is a perceived link between quality care, sophisticated technology and knowledge access.

Knowledge and skills

The second or middle concentric circle portrays technology as knowledge and skills. Our care is in many ways determined by the knowledge and skills we develop and as such we have to include knowledge and skills as part of technology. Without required knowledge and skills we have limited ability to meet the needs of patients. For example, without the knowledge and skills to use an intravenous pump correctly it is of no use as a piece of equipment for your care delivery and consequentially becomes a technology of potential danger for a patient. Nursing is a practical occupation and our knowledge is expressed most often through the way we perform our work. Failure to establish and develop knowledge and skills is inadequate for the quality of nursing practice, your patients, the colleagues with whom you work, the requirements of the healthcare sector and the equipment you hope to use. Technological knowledge takes many forms and relates not only to hands-on competency but also to knowledge of organisational policy, current research and changing evidence.

Technique

The influence of technology on nursing practice is illustrated and described in a broader sense by the third and most inclusive concentric circle, entitled technique. The third concentric circle extends our characterology of technology to include the way policy, politics, economics, ethics, culture, organisational management and human behaviour are organised for the benefit of technology. The way nursing practice is organised for, as well as by artifacts and resources, is as much technology as the first and second levels of meaning. Technique is not a specific thing. Technique describes a way of thinking about the way we do things and go about our daily care. It describes an attitude in which many aspects of our clinical practice that were once instinctive, reflexive, natural and particular to individuals and cultures are being transformed into organised method, behaviour and instruction. In automated and tightly regulated technological environments differing cultural and social values have a tendency to be replaced by a dependency on predetermined actions and protocols and this is increasingly the case with nursing practice.

Technique is complex and has three subtle yet important characteristics. First, technique adheres to a primacy of reason to govern practice. It is a way of thinking, acting and living by which people attempt to control the internal, passionate and emotional world of everyday life via protocols, rules, evidence and general observance to a logical order.

Second, it requires a desire for efficiency in order to assist its goal and to justify its activity. The desire for efficiency is akin to the inventor or factory owner who seeks to streamline methods and actions in order to obtain certain outcomes that simplify and make predictable previously uncontrolled or random activity. It must be stressed that there is nothing wrong or dangerous per se with a desire for planned activity or efficiency. In fact, there is nothing new about efficiency as a reasonable and worthwhile goal. The desire for efficiency and systems to control actions and activity has guided invention throughout human history, and after all, who wants to be exposed to ineffective care? However, the third characteristic of technique brings about new and different experience because it stresses primacy of efficiency in every realm of human activity and thinking.

Technique has become so prevalent in nursing that people are increasingly incapable of thinking outside its boundaries in their search for meaning. The importance of subjectivity and human experience can become marginalised by an emphasis on control, efficiency and logical order.[5-9] Technique reduces human-centred activities such as nursing to measurable and predictable outcomes. That is, technique brings about qualitative transformation(s) in care.

Together all the concentric circles highlight that technology is as much about, for example, pieces of equipment, as it is about our knowledge and skills and how we organise care. The concentric circles highlight that a full understanding of technology must include understanding that it can have a direct impact on, for example, cultural differences and how we each express our nursing practice. There is a growing reliance on efficiency and logical order, sometimes at the cost of advancing human-centred care.

NURSING AND TECHNOLOGY

Nurses have always used tools, chemicals, potions, equipment and machines to provide care for people. Nursing technology includes any technology that we use and/or claim to be fundamental to our daily practice. Depending on context, there are at least 12 different types of nursing technologies (Table 16.1), even though a lot of nursing technology is not immediately evident to us. That is, it lacks recognition

Table 16.1 Examples of types of technology associated with nursing practice[24]	
Types of technology	**Examples**
Clothes	Shroud Pyjamas
Utensils	Bedpan Kidney dish
Structures	Hospital ward Isolation room
Apparatus	Jordan frame Patient transport trolley
Utilities	Electrical power Gas services
Tools	Wheelchair Urinary catheter Sphygmomanometer
Resources	Pharmaceuticals Sterile dressing
Machines	Intravenous infusion pump Mechanical ventilator
Automata	Computer Call bell Refrigerator
Tools of doing used to enact clinical practice	Nurse's watch Stethoscope
Objects of art or religion	Nurse's uniform
Toys (e.g. diversional therapy)	Chessboard

as technology by nurses both in clinical practice and in nursing literature. For example, there is sometimes in the literature an overemphasis on sophisticated technology and an uncritical lack of emphasis of technology associated with the 'dirty work' of nurses. The reasons for this lack of recognition include: excitement about new and sophisticated machinery and equipment, our inclination to focus on new technology and underemphasis of older and simpler technologies, and lack of research and scholarship examining technology within nursing.[10–15] In fact it can be argued that inadequate appreciation of the breadth of technology in nursing has restricted our capacity to interpret the influence of technology on our profession and healthcare more generally.

The 12 types of technology listed in Table 16.1 emphasise technologies that are simple, sophisticated, old, new, unique and commonplace. Given that nursing technologies have not been examined adequately,[6,16–18] the types of nursing technology proposed highlight both the strongly technological basis of nursing and the diverse range of technologies that come together to assist practice. Over time, many types of technology (e.g. tools) evolve from being external and hand-held to becoming machinery and/or automata that operate independently. Witness for example the evolution of blood pressure monitoring from the hand-held sphygmomanometer to electronic devices. Technology often evolves from being human-powered to being controlled by alternative power sources such as electricity and computerisation. The hospital bed can now be adjusted automatically, and nursing/medical records are computer-based and accessible at distance.

Whilst an extended debate could be undertaken to examine what technologies are specific to nursing, it must be recognised that a lot of commonplace and simple nursing technology needs to be better acknowledged as significant to nursing practice (e.g. bedpan), in order to increase clarity and understanding.[19,20] There remains a lack of recognition of the types of technology in clinical practice and this lack of recognition affects how we think about and understand nursing practice.

EXERCISE 16.1

What types of technologies are part of your clinical area? Next time you are engaged in clinical practice, make a mental note of the various technologies you use in your clinical practice.

EXERCISE 16.2

Reflecting on your experience, do you think technologies such as tools, machines and automata are more highly valued than technologies that are less sophisticated? Why do you get this impression? What does this tell you about nursing and healthcare? Make a list of how these values might influence nursing research, practice and professional goals.

READINESS FOR CLINICAL PRACTICE: SKILLS AND KNOWLEDGE

The seminal work of Patricia Benner[21] described different levels of clinical perform-ance and expertise among nurses. Her work, together with that of Bondy[22] and Krichbaum,[23] provided an understanding that at different stages in our careers, nurses approach the delivery of care in different ways. For a beginning registered nurse in Australia, a systematic approach where goals and stages of care provision are explained is beneficial for safety as they assist to guide the completion of less familiar roles and responsibilities, whereas the more experienced nurse in the same context may require less direction to assess practice principles and priorities of practice quickly. This is normal, but both instances emphasise that it is essential in practice to direct our nursing gaze to the principles that underpin a skill or procedure.

Advancement of competency needed for the use of technology in patient care is crucial to foster clinical excellence. Beginning nurses often find that they lack the experience, skills and knowledge required to practise with technology in specialist areas. In addition, beginning nurses are often required to be at ease with the use of technical equipment before they have developed higher-level critical thinking and decision-making skills. As we saw in our characterology of technology, the need to integrate technology in our care before developing skills and knowledge to employ it thoughtfully can compromise quality of care. For example, it is easy to turn on an oxygen saturation monitor, place it on a finger and read the number. Higher-level skills include interpreting the information, knowing whether the information being received is accurate, and responding to it in an appropriate manner. Ongoing education and a commitment to personal development are essential for effective clinical practice. It is not good enough to know how to use the machinery if the nurse cannot also use the information obtained accurately, safely and with appropriate effect.

Knowledge and skills alter regularly and thus an active commitment to maintaining and advancing competence is a sign of a caring and responsible nurse. Attitudes that reflect an offhand and neglectful interest in updating knowledge and skills are inadequate and reflect a failure to value the profession. Competence reduces anxiety and fear, and increases the likelihood of successful care. Technological advances such microsurgery, eHealth and tele-health are exciting, but place unprecedented demands on each nurse to maintain and foster new knowledge and competence.

Competency standards associated with technology in general and advanced practice are part of, for example, the current Australian Nurses Federation Competency Standards for registered nurses.[21] Technology-related knowledge and skills are clearly a major focus and the standards are a useful framework that describes appropriate nursing practice related to, for example, decision making, communication, assessment and ethical behaviour.[24] Achieving and maintaining Australian standards need to be the goals of each nurse.

The standards highlight the central importance of developing skills and knowledge and, according to the Australian Nurses Federation Competency Standards, a registered nurse in general practice, for example (standard 1.4), must recognise and respond to the need for ongoing education and training to maintain competence for nursing practice. For the advanced registered nurse practice competency (standard 6) highlights, for example, that each nurse must seek out and integrate evidence from a range of sources to improve healthcare outcomes based on experience, clinical judgment and statutory and common-law requirements where a decision by an individual or group contravenes safe practice.[24] Numerous standards emphasise the central role and responsibility of nurses in appropriate skill development and knowledge acquisition and a significant part of this development has a direct association with technology.

Even though specialist knowledge and skills are needed in a lot of nursing contexts, there are many technologies that are commonplace and integral to the complex practices of all nurses (e.g. stethoscope, bedpan). As a beginning nurse it is worth remembering that there was a time when even these technologies were challenging (e.g. taking a blood pressure manually for the first time). As a registered nurse you have, and must acquire, knowledge and skills necessary to practise using the commonplace machinery, equipment and resources of nursing. Whilst a personal goal to develop the necessary ability to practise with advanced technology is appropriate, this goal should be balanced with suitable appreciation of your existing capabilities and competency. Technology provides new options in clinical practice and acts to extend skills. You must acknowledge and apply existing knowledge and skills to all technology in a capable and appropriate manner in addition to seeking to foster new clinical skills and knowledge.

'They do things different to the way I was taught'

A beginning registered nurse will witness variation in how different nurses complete clinical activities and on first experience you might think that perhaps you were not taught correctly during your undergraduate degree. You may witness slight differences in the way a simple dressing technique is performed and ask yourself: are these differences important? Is my practice adequate? Do these differences breach nursing standards?

There will be differences and in most cases this is not a problem. One reason for difference can, however, be an overemphasis on behavioural action rather than principles of practice. Fuszard[25] suggested that nurses have tended historically to perform clinical skills based on behavioural rules learnt from teachers and mentors during the formative phase of a career. During formative years nurses learnt rules through a process of modelling that was often based on cultural traditions of an institution, teacher or mentor.[26] For example, there are practice principles such as asepsis that are central when performing a simple dressing. These principles have at times been overshadowed by the traditions of specific employers and institutions, spawning an emphasis on behavioural steps based on preference and context rather than research evidence.

Many generations of nurses have accepted institutional preference as the way to execute skills and complete procedures. An often-heard observation expressed by a registered nurse might be: 'That's not how we do it here'. Non-divergence from behavioural steps was interpreted as the right way to perform a nursing task and clinical assessment of students based on rules tended to reinforce confusion between rules and practice principles. In addition, many nursing procedure manuals utilised expert opinion but lacked the advantage of nursing research. Tradition and personal experience tended to be the primary foundation for the establishment of procedural steps, in association with the preferences of employers, medicine, individuals and other professional groups. These influences need to be critically considered when establishing how practice principles should be applied in practice, especially since our professional environment now emphasises personal responsibility, evidence-based practice and awareness of litigation.

From rules to evidence

In reality there may be no single correct behavioural rule for performing a range of skills and/or procedures, but there are principles of practice embedded in actions that need to be understood and enacted for safe care. In fact, behavioural rules as a basis for your action without equal clarity about the principles that inform action are potentially unsafe and unhelpful. When principles are clearly explained and understood it becomes easier to differentiate practice principles from procedural rules and accept variation in ways of doing a procedure. Preferences when performing (doing) a simple dressing can be adopted but make sure that, embedded in the preferred procedural steps, the principle of asepsis (for example) is maintained at all times. On this basis, performance of actions by different nurses associated with a procedure can vary with no real problem.[27]

In recent years, healthcare providers often seek external accreditation from groups such as the Australian Council on Healthcare Standards (ACHS)[28] and this development is to your advantage because the process of accreditation helps to clarify and improve clinical practice. In Australia the ACHS Evaluation and Quality Improvement Program (EQuIP 4) standards provide a clear indication that procedures and clinical practice more broadly need to be evidence-based,[28] and highlight the need to move away from behavioural rules applied simply as procedural steps. In practice you must think critically and make best judgment based on evidence, reflection and the advice of experienced colleagues. A beginning point to obtain excellence in your practice is to think through the reasons for a specific clinical intervention being undertaken, contrast practice(s) with known evidence and decide on the legitimacy of actions in line with the principles that should be employed.

EXERCISE 16.3

Student nurses are taught principles of wound management during their educational preparation. Can the principle of asepsis be applied absolutely in a practice environment? Think about managing a large sacral pressure area for a patient who is incontinent of faeces. Is asepsis likely to be possible when cleaning the wound? The context of your practice and the presentation of each person's health condition will dictate the best use of technology.

Experience teaches nurses to adapt practice by critically engaging principles in specific situations.

Reflect for a moment on your practice. Can you think of instances where behaviours and practice principles were adapted for a particular situation? What were the reasons for the modification to clinical practice, and what has this type of experience taught you?

Troubleshooting: problem-solving technology

When technology functions inadequately and does not operate in the way it should, the experience of using technology can be one of frustration. If not resolved quickly and with competence, inadequate patient care can occur as a result of decreased efficiency and clinical effectiveness.[17,29–33] Technology can become a burden and is potentially unsafe if it is not maintained well, is inadequate for the job at hand or is inappropriate for a practice environment. The following quotation from an experienced nurse highlights a typical clinical scenario when technology is not well maintained:

you wonder sometimes – like, some machines need to have more time spent with them because they're just not the right design. Some machines are easier and more useful than others, obviously . . . just even yesterday . . . we had to use a pulse oximeter in a medical ward – a guy with COAD [chronic obstructive airways disease], asthma and a chest infection; they [doctors] wanted to know what his oxygen sats were going to be. You know they're not going to be fantastic but, anyway, they want to know what it is now, and the machine, well, I put it on and they [other nurses] said, 'Well, you've got to fiddle with the thing to make it go' and of course I'm fiddling with the thing – 10 minutes I think I fiddled with it. I couldn't get the signal properly, and they said, 'Well, you've got to do it like this' and then I got somebody else and they had a go and they couldn't do it, and then another girl came and finally she said, 'Yes, I got it.' That's great, but that took half an hour to get one reading, and I said, 'Can't you send it down to the workshop to get it fixed?' He said, 'It spends all its life down at the workshop getting fixed.' And then they said, 'Well, you can go and borrow the one from the ward next door,' and I thought oh, no. You know. In that way I think it would make life more difficult. I mean, I spent a lot of time trying to get the machine to work. I got two other people involved in it. I could have had another ward involved in it [as well].[20]

Technology needs appropriate resources to function in an efficient and effective manner (e.g. space, power supply) and when technology is defective or deficient, the practice of nursing can become time-consuming, difficult and distracted.[10,34] Immediate reporting of faulty equipment and replacement of inadequate technology are essential, as is clear understanding of the ways that each specific technology operates. It is essential to develop the necessary skills to manipulate machinery and equipment and problem-solve their operation. Problem-solving the efficient operation of technology is a prerequisite skill for practice and it is the case that many of these skills can only be learnt 'on the job'. The activity of fixing technology such as machinery and equipment whilst they are in use within a clinical area is commonly known as troubleshooting. The following nurse explained her role when troubleshooting technology:

you end up being the trouble-shooter, Miss [Mr] Fix-it-type person, and you're supposed to have a competency to look after, say, somebody with an epidural or to change the PCA [patient-controlled analgesia] syringe. Sometimes you might be the only person on the ward who knows how to fix it, who is allowed to do it or who does really know how to work the machinery. You spend quite a lot of time with them.[20]

It is important to learn from experienced colleagues but not to develop an unhealthy reliance on the Miss/Mr Fix-it in your clinical environment. As explained by the nurse above, reliance creates a significant burden. Time spent managing technology leaves less time to be with people[34] and consumes the time and expertise of those nurses who have to assist you. An inability to troubleshoot technology leaves less time to manage other aspects of care and can compromise patient care. Merely hoping to solve problems without a clear understanding of the technology does not foster the behavioural patterns needed to face future challenges, and will not advance your professional reputation or trust. Table 16.2 outlines strategies you can employ to develop troubleshooting skills and knowledge.

Solving technical problems appropriately ensures that clinical treatment is delivered in a timely manner, a patient's condition is monitored properly, patients do not become anxious about their care because they trust you, safety standards are maintained because you know what you are doing and excessive time is not taken away from you attending to your other roles and responsibilities. Technology will operate incorrectly due to factors such as inadequate resources, incorrect settings, inexperienced staff and malfunction. Failure to develop troubleshooting skills and knowledge will not foster autonomy in your practice. For this reason, although there will probably be a Miss or Mr Fix-it in your clinical area, it is best to view this person as a

Table 16.2 Strategies to develop troubleshooting skills

Activity	Strategies
Education prior to using technology	Identify technologies common to clinical context Read operating manuals/other relevant resources Observe expert nurses Attend in-service sessions Ask a lot of questions
Practise using technology	Operate first when it is not in clinical use Identify clinical opportunities to employ it Seek supervision and feedback in the initial phase
Reflect on technologies employed	Keep a diary of things to remember Reflect on the effectiveness of technologies Identify benefits of correct usage

mentor who can foster the development of your own troubleshooting skills rather than as a long-term solution to your technology problems.

EXERCISE 16.4

Make a note of any unfamiliar technology that you have come across in clinical areas. Increase your knowledge and skills by talking with an expert nurse about his or her use of the technology. Take time to practise the operation of any unfamiliar machinery, automata or equipment, read relevant literature and observe nurses troubleshooting. Don't forget to ask questions, watch every step, and make notes for you to review at a later time.

We work in changing and demanding environments, often with patients who have a high acuity (i.e. a high level of care requirement in terms of symptom management, care needs and healthcare condition). Increasing roles and responsibility require you continually to improve your skills, knowledge and clinical expertise. Knowledge takes many forms and relates to organisational policies, research evidence, scope of practice, ethical standards and hands-on knowledge such as troubleshooting technology. Growing your experience through ongoing education, personal reflection and assistance from colleagues is valued highly in healthcare.[29,32] In contrast, failure to establish and develop knowledge and skills is inadequate for your practice and unhelpful to patient care and the team with which you work.

EXERCISE 16.5

Nurses can sometimes be seen pressing buttons in the hope that a machine will eventually do what they want it to do. If the same problems arise again and the nurse employs the same behaviour, how should this form of troubleshooting be interpreted? Is it always easier to read the manual first? What management strategies could you implement in clinical settings to ensure that all nurses can learn to troubleshoot?

TECHNOLOGY AND CLINICAL ASSESSMENT

As outlined in our characterology (Fig 16.1), technology is more than pieces of equipment, machinery and related resources. As a registered nurse you must focus not only on the skills and knowledge of technology usage, but also on the patients within the healthcare organisation.[10,32,35] Numerous nurses have highlighted problems that arise as a result of the relationship between technology and nursing behaviour.[36–39] Technology will influence professional values, practices, skills, knowledge and the environment of care. For example, clinical environments such as intensive care and medical units are noteworthy for their use of technology and constant demands on your skills and knowledge.

Nurse clinicians and academics continue to stress the importance of achieving an appropriate balance between nursing the patient and integrating technology into daily care. It is the case that nurses sometimes can be distracted by the demands of machinery and equipment. On busy days, basic patient needs such as daily living requirements can become secondary to a focus on maintaining and using technology and, in extreme cases, the experience of a patient can seem less important than information obtained from technology. Subjective experience and clinical presentation of the patient can become secondary to evidence obtained from technology.[2,5,7,32,34,35,40–42] It is easy to be caught up in attending to technology rather than with the experience and presentation of a person. One nurse explained a typical clinical situation she had experienced as follows:

> you have a baby in the nursery on monitors and some people, when the alarm goes off, go and check the monitor to see what it is doing, but with the pulse oximeter and a baby, if they move, shake, rattle or roll, they will set it off [pulse oximeter alarm], so it's more important to go and check what the baby is doing. Is it breathing or shallow breathing? . . . it is more important to go and look at the baby than look at the machine. Yes, the monitor can say, come and see what is happening, but you should see what is happening with the baby, not what is happening with the machine . . . we forget that they are here to alert us to the patient.[20]

Machinery and equipment do not always provide the irrefutable evidence necessary for diagnostic accuracy and best nursing intervention. It is you − not technology − that is responsible for clinical assessment and decision making, even though at times technology assists you in the process. In fact, confounding processes in the body can mask the information provided by technology to you as evidence. It is not appropriate for any healthcare professional to replace, justify or bolster assessment skills through reliance on information from machinery and equipment. The following nurse explained her experience:

> I have seen younger, newer nurses who have gone, oh, that patient is in atrial fibrillation, and you say, well, are they? And they say, the machine [said it], you know (rather than because they had completed a full patient assessment). And particularly, I think, in the ward area, if a patient has chest pain and people do not feel really comfortable with the technology, or with what's happening to the patient because they're unstable, they may tend to rely on the technology a little bit.[20]

Clinical evidence to inform practice choice and clinical judgment that is based on your assessment of the whole person are equally important to care. Assessment based on a patient's symptoms, signs and clinical history needs to be balanced with information from technology and consultation with colleagues. There can be a tendency to respond to information from technology alone rather than integrate it into a comprehensive assessment structure. Interpreting information provided by technology involves ensuring it is accurate and responding to it in an appropriate manner. For example, a pulse oximeter may indicate that the oxygen saturation for a person is only 78% when physical assessment demonstrates no shortness of breath or evidence of cyanosis. In this case it is not appropriate to record the oxygen saturation unthinkingly as 78%. Making a clinical assessment in isolation from other assessment findings will lead to inappropriate conclusions and care. Indeed, physical assessment of the person should cause you to consider why the information from the equipment did not fit (align) with the clinical presentation of the patient.

Information from technology is of benefit and is effective when evaluated in relation to the experience, needs, physical condition, cultural background and desires of the patient. Technology used appropriately can help to reduce suffering and assist to bring about humane care and excellence in clinical practice. Locsin[39] states that technological competence, as a form of caring, is expressed as an authentic desire and intention to use technology expertly for the betterment of each individual. What determines whether a technology depersonalises care or marginalises the person being treated is not the technology per se, but rather how individual technology is used in specific contexts, the meanings attributed to information gained from the technology, the skills and knowledge of the healthcare worker(s).[43] Your nursing intervention and treatment must be guided by compassion, skill, knowledge, appropriate assessment and an understanding of each person's experience and physical condition.

EXERCISE 16.6

Registered nurses who are new to a clinical area can sometimes place their clinical trust in technology rather than in other forms of patient assessment. In addition, a great deal of time may be spent examining and responding to the operation of technology. Over time, as familiarity with technology improves, there is a (re)focus on human (patient) experience. However, when new technologies are introduced we once more focus on their use.

With your colleagues discuss and make a list of strategies that could be implemented to assist student and registered nurses to familiarise themselves better with technology and encourage holistic patient assessment skills.

NURSING PRACTICE WITH TECHNOLOGY

Nurses are often the only healthcare workers who possess the skills required to use technology in clinical environments. Your expertise can lead to increasing involvement in decision making, autonomous practice, professional recognition and collegiality. Technology is of value to the healthcare sector and society, and this quality of value transfers to those individuals who use it.[10,12,15,44] However, true expertise and quality of value are achieved when all aspects of our care are enhanced and balanced as part of our clinical role. For example, if you use technology efficiently but fail to ensure adequate care (e.g. mouth care) for your patient, you have missed the point of nursing. Nurse authors have argued consistently for the centrality of the person in nursing practice.[10,12,34,43] Failure to focus on the person is not necessarily caused by technology, and may more accurately reflect the way nursing is organised and the priorities that are rated most highly at any one time. Authentic respect and autonomy come from a consistent excellence in nursing practice, appropriate use of technology and a willingness to resolve challenges that lead to unacceptable standards of care.

For example, whilst education, experience and commitment will focus your attention on professional responsibility, the push for new or increased skills and knowledge will not always make clinical practice less busy or demanding. It is a fact that, on some days, an outcome of increasing technology will mean that your clinical environment can be so demanding that the human focus of nursing is subsumed in a haze of activity. Under these conditions, it is difficult to focus on human experience and nurses develop various strategies to compensate for the challenge, as described by the following registered nurse:

> Other days you work your butt off, get through the day and you know. Sometimes I'll stay back after work, in my own time, just to talk to someone because I felt like I cheated them a bit, I wasn't there for all their needs.[20]

Whilst it is noteworthy that this specific nurse gave her own time back to her patients because she could not give it during her working hours, there are other ways of meeting the needs of patients without having to stay late at work. A less desired strategy that nurses sometimes employ to complete their day's work when technology places high demands on their energies includes adopting a task-based approach to care. There is a focus primarily on those patients who are most in need of physical assistance. More often than not this strategy will relieve a demanding work situation, but does not lead to excellence in care. Alternative strategies to address the issue are listed in Table 16.3 and may help to manage and improve your practice.

Table 16.3 Strategies to manage technology during your working day

Activity	Strategies
Maintain knowledge base	Actively seek education on technology Develop skills in utilising technology Establish troubleshooting capacity

Choose wisely	Assess the usefulness of technology
	Consider the practice environment
	Only employ technologies if they definitely:
	  – help to provide care
	  – save time

Maintain environment	Lobby[10,32] for a clinically relevant resource base which considers:
	  – appropriately trained staff
	  – patient acuity
	  – agreed standards of care
	Replace inefficient technology
	Remove non-essential technology

Increasing technology in the workplace acts to organise our labour. It is important to be involved in decision-making processes that influence the purchase, assessment, research and future use of technology since it directly influences your practice. Technology purchase, use and integration are influenced by political and economic agendas and decisions. Therefore an important activity for nurses is to become actively involved in assessing the safety skills and knowledge implications of new technology.[32,33,45–48] For example, one way of engaging in this activity is through involvement in economic and organisational decisions related to the ongoing use and purchase of technology. A starting point is to make known your interest in helping to integrate useful technology better into the clinical practice environment.

EXERCISE 16.7

Reflect on your nursing experience. Do you have any recommendations for integrating technology with nursing practice that would improve care? Think of an example from your own experience and discuss what changes are needed to nursing policy.

CONCLUSION

Technology has a direct influence on the knowledge, skills, practice, values, ethics and politics of nursing. As such, the meaning and implications of technology for your nursing practice must be considered in relation to all aspects of nursing and healthcare. As the contexts of nursing practice alter with the needs of a changing society, your roles and responsibilities will change. New graduates and more experienced nurses need to foster insight into the ongoing challenges that technology brings to nursing practice, skills development, knowledge and standards of patient care. Nursing practice has altered as much, and as quickly, as the types of technology that are now integrated into care. You must be diligent to use all your skills and knowledge in order to advance clinical excellence and the best care outcomes for each person.

CASE STUDY 16.1

John is a 3-year-old boy with severe cerebral palsy. He has been in hospital for an extended period of time but is now being discharged home, with his family providing his primary care. He is in a permanent wheelchair and has partial ventilator support. Sarah is new to her registered nurse position in her ward and wants to ensure John and his family are supported to provide best care.

REFLECTIVE QUESTION

To ensure both John and his family are supported, what predischarge considerations and discharge plans should Sarah put into place so that this family can best provide care at home for this ventilator-dependent child?

CASE STUDY 16.2

During Greg's second rotation in his transition year he is assigned to an acute 32-bed respiratory medical ward in a large metropolitan hospital. On arrival for duty he is unsure of a lot of the equipment used for care on the ward. Greg decides it is an opportunity to set about familiarising himself with all the available technology. He finds also that most of the registered nurses employed on the ward have limited experience.

REFLECTIVE QUESTION

What strategies and resources could assist Greg to prepare for this clinical role and his responsibilities?

CASE STUDY 16.3

After completing her new graduate program, Amal secures a permanent position in the intensive care unit. Many of the patients admitted to the unit require management of acute and chronic medical conditions. After witnessing a number of events that occurred in the unit, Amal believes that a lot of the healthcare team tend to rely too much on information from technology when undertaking patient assessment, rather than also seeking evidence directly from their patients. Amal is eager to encourage a more holistic approach to the management of patients and to improve the level of patient-focused care.

REFLECTIVE QUESTIONS

- How could Amal begin to express her views in a supportive and constructive manner?
- Who should she speak to about her perception of patient care in the unit?

REFLECTIVE QUESTIONS

1. In a small group, discuss your experiences of technology. List strategies to improve understanding and appropriate use of technology in clinical practice and discuss with others.
2. In small groups, list three potential technology- and nursing-related research studies. In a larger group report on your proposed studies. Rank the accumulative list for their relative priority. Why have certain research studies been ranked above others?

RECOMMENDED READING

Australian Nurses Federation. Competency standards for nurses in general practice. Retrieved 2 September 2011. http://www.anf.org.au/nurses_gp/.

Barnard A, Sandelowski M. Technology and humane nursing care: a(n) (ir)reconcilable or invented difference? Journal of Advanced Nursing 2001;34:367–75.

Locsin R. Advancing technology, caring, and nursing. Westport, CT: Auburn House; 2001.

Marck PB. Recovering ethics after 'technics': developing critical text on technology. Nursing Ethics 2000;7:5–14.

Rinard R. Technology, deskilling, and nurses: the impact of the technologically changing environment. Advances in Nursing Science 1996;18:60–70.

REFERENCES

1. Feenberg A. Questioning technology. New York: Routledge; 1999.
2. Pacey A. Meaning in technology. Massachusetts: MIT Press; 1999.
3. Winner L. Autonomous technology. Massachusetts: MIT Press; 1977.
4. Rinard R. Technology, deskilling, and nurses: the impact of the technologically changing environment. Advances in Nursing Science 1996;18:60–70.
5. Barnard A. On the relationship between technique and dehumanization. In: Locsin R, editor. Technology, caring and nursing. Westport: Greenwood; 2001. p. 96–105.
6. Barnard, A, Locsin RC, editors. Technology and nursing practice. London: Palgrave-Macmillan; 2007.
7. Clifford C. Patients, relatives and nurses in a technological environment. Intensive Care Nursing 1986;2:67–72.
8. Fairman J, D'Antonio P. Virtual power: gendering the nurse–technology relationship. Nursing Inquiry 1999;6:178–86.
9. Purcell C. White heat: people and technology. London: BBC Publications; 1994.
10. Barnard, A, Locsin RC, editors. Technology and nursing practice. London: Palgrave-Macmillan; 2007.
11. Barnard A, Cushing A. Technology and historical inquiry in nursing. In: Locsin R, editor. Technology, caring and nursing. Westport: Greenwood; 2001. p. 12–21.
12. Fairman J. Watchful vigilance: nursing care, technology, and the development of intensive care units. Nursing Research 1992;41:56–60.
13. Pelletier D. Health care technology: sharpening the definition and establishing aspects of the social context. Australian Health Review 1989;12:56–64.
14. Reverby S. Ordered to care: the dilemma of American nursing, 1850–1945. Cambridge: Cambridge University Press; 1987.
15. Sandelowski M. Devices and desires: gender, technology and American nursing. Chapel Hill: University of North Carolina; 2000.
16. Fairman J. Response to tools of the trade: analysing technology as object in nursing. Scholarly Inquiry for Nursing Practice 1996;10:17–21.
17. McConnell EA. The impact of machines on the work of critical care nurses. Critical Care Nursing Quarterly 1990;12:45–52.
18. Sandelowski M. Tools of the trade: analysing technology as object in nursing. Scholarly Inquiry for Nursing Practice 1996;10:5–16.
19. Barnard A. Technology and nursing: an anatomy of definition. International Journal of Nursing Studies 1996;3:433–41.
20. Barnard A. Understanding technology in contemporary surgical nursing: a phenomenographic examination. PhD thesis. Armidale: University of New England; 1998.
21. Benner P. From novice to expert: excellence and power in clinical nursing practice. Menlo Park: Addison-Wesley; 1984.

22. Bondy KN. Criterion-referenced definitions for rating scales in clinical evaluation. Journal of Nursing Education 1983;22:376–82.

23. Krichbaum K. Clinical teaching effectiveness described in relation to learning outcomes of baccalaureate nursing students. Journal of Nursing Education 1994;33:306–16.

24. Australian Nurses Federation. Competency standards for nurses in general practice. 2011. Online. Available: http://www.anf.org.au/nurses_gp/ 15 Feb 2011.

25. Fuszard B. Innovative teaching strategies in nursing. Gaithersburg: Aspen; 1995.

26. Aviram M, Ophir R, Raviv D et al. Research briefs. Experiential learning of clinical skill by beginning nursing students. 'Coaching' project by fourth-year student interns. Journal of Nursing Education 1998;37:228–31.

27. Potter PA, Perry AG. Fundamentals of nursing: concepts, process, and practice. St Louis: Mosby; 1997.

28. Australian Council on Healthcare Standards (ACHS). EQuIP 4: Standards and guidelines for the ACHS. Sydney: ACHS; 2007.

29. Barnard A, Gerber R. Understanding technology in contemporary surgical nursing: a phenomenographic examination. Nursing Inquiry 1999;6:157–70.

30. Carnevali DL. Nursing perspectives in health care technology. Nursing Administration Quarterly 1985;9:10–8.

31. Pelletier D. Technology. In: Romanini J, Daly J, editors. Critical care nursing. Sydney: Harcourt Brace; 1994. p. 1039–63.

32. Pelletier D, Duffield C, Mitten-Lewis S, et al. Australian nurses and device use: the ideal and the real in clinical practice. Australian Critical Care 1998;11: 10–14.

33. Pillar B, Jacox AD, Redman BK. Technology, its assessment, and nursing. Nursing Outlook 1992;38:16–19.

34. Barnard A. Alteration to will as an experience of technology and nursing. Journal of Advanced Nursing 2000;31:1136–44.

35. Pelletier D. Diploma-prepared nurses' use of technological equipment in clinical practice. Journal of Advanced Nursing 1995;21:6–14.

36. Brown J. Nurses or technicians? The impact of technology on oncology nursing. Canadian Oncology Nursing Journal 1992;2:12–17.

37. Cooper MC. Care: antidote for nurses' love–hate relationship with technology. American Journal of Critical Care 1994;3:402–3.

38. Locsin R. Machine technologies and caring in nursing. Image: Journal of Nursing Scholarship 1995;27:201–3.

39. Locsin R. Technologic competence as caring in critical care. Holistic Nursing Practice 1998;12:50–6.

40. Green A. How nurses can ensure the sounds patients hear have a positive rather than negative effect upon recovery and quality of care. Intensive and Critical Care 1992;8:245–8.

41. Merideth C, Edworthy J. Are there too many alarms in the intensive care unit? An overview of the problems. Journal of Advanced Nursing 1995;21:15–20.

42. Sandelowski M. A case of conflicting paradigms: nursing and reproductive technology. Advances in Nursing Science 1988;10:35–45.

43. Barnard A, Sandelowski M. Technology and humane nursing care: (ir)reconcilable or invented difference? Journal of Advanced Nursing 2001;34:367–75.

44. Barnard A. Towards an understanding of technology and nursing practice. In: Greenwood J, editor. Nursing theory in Australia: development and application. 2nd ed. Sydney: Prentice Hall; 2000. p. 377–95.

45. McConnell E. How and what staff nurses learn about the medical devices they use in direct patient care. Research in Nursing and Health 1995;18:165–72.

46. Darbyshire P. Rage against the machine? Nurses and midwives' experiences of using computerized patient information systems for clinical information. Journal of Clinical Nursing 2003;13:17–25.

47. Keefe-McCarthy SO. Technologically-mediated nursing care: the impact on moral agency. Nursing Ethics 2009;16: 786–96.

48. Henderson A. The evolving relationship of technology and nursing practice: negotiating the provision of care in a high tech environment. Contemporary Nurse 2006;22: 59–65.

Establishing and maintaining a professional profile: issues in the first year of practice

Judy Mannix and Lyn Stewart

LEARNING OBJECTIVES

By the end of this chapter you will be able to:

- discuss the necessity for having an up-to-date professional profile
- demonstrate an understanding of the importance of ongoing professional development
- develop and maintain a professional portfolio
- clearly explain the preparation needed for a job interview
- debate the significance of lifelong learning in career planning and development.

Keywords: professional portfolio, curriculum vitae (CV), interview, career planning, lifelong learning

---

INTRODUCTION

As student nurses near the end of their preregistration education, thoughts focus on gaining entry into the workforce as a registered nurse and securing employment in an area of choice. Few student nurses tend to contemplate further education at this point. However, the reality is that completing a Bachelor of Nursing degree is not the end of a registered nurse's education; it is merely a foundation qualification to further studies in the postgraduate area. Opportunities in this area range from graduate certificates in clinical specialties through to Masters-level study and research higher degrees. Registered nurses can practise in a variety of clinical settings and within many clinical specialties. The possibility also exists for registered nurses to work outside the clinical genre, pursuing a management career in areas as diverse as the public sector, human resources, healthcare, industrial organisations or the private sector. As well, registered nurses can establish themselves in the education sector, within the health-care system or in the tertiary sector in universities, technical and further education institutes, polytechnics or institutes of technology.

To maximise choices from the range of experiences available in nursing and to develop a successful career, you, as a beginning registered nurse, need to have a plan that involves capitalising on opportunities to develop skills and expertise available in the workplace, or as part of a postregistration education course. Either way, the acquisition of skills and expertise is an important aspect in your development as a competent registered nurse and is reflective of self-regulation and autonomy, dimensions of professionalism in nursing.[1]

One strategy to assist with your successful career planning is to set about establishing a repository to house relevant details and information about your professional development. This type of repository may be referred to as a professional portfolio or a professional profile, depending on the situation. As Bowers and Jinks[2] explain, a professional portfolio is a private collection of evidence of professional development whereas a professional profile is a collection of evidence from your portfolio selected for a specific intention, e.g. to present at a job interview.

This chapter presents specific information to assist you in establishing a professional profile, including the development of a professional portfolio, preparing a CV and cover letter, applying for positions and preparing for an interview. We also examine aspects of lifelong learning and its importance in maintaining a professional profile.

DEVELOPING A PROFESSIONAL PORTFOLIO

Establishing a professional portfolio can occur quite early in your career, In fact, you may be familiar with portfolios because of their use as a way of assessing competence and learning during your undergraduate nursing course.[3] In this context portfolios can facilitate the integration of theory and practice through reflection.[4] Limiting their use to formal assessments is not the case in your working life as having a portfolio to reflect your professional and personal development will be an important aspect of your professional working life.

As a registered nurse and lifelong learner you can develop a comprehensive professional portfolio that comprises three different, yet related, categories:
1. an assessment portfolio
2. a learning or working portfolio
3. a portfolio for presentations.[5]

Each category of portfolio may be a focus at different times in your professional life, depending on the circumstances. For example, at some point you may engage in postgraduate studies where the development of an assessment portfolio is a requirement.[6] In terms of your day-to-day working life you are more likely to engage with a learning portfolio, particularly as a place to collect and record evidence of your critical reflections and your self-assessment of your practice against professional competency standards.[5] In a profession that demands the ability of nurses to integrate lifelong learning into the safe execution of patient care, a professional portfolio is a way of showing your increasing clinical practice expertise in a complete and holistic manner.[7] In addition, portfolios can serve as a repository for the documentation of lifelong learning, encompassing critical reflection, professional accomplishments and other professional experiences such as conference attendance.[7]

Increasingly, professional portfolios are being used or considered for use by regulatory authorities, as a way of nurses demonstrating continuing competency in their practice when applying or renewing their registration to practise.[5,7–11] For example, the New Zealand Nursing Council[10] expects all nurses applying for a practising certificate to be able to produce substantiated evidence of practice hours, professional development hours and assessment of competence. Similarly, in 2010 the Nursing and Midwifery Board of Australia[9] introduced standards requiring nurses and midwives to complete 20 hours of continuing professional development annually in order to ensure an authority to practise.

EXERCISE 17.1

Access a copy of the relevant competency framework for registered nurses (e.g. in Australia the Australian Nursing and Midwifery Council National Competency Standards for the Registered Nurse[8]; in New Zealand the Nursing Council of New Zealand Competency Framework[10]) and list how you think you can provide evidence of beginning competency in each of the areas. Also consider how you could plan to meet the competencies once you have completed your graduate year as a registered nurse.

How you design and structure your portfolio is a personal choice. You may elect to develop either a paper-based portfolio or an electronic portfolio. In an increasingly paperless workplace, e-portfolios are becoming more accessible, especially with the development of commercial e-portfolio software programs.[12] Anderson et al.[13] argue that the structure of the portfolio depends on the purpose of the portfolio. For example, to satisfy registering authorities one could use competency standards as a vertical scaffolding or spinal column and align evidence and critical reflections against relevant competencies.[13] Irrespective of how you present your portfolio, it is important that your portfolio evidence is relevant and reflects your continuing professional development. This may include:

- CV
- record of formal qualifications and practising certificate(s)
- copies of appraisals, including self-assessment, peer appraisal and performance appraisals
- review of competencies and career objectives
- evidence of achievement of competencies and objectives, e.g. outcomes of any committee work, attendance at study days, journal subscription
- plans to meet unmet competencies and objectives, e.g. mapping of learning opportunities for the coming year such as conference attendance and short courses.[14]

In some areas of your portfolio, for example your appraisals, it is advisable to keep one or two examples of evidence rather than every piece of evidence. As Mills[5] argues, the process of establishing and maintaining your portfolio involves reviewing, reflecting and recording. Your portfolio needs to be a catalyst for reflection and evaluation on your professional achievements and not merely a compilation of useful documents. By establishing and maintaining a professional portfolio to showcase your professional development you demonstrate your commitment to continuing education and life-long learning.[15]

EXERCISE 17.2

Take some time to consider how you might compile your own professional portfolio. In doing so, gather and organise all documents you think are relevant to your professional profile.

PREPARING YOUR CURRICULUM VITAE

A key aspect of your career development involves keeping an up-to-date record of your employment history, education and qualifications. This information is kept in your CV, or, as it is sometimes referred to, your résumé. Although it is not uncommon for the terms to be used interchangeably, a CV includes detailed information about your education, employment, research, publication and professional development history, while a résumé is a summary of your professional history, often limited to one or two pages in length, and tailored for a specific purpose, e.g. a promotion. You can develop your résumé from information contained in your CV.

As a registered nurse beginning your professional life, your CV will likely be brief in relation to clinical nursing experiences. However, it is important to note that some preregistration experiences, such as employment in a service-based position necessitating teamwork and competent communication skills, can be included in your CV to add to your profile. This will inform prospective employers of any transferable knowledge and skills that will enhance your capacity for a position. Nonetheless, you need to ensure that you have a CV and use it to keep an updated record (in an electronic format) of the roles, responsibilities and achievements of your professional life. Your CV is generally the first opportunity to impress potential employers, and, as such, needs to showcase your capabilities in relation to the position on offer. Therefore, in presenting your CV remember to highlight your strengths and key qualifications in relation to the position you are seeking.[16] Regardless of the format, your CV should be succinct, factual, clear and free of grammatical and spelling errors.[16] Providing personal information such as your age, marital status and country of birth is unnecessary in your CV; in fact, providing such information may detract from giving potential employers a professional impression.

When developing your CV it is suggested that you should present your information in the following order, ensuring that the most recent information is listed first in each section:

- Name and contact details (including phone and email addresses)
- Details of professional registration

- Education qualifications can follow. When showcasing your qualifications name the academic award, e.g., Bachelor of Nursing, the university or polytechnic and date of graduation
- List any professional prizes or awards you have received
- Professional employment history, beginning with your current position. If you have experience outside nursing it can also be included. In this section include position title, organisation, dates of employment and a brief descriptor of the role and associated responsibilities and achievements
- Professional development, including professional memberships, professional presentations, publications and research projects. You may also include in this section any continuing education that you have completed that did not lead to a formal educational qualification
- Specific skills and attributes that will assist you in a professional setting, e.g. fluency in a second language, advanced computing skills
- Referees: a list of referees comprises the final section of a CV. Most employers contact referees directly, either by phone or email. Therefore, it is imperative to provide accurate referee contact details. Ensure that before you submit a CV you ask potential referees if they agree to provide a reference. It is also important to select suitable referees, e.g. your nurse manager rather than a colleague of a similar level.

APPLYING FOR NURSING POSITIONS

In an employment environment where legislative requirements around equity and fairness guide employment practices, employers cannot discriminate on the basis of ethnicity, gender, age, sexual orientation, marital status, disability or religious beliefs.[17] The few exceptions to this relate to the nature of the position requirements, e.g. where a person of a particular ethnicity is deemed essential and appropriate for the provision of healthcare to a particular ethnic group. In these types of situation, employers can apply for exemptions from the legislation and this exemption would be stated in the position advertisement.

When you apply for a position you need to have a clear understanding of the process of staff selection procedures so that you maximise your chances in what is usually a competitive process. Begin with the job advertisement where the essential and desirable selection criteria are usually stated (Fig 17.1). The essential criteria listed will give you an indication of the qualities and background of the person being sought for the position. The selection criteria provide the key to obtaining an interview for a position, as they are the essential and desirable attributes used to determine the eligibility of an applicant for an interview.

In applying for a position in response to an advertisement, you need to show your capacity to meet all of the essential criteria and as many of the desirable attributes as possible. This is achieved using a cover letter (Fig 17.2) that accompanies your CV when applying for a position. The purpose of a cover letter is to introduce and showcase yourself as an applicant, and to indicate that you are awaiting confirmation of an interview for the position. Failure to showcase your ability to meet all essential criteria will usually result in being culled from the interview process. Therefore, if

Registered nurses (ref no. 08/04-06)
Surgical Unit, Westdown Hospital

The Division of Nursing, Westdown Hospital, invites registered nurses to apply for a full-time position on the surgical ward.

Essential

1. Current Nursing and Midwifery Board of Australia (NMBA) registration
2. Proof of works rights or citizenship within Australia or New Zealand
3. Recent clinical experience in an acute care setting
4. Commitment to quality improvement principles
5. Ability to work effectively within a multidisciplinary team
6. Documented evidence of ongoing professional development

Desirable

1. Effective written and verbal communication skills
2. Appropriate postgraduate qualifications
3. Computer competence

Closing date: 1 March 2012

Enquiries to: Nurse Unit Manager, Sally Yu 0418555333or sallyyu@westdown.gov.au

Applications to: Simon Saaid, Manager, Human Resources Unit, Westdown Hospital, Locked Bag 2060, Westdown NSW 1678

Fig 17.1 Sample job advertisement.

you are qualified for a position it is important to present yourself on paper so that employers will want you to be part of their organisation.

The application may be lodged by mail or electronically through the internet, requiring the cover letter and CV to be uploaded via a password-protected account. A receipt number as well as email notification (to your personal email account) is usually received once the application has been lodged. You may be required to complete screening questions requesting permission to undergo criminal record, working with children and immunisation checks before your application is uploaded as part of the terms of employment.

PREPARING FOR A PROFESSIONAL JOB INTERVIEW

Being called to an interview is the culmination of your employment-seeking activities. It means that you have successfully written about your suitability for a particular job. Your job application has convinced a selection panel that your qualifications, experience, knowledge and skills match the person specification (selection criteria) for the position for which you have applied. It also means that you have remembered that employers are bound by equal employment legislation.[18] This legislation requires that recruitment and applicant selection are based on clearly articulated, job-related criteria. Consequently your job application has addressed each and every one of the selection criteria and has led to your selection for interview.

Mary-Jo Barwon
Address

Mr Saaid
Address

15 February 2012

Dear Mr Saaid

I wish to apply for the recently advertised position of registered nurse, ref. 08/04-06 in the surgical unit of Westdown Hospital. As demonstrated below I meet all of the essential attributes for the position, as listed in the advertisement.

Current Nursing and Midwifery Board of Australia registration
I hold a current authority to practise in Australia (RN 00005).

Recent clinical experience in an acute care setting
Since completing my Bachelor of Nursing in 2008 I have worked in a variety of different medical, surgical and rehabilitation wards in acute hospitals. In my current position I work in a busy surgical unit, specialising in gynaecology and urology. Nursing patients in this setting has enabled me to develop my clinical skills in acute surgical nursing further.

Commitment to quality improvement principles
In my practice I am committed to delivering quality care to all patients. I am currently one of two elected nursing representatives on the hospital's Quality Management Committee, having served on the committee for 12 months.

Ability to work effectively within a multidisciplinary team
During my career I have found that working in multidisciplinary teams is an effective method of ensuring the delivery of holistic care to patients. In my previous position in the rehabilita-tion unit at Gracelands Community Hospital, patient care was managed effectively using a multidisciplinary team approach with input from nurses, medical officers and allied health professionals.

Demonstrated commitment to professional development
Throughout my career I have regularly attended relevant in-service education sessions and have achieved hospital accreditation in a number of clinical skills and procedures, docu-mented in my professional portfolio. Furthermore, I am currently enrolled as a part-time student in a Master of Nursing degree at Downtown University and am due to complete this course in the next 12 months. I have also recently presented a clinical paper at a national conference on renal nursing.

I believe that I am suitably qualified to fulfil the position and look forward to discussing this further at interview. Please find attached my curriculum vitae for your consideration.

Yours sincerely

Mary-Jo Barwon RN BN

Fig 17.2 Sample cover letter.

The preparation of your application, including a cover letter that addresses the person specification details (essential and desirable selection criteria) and your CV, will have given you the opportunity to consider carefully all requirements for the job and to explain exactly how you satisfy each one. This is an ideal beginning to your interview preparation.

It is likely that when you are notified of the success of your application, and have put an interview date in your diary, you will experience a level of anxiety and nervousness.[19] Adequate and strategic preparation for the interview can help you manage some of the anxiety you will be feeling. Confidence in your capacity to explain how your strengths, qualities and expertise make you the right person for the job will increase as you project yourself into the job for which you are being interviewed. Begin the preparation process immediately you are informed that you have been selected for interview.

Preparation checklist

1. Do some research into the hospital, organisation or area health centre where you are hoping to work. If there is a website available it will be a valuable source of information about the visionary statements of the organisation.
2. Learn as much as possible about the position and what the job entails.
3. Be clear about why you are interested in the job and what made you apply. Think through how it suits your professional interests. Will it provide you with the opportunity to work in an area you find stimulating and satisfying?
4. Think about the interview process. Anticipate the questions that may be asked for each of the selection criteria and rehearse your answers.
5. Ensure that the date and time of interview as well as the venue are in your diary.

RESEARCH INTO THE HOSPITAL, ORGANISATION OR AREA HEALTH SERVICE

Find out as much as you can about the values and mission statement of the organisation and then think about how they fit with the job for which you have applied. Reflect on your own values and interests and understand how they could enhance the organisation. Many organisations now have a website so this is a good place to start your research. You may know people who already work in the organisation and they would be an invaluable source of information about the structure of the organisation.

REVIEW THE POSITION SPECIFICATIONS AND WHAT THE JOB ENTAILS

Learn as much as you can about the job for which you are being interviewed. In the first instance have a detailed look at the job specification and the essential and desirable criteria. In addition seek information from the contact person specified in the job advertisement. This person is very likely to be a senior person, like a line manager, in the area for which the position has been advertised. You can expect this person to be very knowledgeable about the position and its associated responsibilities. It may also be useful to do some background reading to enhance your knowledge about specific aspects of the position and role.

KNOW WHY YOU ARE INTERESTED IN THE JOB

It would be usual for a selection panel to ask you why you have applied for the job. This is a question that can be difficult to answer if you have not thought about it in advance. It may require you to talk about the qualities you would bring to the job. Your response should include an explanation of your strengths as appropriate to the job, and a discussion of what you have to offer as a person and as a professional.

THINK ABOUT THE INTERVIEW PROCESS

Human resources departments are able to confirm the number of people who will be present at your interview. This is good information because there may be up to five people interviewing you and this can increase anxiety levels if you are not prepared. The standard format for the interview is for each member of the selection panel to ask one or two questions. The questions are identical for each person being interviewed. Time is usually made available at the end for you to ask questions of the panel, if you wish. Anticipate a venue that may be large and feel sterile so that you are not surprised and discomforted on the day. The chairperson of the selection panel will try to put you at ease and you will be provided with a drink.

ANTICIPATE THE QUESTIONS THAT MAY BE ASKED

Interview questions are based on the position specification and the essential and desirable criteria. Being very familiar with these will enable you to anticipate the topics that will be included in the interview and to give appropriate and detailed responses to questions. Think through the main aspects of each of the criteria and from this write questions that you think could be asked to elicit your knowledge and experience. Sometimes the panel will ask you to give examples to support the claims that you make about your experiences. The question-and-answer approach may sometimes include a request that you pre-prepare a response to a given scenario, or you may be given a scenario during the interview to which you will need to respond spontaneously.

If relevant to the job description, the selection panel may be interested in knowing about your ability to communicate, to work independently and/or in a group, to solve problems and to set goals. The panel may want to ascertain how you will achieve goals that are set and whether you practise critical self-reflection when evaluating your achievements. This will be the case in an organisation that stipulates that the person who is offered the job be someone who is reflective about his or her capacities and clear about professional aspirations. As a result the person specifications, as well as the criteria, may require that the panel ask you questions about your strengths and weaknesses, short- and long-term career goals, approach to interpersonal communication and capacity for managing difficult situations, as well as your familiarity with occupational health and safety and equal employment opportunity legislation.

The selection panel will be interested in whether or not you can give examples of your practice in a certain area. Always know how you know that you have been good at something. Think about what evidence you may need to provide to convince the selection panel that you have detailed knowledge of all aspects of the job.

EXERCISE 17.3

Find a job advertisement for a registered nurse, either from a newspaper or on the internet. Note the essential and desirable attributes listed in the advertisement. From the advertisement, develop at least five questions that could be asked at an interview. Develop written responses to the questions you have developed.

REHEARSE ANSWERS

Once you have decided what questions are likely to be asked, prepare answers that are focused only on the question, and that are always to the point. Be disciplined in your thinking and do background reading if you cannot explain concepts in much detail. Ask friends and work colleagues to run through the questions with you and to give you honest feedback about your answers. Try not to be unsettled if questions for which you have not prepared are asked on the day. Remember your reasons for applying for the job, and the goodness of fit between the job description and your own personal and professional strengths and you will be able to fashion an appropriate answer on the spot.

WRITE THE DATE, TIME AND VENUE OF INTERVIEW IN YOUR DIARY

Ensure that the interview date, time and venue are in your diary. Leave nothing to chance. If you are not familiar with the address or the venue take a trip there before your interview, find the parking lot and make sure you have correct money if parking is not free. This will lead to a worry-free trip on the day of the interview.

Interview day

There are some golden rules that you should follow on the day of the interview. Give yourself sufficient time for travel so that you arrive at the interview with time to spare. If uncertain about what to wear, dress more formally than you would normally, in clothes that look fresh and well groomed. Be courteous when introduced to the panel, maintaining good eye contact and responding to questions with interest and enthusiasm. Careful interview preparation will help you to ensure that your answers are comprehensive and yet succinct. Be thoughtful when responding, but get to the point of your answer quickly. At every opportunity illustrate the point you are making with an example. If you are unsure about what is meant by a question ask the panel to clarify what they are asking. Come to the interview ready to ask one or two questions about the position or the organisation. Take care not to ask questions that may indicate a lack of knowledge about the position or that you have not prepared for the interview. The chair of the panel will inform you of what comes next in the process, and when you are likely to hear the outcome of the interview.

After the interview

Irrespective of your success in gaining the position, critical self-reflection about your performance at interview can help you to develop your interview skills. Jot down how you felt on the day, what questions were asked and your evaluation of the appropriateness of your responses. Inevitably you will think of things you wish you had said. Write these down too so that they can inform your preparation for any subsequent interviews. Seek feedback from the panel, through the chairperson. Compare the panel's feedback with your own reflections and, above all, learn from the experience. This will enable you to develop interview-related skills and strategies that will be useful throughout your career.

MAINTAINING LIFELONG LEARNING THROUGHOUT YOUR NURSING CAREER

Lifelong learning has been recognised as an important component of a skilled and professional workforce. As a new graduate you have experienced a unique learning journey including learning experiences prior to your nursing studies, classroom experiences during the course and the diverse learning experiences gained during clinical practicum. Upon entering a professional workforce you need to embrace opportunities to maintain and enhance your graduate-entry skills.

Lifelong learners have been described as individuals who accept responsibility for their own learning and are willing to make the effort and find the time to involve themselves on a regular and continuous basis in education or training.[20] Lifelong learners are referred to as the 'pillars' of a learning society,[20] acquiring transferable skills as they learn for application to their relevant field of practice (such as nursing). These skills include life skills such as: 'learning to be', to enhance creativity and personal fulfilment; 'learning to know', by acquiring new knowledge and skills to facilitate the development of critical thinking and competence; and 'learning to live [and work] together', thereby 'exercising tolerance, understanding and mutual respect'.[20]

An Australian government report on lifelong learning[20] recognises that a blend of both formal and informal learning occurs as the amount of education and training increases to provide the community with individuals with higher-level skills. Therefore self-motivated learning, either self- or employer-funded, has been highlighted as a necessity in building a skilled workforce. It is important for you to develop strategies to maximise opportunities for both formal and informal learning as you start your transition from student to professional nurse.

Strategies for achieving lifelong learning

As a registered nurse there will be numerous opportunities for professional development and lifelong learning. Table 17.1 outlines key indicators and strategies to facilitate this process in your career.

Lifelong learning resources in the workplace

In the nursing workplace opportunities exist for lifelong learning. As the major employer of nurses the healthcare industry has the capacity to offer countless opportunities for nurses to develop both personal and professional skills for career progression. This infrastructure includes the provision of a library with access to a broad range of journals, periodicals and online resources available to all staff. Spending time accessing and browsing these resources can be an enjoyable and relaxing activity to do on a regular basis, assisting you to stay up to date with professional issues and research.

Table 17.1 Strategies for achieving lifelong learning

Descriptor	Strategy	Rationale
Maintaining contemporary knowledge in nursing	• Postgraduate studies, whether university-, college-or industry-based • Professional development opportunities in your workplace • Regularly reading peer-reviewed journal articles • Maintain currency with policies and procedures at industry, state and national level	Although the major motivation for completing these postgraduate courses may be practice-based to develop higher-level clinical skills, academic scholarship is often enhanced. As a graduate you need to be well informed regarding courses on offer to ensure that the targeted course addresses your learning needs, assists with the development of your chosen career path and maintains your continued professional education (CPE) requirements for NMBA licensure[9] or the Nursing Council of New Zealand.[10] Currently, it is an expectation that graduates enter the healthcare domain with the ability to demonstrate self-reliance and self-directed learning capacity[9,10]
Membership of professional organisations	• Join special-interest groups, reflective of your clinical interest/s – specialty interest groups affiliated with larger organisations such as the Coalition of National Nursing Organisations (CoNNO)[21] • National and international nursing organisations, e.g. Royal College of Nursing, Australia (RCNA), College of Nurses Aotearoa (NZ), Sigma Theta Tau International (STTI)	Access to peer-reviewed journals, bulletins, as well as opportunities to attend seminars, professional days and conferences that enable clinicians to enhance lifelong learning, network, develop collegial relationships (including mentoring), debate professional issues, and keep up to date with current practice and research. Professional organisations continue to support nurses in their pursuit of lifelong learning by offering scholarships for postgraduate study, conference attendance and research
Membership of an industrial organisation	• Engage with industrial media bulletins, press releases and journals • Attend workplace meetings of the organisation • Participate as delegate in the organisation	Industrial organisations are the nurses' advocate, negotiating on our behalf with employers and governments for provision of study days when negotiating industrial awards. Industrial organisations also arrange workplace-related seminars and workshops to keep members informed of safe work practices and other workplace issues. For example, the NSW Nurses' Association[22] conducts, as part of its annual conference, a professional day for members. Similarly, the New Zealand Nurses Organisation[23] provides professional development opportunities for nurses to attend throughout the year. Industrial organisations also provide online CPE opportunities which may be supported by scholarships

NMBA, Nursing and Midwifery Board of Australia.

The majority of industry workplaces have education units to promote ongoing continuous education. Nurse educators can be assigned to wards and units to deliver clinical education and support within the clinical learning environment, thereby enabling nurses to improve their skills. Many larger healthcare institutions are offering clinical support over extended hours to provide support to nurses when it is required, regardless of the time or day. In addition, a more formal style of education is offered through the many in-service education sessions held on a regular basis throughout the institution to improve the quality and standards of care.[24]

The transition period from student to registered nurse encompasses an intense period of on-the-job learning as you move from a formal learning process to a more self-directed informal approach to achieving your own career goals and objectives. Transition is an exciting and invigorating time for most graduates but it can also be a time of critical reflection when your own ideas about nursing may be significantly challenged. Both formal learning obtained from tertiary institutions such as universities and informal learning acquired by workplace experience will assist you to move towards becoming an expert nurse in your chosen field, as described by Benner.[25] Therefore, engaging in strategic lifelong learning will enable you to develop confidence in your ability to perform as a registered nurse in a contemporary nursing workforce.

CONCLUSION

As a registered nurse you will find that nursing presents you with many opportunities for career development. In this chapter we have provided information about establishing your professional profile, including developing your professional portfolio and CV, and preparing for professional job interviews. The discussion of lifelong learning highlights its importance to your professional development. Giving yourself time to showcase your career development through a professional portfolio enables you to reflect on your career strengths and weaknesses, and helps with career planning and achieving career goals.

ACKNOWLEDGMENT

The authors would like to thank and acknowledge Debra Jackson, Nikki Brown and Ana Smith for their contribution to this chapter in previous editions of the text.

CASE STUDY 17.1

During his transition year, one of Joseph's placements is community health within a large metropolitan community health centre. During this placement Joseph will attend an orientation program and work through a series of clinically based modules to prepare for this role. To facilitate his transition from acute to community nursing, Joseph is assigned to an experienced nurse who will act as a mentor during this placement.

REFLECTIVE QUESTION

How will Joseph record this experience in his professional portfolio so that it accurately reflects both educational and clinical opportunities, and also demonstrates his clinical competence?

CASE STUDY 17.2

During Rosie's second rotation in her transition year she is assigned to an acute 28-bed medical ward in a large rural facility. On arrival for an evening duty shift Rosie is informed that the experienced registered nurse who was team leader for this shift has called in sick at short notice. Rosie has been informed by the nursing unit manager that she will be the team leader for this shift. This will be the first opportunity Rosie has had in the role of team leader. Apart from two experienced enrolled nurses rostered on for the evening shift, an experienced replacement registered nurse from the casual list will be available for the 8-hour shift.

REFLECTIVE QUESTION

What strategies and resources could assist Rosie in preparing for this new role and its increased responsibilities?

CASE STUDY 17.3

After completing her new graduate program, Beryl secured a permanent position in the general medical ward of the hospital. Many of the patients admitted to the ward require management of acute and chronic wounds as a consequence of underlying medical conditions. Because of the number of patients requiring wound management, Beryl has attended a number of wound care in-service education sessions and has attended a national wound care conference in the last year. At the conference Beryl joined the Wound Care Association and has attended the quarterly meetings. She is also currently helping in a research project being conducted by the regional clinical nurse consultant in wound management. Beryl has been working in the ward for 2 years and is now considering applying for clinical nurse specialist (CNS) status in the area of wound management.

REFLECTIVE QUESTION

In her application for CNS status, how could Beryl use her membership in the Wound Care Association and her other professional activities to support and strengthen her case?

RECOMMENDED READING

Andre K, Heartfield M. Professional portfolios: evidence of competency for nursing and midwives. Sydney: Elsevier; 2007.

Bright K. Getting a brilliant job: the student's guide; resumes, interview skills and everything you need to know to convince a prospective employer. Sydney: Allen & Unwin; 2005.

Chambers P. From bystander to architect: designing the nursing career you want. Viewpoint 2009; March/April: 4–5. Online. Available: www.aaacn.org.

Howatson-Jones L. Transforming nursing practice: reflective practice in nursing. Exeter: Learning Matters; 2010.

McAllister L, Hallam G, Harper W. The ePortfolio as a tool for lifelong learning: contextualising Australian practice. In: Proceedings International Lifelong Learning Conference 2008; 246-252. Online. Available: http://eprints.qut.edu.au/.

REFERENCES

1. Kim-Godwin Y, Baek H, Wynd C. Factors influencing professionalism in nursing among Korean American registered nurses. Journal of Professional Nursing 2010;26:242–249.
2. Bowers S, Jinks A. Issues surrounding professional portfolio development for nurses. British Journal of Nursing 2004;13:155–159.
3. Taylor C, Stewart L, Bidewell J. Nursing students' appraisal of their professional portfolios in demonstrating clinical competence. Nurse Educator 2009;34: 217–222.
4. McMullan M. Using portfolios for clinical practice learning and assessment: the pre-registration nursing student's perspective. Nurse Education Today 2008;28: 873–879.
5. Mills J. Professional portfolios and Australian registered nurses' requirements for licensure: developing an essential tool. Nursing and Health Sciences 2009;11: 206–210.
6. McCready T. Portfolios and the assessment of competence in nursing: a literature review. International Journal of Nursing Studies 2007;44:143–151.
7. Byrne M, Schroeter K, Carter S, et al. The professional portfolio: an evidence-based assessment method. Journal of Continuing Education in Nursing 2009;40: 545–552.
8. Australian Nursing and Midwifery Council (ANMC). Online. Available: http://www.anmc.org.au 1 November 2010.
9. Nursing and Midwifery Board of Australia (NMBA). Registration standards. Online. Available: http://www.nursingandmidwiferyboard.gov.au/Registration-Standards.aspx 1 November 2010.
10. Nursing Council of New Zealand Te Kaunihera Tapuhi o Aotearoa. Continuing competence framework. Online. Available: http://www.nursingcouncil.org.nz 1 November 2010.
11. College of Registered Nurses of British Columbia. Online. Available: https://www.crnbc.ca/Pages/Default.aspx 1 November 2010.
12. Parslow G. Multimedia in biochemistry and molecular biology education, Commentary: ePortfolios, beyond the curriculum vitae. Biochemistry and Molecular Biology Education 2009;37:131–132.
13. Anderson D, Gardner G, Ramsbotham J, et al. E-portfolios: developing nurse practitioner competence and capability. Australian Journal of Advanced Nursing 2009;26:70–76.
14. Andre K, Heartfield M. Professional portfolios: evidence of competency for nursing and midwives. Sydney: Elsevier; 2007.
15. Billings D, Kowalski K. Learning portfolios. Journal of Continuing Education in Nursing 2005;36:149–150.
16. Grogan L, Gelman J. How to write a killer CV. Intheblack 2009;79:32–35.
17. Department of Labour Te Tari Mahi. Guide to hiring for employers. Online. Available: http://ers.govt.nz/relationships/hiringguide/index.html 1 November 2010.
18. Department of Premier and Cabinet. New South Wales Government. What is EEO? Online. Available: http://www.eeo.nsw.gov.au/ 1 November 2010.

19. Sieverding M. 'Be cool!' Emotional costs of hiding feelings in a job interview. International Journal of Selection and Assessment 2009;17:391–401.

20. Department of Education, Science & Training (DEST). Lifelong learning in Australia. Canberra: Commonwealth of Australia; 2003.

21. Coalition of National Nursing Organisations (CoNNO). Online. Available: http://www.conno.org.au/ 1 November 2010.

22. NSW Nurses' Association (NSWNA). Online. Available: http://www.nswnurses.asn.au/ 1 November 2010.

23. New Zealand Nurses Organisation (NZNO). Online. Available: http://www.nzno.org.nz/ 1 November 2010.

24. Bahn D. Orientation of nurses towards formal and informal learning: motives and perceptions. Nurse Education Today 2007;27:723–730.

25. Benner P. From novice to expert: excellence and power in clinical nursing practice. Menlo Park: Addison-Wesley; 1984.

CHAPTER 18

Dealing with the theory–practice gap in clinical practice

Maxine Duke and Helen Forbes

LEARNING OBJECTIVES

When you have completed this chapter, you will be aware of the:

- expectations facing new graduates entering the workforce
- imperative of a sound theoretical preparation for safe practice
- potential challenges faced by new graduates
- strategies to deal with the transition from student to registered nurse
- strategies to provide optimal patient care.

Keywords: theory–practice, evidence-based practice, reflection, critical thinking, confidence

---

INTRODUCTION

The nexus between theory and practice has been a topic of debate in the nursing literature since the time of Florence Nightingale. The amount of literature and discussion afforded the topic increased significantly in Australia with the commencement of the transfer of nursing education to the tertiary setting in the 1970s. Most observations conclude that a theory–practice gap exists in nursing and it is most often described as problematic.

Certainly, it was a well-held belief that there is a gap between what was taught in the classroom and what is needed in day-to-day practice.[1] Walker[2] argued that there are tensions between those who theorise about nursing and those who actually provide care. This kind of debate implied that either theory or practice was more valuable. Clearly this was a naïve understanding of what is an inextricable relationship and was divisive and unhelpful to those entering the profession for the first time. In this chapter, we explore some of the expectations ahead of you as newly registered nurses. The literature related to transition issues and strategies for management are designed to help you to integrate and apply your knowledge in practice as you develop your professional identity.

WHAT WILL IT BE LIKE?

Exhilarating, dynamic, scary, exhausting and a massive learning curve are some of the myriad of emotions and feelings that graduates mention when describing their initial experiences as newly registered nurses.[3] Undoubtedly, you will share some of these opinions when dealing with your new status. Some experiences you will approach with confidence and pleasure, while others may cause you to reflect upon your own knowledge and skill as you come to grips with the adjustment to your new role and responsibilities.[4]

Duchscher[3] argues that the variations and unpredictability of clinical contexts may contribute to newly graduated nurses feeling underconfident and anxious. Importantly, though, within a few short months there is a rapid increase in thinking, knowledge and skill competence. Schoessler and Waldo[5] suggest that during this process of adjustment it is important to recognise that you are in an evolutionary process. This acceptance can ease your transition and allow you to reinforce what you do know and identify what may be missing from your experience thus far. Dealing with your anxiety will be an important aspect of managing your emotions and thus we ask you to complete Exercise 18.1.

EXERCISE 18.1

The opening sentiments in the previous paragraphs are those that new registered nurses have used to express their feelings in the first few weeks of their practice.

- Do the feelings mentioned above strike a chord with you?
- Have you had similar feelings in other facets of your life? First date? Examinations? Becoming a parent? New job? University assessment? Clinical placements?

    Jot down some of the strategies you use to deal with anxiety-producing situations in your life. Some that we have found to be useful include:

- deep breathing
- counting to 10
- positive self-talk:
    - 'I have had a sound education'
    - 'I do know a lot'
    - 'I am not alone here'
    - 'I can find out what I don't know'
    - 'There are people to help me'
- preparing well for anticipated events by practising and reading
- checking for accuracy before proceeding
- debriefing with someone who has had similar experiences.

    Can you use any of these coping strategies to meet the challenges of being a registered nurse?

Armed with familiar coping strategies you may feel better prepared to deal with the clinical day and the many new challenges it presents. Cheeks and Dunn[6] assert that uneasiness and feelings of inadequacy can lead to new graduates reproaching themselves for not coping, when what they are experiencing is part of the normal transition phase. Likewise, Schoessler and Waldo[5] point out that this phase is difficult and must not be mistaken as failure on the new nurse's part or a sign that the nurse is in the wrong profession. They further caution that there is no way to 'leap over' this stage of development, no matter how disconcerting it may be. It is important to assure yourself that these feelings are normal and will pass as you develop confidence and become comfortable in your role.

WHAT WILL BE EXPECTED OF YOU?

You will be expected to do the job! So, what does the job entail? You are well aware that nurses are concerned with health promotion, recuperation from illness and facilitating death with dignity. Nursing is said to be both art and science, the essence of which involves the interplay of knowledge, intuition, critical thinking and compassion for others.[7] You will also be conscious of competencies that are expected of beginning practitioners. These competencies are clustered under four domains of practice: (1) professional practice; (2) critical thinking and analysis; (3) provision and coordination of care; and (4) collaborative and therapeutic practice, and provide a framework to guide beginning-level practice.[7] However, Hinds and Harley[8] found that new graduates often perceive competence to be more related to their ability to cope with every given situation rather than the attainment of the professional body's competencies. It is important to appreciate that the hallmark of professional practice is the continuous development of knowledge and skills over time and that it is therefore unrealistic to expect to feel capable in every circumstance. Fox et al.[9] conducted a two-phase longitudinal study to explore new staff perceptions of support during transition. The study involved 16 newly qualified nurses and concluded that there is a connection between successful socialisation, that is, 'getting to know the place' (p 197), and confidence levels about personal knowledge and skill.

You, may however, find that other registered nurses have expectations of your performance that do not take into account your need to adapt your knowledge and skill from that of student to registered nurse in an environment that is supportive and encouraging. You may hear discussions about the need for evidence-based practice to ensure quality and safe care and this may lead you to consider whether you have been provided with the skills and knowledge to deliver this objective.

We would argue that for the most part you will have had an excellent preparation for your chosen career. In particular you will have a sound understanding of evidence-based practice. Nevertheless, Duchscher[3] suggests that the gap between what you know and how you use what you know will narrow only as your expertise develops. Speedy[10] warns that expertise and experience are not the same as length of time in the job, or seniority of position. Thus there is a relationship between what you know and how skill develops in practice. Nurses gain expertise by virtue of their knowledge and their ability to observe, reflect upon and analyse the essence of nursing care. Therefore, we encourage you to respect your current levels of knowledge and skill at the same time as you commit to continuing your learning by using the best available evidence every time you plan and deliver patient care. This approach provides not only optimal outcomes for patients but personal job satisfaction.

A study by Daehlen[11] compared Norwegian nursing graduates' levels of job satisfaction, perceived rewards and values with medical and teaching graduates, firstly, as they commenced their new roles and again 3 years later. While all graduates were 'fairly satisfied', the degree to which their job was thought to be interesting appeared to be related to the level of job satisfaction. Therefore we encourage you to take advantage of the people around you who can guide your development. This will help build your confidence and thus ensure the quality of the care you deliver, your satisfaction with your work and ultimately patient safety.

WHO WILL HELP YOU?

Transition (graduate-year) programs are considered one way of supporting new graduates. Although there is a perception that transition programs are necessary before proceeding to independent practice, remember that this is not so — the programs are not compulsory but are one formalised means of supporting new graduates. Transition programs evolved to meet a perceived need to support registered nurses in their first year of practice. With the advent of more sophisticated clinical models developed collaboratively between universities and healthcare agencies, some hospitals believe there is less need for this formalised year as transition is occurring more rapidly. In some Australian states, however, these programs are supported financially through government initiatives to meet the needs of beginning registered nurses and to provide an incentive for hospitals to employ graduates.[12] Although, as a beginning graduate, you have accumulated a body of knowledge, Kolb[13] asserts that such knowledge is awaiting transformation through clinical experience. Transition programs are generally designed to facilitate this transformation.

The crucial component of these programs, however they are organised, is the provision of support for the nurse in the clinical setting. This support may come from a variety of sources, and will vary according to how the program is structured and the range of resources available. Clinical educators, preceptors and experienced clinical nurses all provide support as they work with graduates in various capacities.

Clinical educators in this context are registered nurses with a wealth of clinical experience, who also have educational skills and have developed a high level of expertise in facilitating learning in the clinical setting. Because they are not a part of the management structure of the ward and, in many hospitals, are not attached to a specific ward, they are able to provide an objective unbiased view of any clinical issue that may arise. They are also aware of other resources and support systems that may be available to assist you through the period of transition.

Where a preceptorship program is in place, the new nurse is assigned a preceptor for a specified period. This nurse acts as a role model and support person throughout the period of orientation to the clinical area. A useful guideline is provided by

Johnstone et al.,[14] who recommend that support be provided for a minimum of 4 weeks. Programs where mentorship or preceptorship is provided have been found to increase new graduate confidence and lead to independent practice more quickly.[15] Maben et al.[16] argue that high-quality mentors/preceptors are essential in helping the new graduate to manage the transition from university to work and to negotiate the inherent differences between the two. Hopefully, the relationship between you and your preceptor, if you are in such a program, is close and supportive, to allow you to begin to transfer your theoretical knowledge to practice, gain confidence and become a member of the team. Many graduates report that their preceptor becomes a mentor over a long period of time, as a high level of trust and confidence develops between the two. (Preceptorship and mentorship are covered in detail in other chapters in this book.) All nurses in the wards are potentially excellent resources for you.

The most important aspect of a transition program is the clinical support and resources it offers. In selecting a program, it is well worth spending time gathering information so that you can compare the day-to-day support offered by a range of programs. Individual hospitals may offer opportunities to speak with graduates already in programs regarding support in the clinical environment. Nursing 'expos' or trade fairs, if available, provide a valuable means of gathering information about graduate programs in a range of hospitals and other health facilities. It is worth considering whether stability in one placement will benefit consolidation of theory and practice and eliminate the need for repeated orientation and team building.

DEVELOPING PRACTICE EXPERTISE BY THINKING, DOING, REFLECTING

Despite the obvious constraints of the current healthcare system you will have noted experienced nurses who seem like magicians, juggling several patient care activities at once. You have probably admired these abilities whenever you have witnessed them and long for the day when it flows as easily for you. Consider one such nurse in Exercise 18.2.

EXERCISE 18.2

A registered nurse caring for 5 patients on a busy ward was observed carrying out the following activities: first, she placed an oximeter on one patient's finger, then hurried off to assist an unsteady elderly patient to walk to the toilet. Leaving the patient in the toilet, she returned, filled an intravenous burette after an antibiotic had been completed, recorded the first patient's oxygen saturation and heart rate and returned to collect the patient from the toilet.

Consider these actions:

1. Were they time-efficient?
2. Did they meet the needs of the patients?
3. Were they safe?
4. Did they provide accurate patient information?

Over the years of working in education and practice we have noticed that new graduates often attempt to mimic the efficient behaviour of more experienced nurses without due thought to the elements of the activities. While the registed nurse in Exercise 18.2 is obviously time- and task-efficient, it was not obvious that the patients' needs were met. Was it important to know the character and regularity of the heart rate? Was the integrity of the intravenous site maintained after the administration of the antibiotic? Was it safe to leave the unsteady patient alone in the bathroom? While the answer to all these questions may be 'yes', there are those who would argue that the care provided was task-oriented rather than person-centred. Certainly, there are traps for new players who imitate such an approach without carefully considering the detail of patient care.

It has been reported that newly registered nurses use incorrect techniques which they justify as 'short cuts' in order to 'get through' their workload,[17] believing this to be real nursing as they see it performed by experienced nurses. What is not often apparent to them is that those with experience have finetuned their judgment to such an extent that they only appear to be taking short cuts. Their expertise allows them to make quick assessments with minimal fuss, anticipate outcomes and, as a result, efficiently manipulate a number of tasks at the same time without compromising patient safety.

This capacity is not easily achieved without experience but the development of this ability begins in the educational system. The aim of nursing educational programs is to teach the principles of nursing practice based on research findings. This is done within a theoretical framework that honours the central concept of nursing and patient-centred care. To achieve this aim, students are given many clinical learning opportunities to develop their understanding of these principles and concepts. However, once you are working as a registered nurse you may find it difficult to maintain the person-centred approach because adhering to the routine and getting through the work will be much more the focus of your attention. Exercise 18.3 will encourage you to look beyond the tasks to the principles and knowledge embedded in the actions.

EXERCISE 18.3

Describe the activities you have seen 'juggled' simultaneously by experienced nurses. Try to 'tease out' how they were able to do this.
1. Could the nurse explain the theory behind the actions?
2. Have you considered the role of accurate assessment skills?
3. Is it safe for you to mimic the behaviour of experienced nurses in terms of task performance?

THE REGISTERED NURSE AS LEARNER

Despite the likelihood that you will spend the first few months as a registered nurse in a supportive transition program and that your learning curve will be steep, the expectation of all nurses, at all levels and spheres of practice, is that they will identify and seek out appropriate learning experiences. This pattern of self-directed learning was probably encouraged in your undergraduate education and continues to be an expectation of you as a professional. An important aspect of self-directed learning is the ability to identify knowledge deficits – that is, to 'know what you don't know'. The awareness of gaps in knowledge, linked to the ability to reflect on practice, is essential for the nurse to be a safe practitioner. Accountability for your actions includes the ability to recognise when knowledge is insufficient, resulting in the need to consult with a resource or support person before proceeding. Safe practitioners know their limitations, in both knowledge and in experience.

It is important from the first day of your professional career to establish personal standards and systems for identifying learning deficits, and gathering and maintaining knowledge and skills, so as to ensure your clinical practice remains contemporary. A whole range of resources is available to assist in this process. Most hospitals have libraries, or ready access to library facilities, that include resources focused on clinical practice and specialties of the hospital. Libraries are usually multidisciplinary and provide the opportunity to access medical and allied health journals and books as well as those published for nurses. Setting aside a regular time, even a short period, provides the opportunity to browse through current journals and new books in the library. It can be extremely valuable to purchase a reference text if you are working in a specialty, or to subscribe to a highly relevant journal.

It is important that all registered nurses, including beginning graduates, take advantage of the many learning opportunities available in the clinical setting. Many clinical areas conduct in-service education sessions on a regular basis; these usually relate to topics of particular interest to the staff in those areas but may also include broader topics of interest to all, such as occupational health and safety issues, and quality improvement. Most hospitals and healthcare agencies provide opportunities for continuing your learning. These programs or sessions cover a range of topics, including clinical development, professional development, management and interpersonal skills. It is important to select relevant, pertinent sessions that have application to your current area of employment. Many conferences and short courses offer opportunities for nurses to extend and expand their knowledge so that they remain abreast of contemporary practice. It is important that you document the various activities that you undertake in your professional portfolio to demonstrate your ongoing development. The portfolio will become important to verify your contemporary practice when you apply to re-register each year.

REFLECTION

You will no doubt recognise learning activities 18.2 and 18.3 as a way of promoting reflection. Rolfe[18] suggests that nurses develop their own informal theories as a result of drawing from their scientific and nursing theory base. This is then combined with their own knowledge of the patient and of similar cases. This process of theory development is called 'reflection in action' and is described as combining scientific and personal knowledge by reflecting on practice to understand the principles and processes involved.[19] Rolfe[20] claims that this type of reflection leads to improvement in professional judgment and the emergence of a personal theory of practice. Forneris and Peden-McAlpine[21] suggest that nurses develop their knowledge and critical thinking ability as a result of reflecting on practice. The process of evaluating beliefs and assumptions within the clinical context assists you to understand the specific situation better. You may find your own theory will develop from drawing on your past experience, from the feedback you receive, and by reflection on things that you did very well and the things that didn't go so well.

EXERCISE 18.4

Think about how doctors learn. Do you ever see medical students on their own? Your answer is probably, 'no, not usually'. Medical students travel in groups, talking to each other and to doctors who are more experienced than themselves as well as those who have specialised knowledge. Doctors present cases to each other at morbidity and mortality meetings. Is there anything in this approach that nurses can emulate?

Develop a network with peers in which you either share or listen to accounts of care decisions that had to be made. Ask:
- What were the facts of the situation?
- What did you think was happening?
- How did you check your perceptions?
- Which alternatives did you generate?
- What resources did you use to assist the decision making?
- What decisions were made?
- What did you learn from the situation?
- Can this information be transferred to other situations?

In developing your personal theory and expertise it may be that mistakes will be made. The need for reflection is often triggered by a 'near miss' such as a potential medication error. Regardless of their level of experience, most nurses can recall making a mistake. If you discuss this with other nurses you will find that, overwhelmingly, they report having learned from the mistake and never allowing it to happen again. In other words, they are developing a personal theory of practice derived from experience.

For most of us, making a mistake will precipitate some soul searching, especially when we suffer from a loss of confidence. However, the reason nurses rarely repeat their mistakes is that they reflect upon them. Often this activity is not recognised as reflection, as it can be a self-conscious and shamefaced experience. Nevertheless, it is usually true that a mistake made in practice is accompanied by a period in which the nurse consciously considers how it happened, who was involved, who said what and who did what, and asks: What was my role? What could I have done differently? Importantly, healthcare agencies now recognise that, when errors occur, proper investigation of the systems involved is more helpful than blaming individuals. If you make a mistake it is highly likely others like you in similar situations will make similar mistakes. Therefore, your hospital will have a reporting system such as RiskMan and processes that include root cause analysis aimed at identifying gaps in the system to prevent similar occurrences.

EXERCISE 18.5

Describe an incident from your clinical practice that demonstrates the difference between your ideal of care and what can actually be achieved. It may have occurred when you were a student, or as a new graduate.

Describe as objectively as possible what took place. At this point avoid interpretations and analysis. Just give a detailed account of what happened.

- What was your role?
- What was the flow of events?
- What was the result?
- What did you feel about what you did?
- Now think about what you are concerned about in regard to this incident. What do you think is the underlying issue that needs to be addressed?

ETHICAL AND OTHER DILEMMAS

Ethical dilemmas that arise in practice may also provide an impetus for reflection and the generation of a personal theory of nursing. Ethical knowledge, as described by Carper[22] in a seminal work, is the moral component of knowledge; it involves understanding what is right and wrong and being responsible for the choices we make. It seems from the literature that it is in this area that the theory–practice gap will be most noticeable to you. A past student once commented to us that her education had taught her to be like a 'god' to the patient, yet she always felt that she fell short of this ideal in practice. You too may have periods of disappointment about your ability to provide for all the patient's needs, psychological as well as physical. Like the student mentioned, you may feel that you can never be the kind of nurse you aspire to be. Yet others may insist that the standard of patient care provided is acceptable and that perhaps your ideals are too high. In coming to terms with this you will note the different ways that individual nurses understand philosophical positions regarding what is good and what constitutes quality care, what ought to be desired, what is right and what is responsible practice. It is this difference between individual nurses, nurses and doctors, nurses and institutions and even nurses and patients that may lead to value conflicts for you because you have not yet attained confidence in your expertise.

Another dilemma may be generated by your desire to fit in. It appears that one of the most important elements that aids integration of new graduates is to feel that they are welcome as part of the team. The price some new nurses have to pay to be accepted is to fit in with the moral philosophies of others rather than their own personal values and sometimes those held jointly by the profession. How do you deal with situations such as caring for a patient who refuses treatment that could be life-saving, or the doctor or nursing colleague who consistently neglects to wash hands between patients? Clearly, when these conflicts arise you will need support and guidance in order to develop confidence in your own ethical stance.

PRIORITISING CARE

It is important for you to keep a clear perspective about what is considered optimal patient care and what is achievable. You may have had the opportunity to study or discuss the work of Abraham Maslow,[23] a humanist psychologist. If so, you will recall the hierarchy, or ordering, of human needs that he described and depicted in the form of a pyramid (Fig 18.1). The most basic needs are physiological, as they are necessary for survival, with the need for safety and security also seen as basic. When these are met, it is possible to move attention to the higher growth needs, which include love and belonging, esteem and self-esteem and, at the top of the pyramid, the need for self-actualisation, which may be easily disrupted by the lower or basic needs.[25]

Because of the familiarity of the pyramid shape it remains a useful way for you to organise your thoughts as you prioritise your work for the next few hours, or for the day. When faced with the competing needs of several patients it may seem impossible to accomplish the day's work but, however pressing or urgent, physiological needs will always take precedence over higher needs.

Your focus will be on the needs of individual patients, rather than a rigid application of Maslow's hierarchy as you work through the day. Priorities for patients will

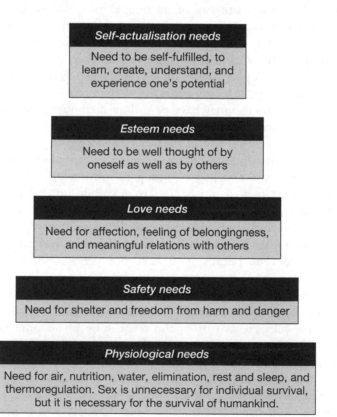

Self-actualisation needs
Need to be self-fulfilled, to learn, create, understand, and experience one's potential

Esteem needs
Need to be well thought of by oneself as well as by others

Love needs
Need for affection, feeling of belongingness, and meaningful relations with others

Safety needs
Need for shelter and freedom from harm and danger

Physiological needs
Need for air, nutrition, water, elimination, rest and sleep, and thermoregulation. Sex is unnecessary for individual survival, but it is necessary for the survival of humankind.

Fig 18.1 Maslow's hierarchy of human needs. (Craven & Hirlne:[25] 62; as adapted in Brooks N (ed.) *Kozier and Erb's Fundamentals of Nursing.* Australia: Pearson, 2010: 282.[24])

vary, as there will be a range of factors influencing the needs they perceive as most important for themselves, and you will also develop an awareness of their individual needs. You may be able to meet several needs at the same time. For example, the need for safety and security, and the higher need for self-esteem, may both be met as you care for physiological needs. If you are showering a patient, you will ensure that safety is maintained, and that dignity and privacy are respected. The application of Maslow's theory of the hierarchy of human needs to your prioritisation of care for patients demonstrates a way in which you are able to apply a theoretical concept directly to your nursing practice. Exercise 18.6 allows you to test this theory.

EXERCISE 18.6

One of your patients is receiving intermittent nasogastric feeds following a left-sided cerebrovascular accident. You are preparing to start a flask of feeding supplement when a colleague enters the room and asks you to help him to change the soiled bed of another frail elderly patient. You tell him you will be with him as soon as you test the position of the tube and hang the flask but he tells you to 'just hang the flask and come quickly. Mr Smith is very upset and embarrassed and needs changing right away'.

Using the hierarchy of needs as a guide, list the order in which you would attend to these competing demands on your time.

Prioritisation is vital to ensure safe patient care but it is also an important component of efficient time management. Seminal articles by Siviter[26] and Waterworth[27] provide further strategies to assist with time management.

CRITICAL THINKING AND PROBLEM SOLVING

Critical thinking ability will be foremost in helping you deal with any potential gaps in your ability to use knowledge to guide practice. However, Duchscher[3] identifies that this is more likely to happen once you have moved out of the postorientation phase of your transition to practice. She reports that new graduates enter a stage called 'being' where the nurse searches, examines, doubts and questions the rationales and effectiveness of nursing and medical care. This requires the ability to think critically. Critical thinking is thinking that is rational and reasonable – that is, it is thinking based on reason rather than preference, fear, self-interest or prejudice. It is reflective, in that the critical thinker does not jump to conclusions but takes time to collect and link information in a systematic manner.

Critical thinkers are autonomous. They do not accept the beliefs of others but analyse issues and decide which authorities are credible. They are creative rather than traditional; they question the status quo and find new ways of doing things. Consequently, critical thinkers need knowledge. What does this mean in practice? Does it mean knowing 'about' something or knowing the 'how' of it? Today's nursing practice must encompass both. Historically, nurses have been receivers of information from others, namely physicians. In more recent times we are developing a knowledge base specific to nursing, incorporating knowledge from other sciences. The knowing 'how' entails the cognitive processes of concept learning, problem solving, critical thinking and clinical judgment. Experience as well as knowledge has been identified as being the most influential factor in developing clinical reasoning skills. It is therefore imperative that learners are facilitated to practise reasoning and decision making.

In Exercise 18.6, what was your decision? Did the hierarchy of needs assist your critical thinking process? Certainly, it would be detrimental to Mr Smith's self-esteem to stay in a soiled bed and his skin would be damaged from prolonged contact with urine and faecal material, but hanging a flask without testing the position of the nasogastric tube in the stomach could lead to aspiration and death.

THINKING ALOUD

Since experience is positively related to effective decision making,[28] it would be fair to expect that as a beginning practitioner there will be differences in the quality of your clinical decisions when compared with those of a more experienced nurse. Differences have been identified in the amount of information accessed by inexperienced and experienced nurses.[29] Experienced nurses were found to make more accurate choices concerning patient treatments compared to inexperienced nurses and focused on more specific information to make their decisions. A useful strategy to assist you to develop this ability is to consider adopting the 'think aloud' technique. In this context the 'think aloud' technique is used between clinicians to allow one to examine the thought processes of the other.[30] Specifically, nurses can use it by asking a colleague to listen to their thought process as they verbalise their approach to patient care. This may take the form of verbalising their decisions related to the use of assessment data and the prioritisation of patient care needs. Your colleague's role is to listen and reinforce your decisions or make suggestions to improve outcomes. Thinking aloud may help you to have confidence in your clinical decision-making skills and overcome any concerns you may have had about your plan of care.

EXERCISE 18.7

Joseph, aged 43 years, has been admitted to your unit today. He has had an acute myocardial infarction (AMI). He was on the toilet this morning when he experienced severe chest pain. During the bout of chest pain he fell off the toilet and fractured (#) his wrist. He has a past history of prolapsed discs lumbar 1 and 2 (L1, L2), for which he takes Panadeine.

Ask a friend to practise the 'think aloud' technique with you then talk through the key issues you need to address in the scenario above. Think through and verbalise the subjective assessment data you would collect and give your reasons.

The key issues you identified were, we are sure, AMI, # wrist, L1, L2 prolapse, chest pain and Panadeine. You would also, more than likely, have identified the need for thorough assessment of the chest pain, wrist pain and even whether or not he has had any back pain as a result of the fall. Management of the chest pain remains a key priority.

Verbalise the questions you would ask and ask for feedback from your colleague.

You may have considered some of the questions below.

Chest pain	How much Anginine was required at the time? Was other medication such as morphine administered? Has Joseph had more chest pain since? What is the medical plan? What tests were conducted? What did the electrocardiograph show? How much activity can Joseph tolerate now? Will he need assistance with hygiene and toileting?
Fractured wrist	What is the medical plan for treating the fracture? Is the wrist painful? Is it his dominant hand? What effect will this have on his ability to perform activities of daily living?
History of back pain	Is Joseph experiencing back pain since the fall? If Joseph is required to rest in bed because of chest pain, what impact might this have on his back?

What did you learn about this approach? Some additional questions are: Is there a relationship between the AMI and Panadeine? How does Panadeine work? What is the relationship between chest pain and AMI? Is there a relationship between Joseph's gender and age and AMI?

SELF-QUESTIONING

Clearly you need to be able to ask yourself key questions in order to increase the efficiency of your clinical decisions. The ability to self-question as a way of developing thinking skills is very underrated. You may have experienced teaching and learning methods in your course such as inquiry-based learning or problem-based learning. These methods are designed to help you identify what knowledge you have and what gaps need to be followed up through questioning yourself. There has been little written about questioning and little research conducted, but what has been done clearly points to questioning as an extremely useful means of encouraging thinking skills and critical reflection.

Phillips and Duke[31] found that the questions most asked are not those that encourage critical or lateral thinking but tend to be questions that simply require the recall of facts. For critical thinking skills to develop, questions need to be those that encourage synthesis of information, the 'what if?' type of questions. While these research studies investigated the questioning skills of clinical teachers, it is not difficult to imagine that we as individuals may also resort to asking ourselves the easy questions.

In the 'think aloud' exercise (Exercise 18.7), what sort of questions did you ask yourself? Look back at those we presented. Do they require the integration of theoretical concepts or are they those that simply require you to recall memorised facts? What does Panadeine do? is an example of a question that requires low-level recall of information only. However, questioning the relationship between the AMI and

Panadeine requires you to link recalled information about Panadeine to the other concept, AMI; that is, it encourages critical thinking.

Try asking 'what if?' questions of yourself after reading the clinical scenario in Exercise 18.8.

EXERCISE 18.8

You are asked by your preceptor to remove a central venous catheter from a restless patient. You have only ever attempted this skill once before as a student, with your teacher talking you through it.

What questions would you ask of yourself while preparing for the procedure, during it and on its completion to ensure you linked theoretical concepts to skill performance?

One of the first questions you probably asked yourself is, who can I check out the procedure with? This is an excellent first move as checking your plan of action and the major points with another will help increase your confidence as well as ensure patient safety.

Self-questioning is a skill you can develop to improve your problem solving. Another useful technique is to question those who are more experienced than you. Encourage the experienced nurses around you to share their knowledge by asking questions to clarify situations and help you understand their decision making. Many years ago Wolf[32] postulated that the nursing shift-to-shift handover could be used as a means of assisting inexperienced nurses to integrate theory and practice. More recently effective communication at handover has been identified as a key aspect of safe patient care. Handover can be a useful forum for you to note the type of questions nurses ask each other when they want more information about the patient they are to care for, or if they wish to understand the decision making of the medical staff and other nurses. It is often in handover that nurses discuss issues as a way of checking their understanding and thus it is a form of thinking out loud that helps to ensure patient safety.

CONCLUSION

In this chapter we have explored some practical ways to develop your doing and thinking skills to help you cope in the practice setting. It has been identified that, as new graduates begin their professional careers, coupled with the volume of work, they may experience a gap between the high ideals taught in the educational setting and the sometimes low standard of patient care necessitated by the working conditions imposed. Have you had such an experience?

Nursing is a practice discipline and it is practice that will assist you to develop the expertise that you admire in experienced nurses. In the early weeks and months of life as a registered nurse, areas in which support may by sought include prioritising workload, time management related to patient care, becoming a team member, developing and refining clinical skills, being able to assess patients and drawing a clinical picture together in order to plan and implement appropriate nursing care. In this chapter we have provided some strategies to assist you with your transition tasks. The activities will help you to take an active role in your own development now and in the future.

CASE STUDY 18.1

Elizabeth is 3 months into her graduate nurse year and on her first week in a rehabilitation unit where most patients are stable. Her observations of one of the patients indicated that he had deteriorated. Elizabeth presented her observational data, including vital signs and electroencephalogram to the resident medical officer, asking: 'Can you have a look at Mr Schneider?' The resident was unhurried and dismissive and Elizabeth felt that because she was not known to the resident and not yet trusted that the physician took the attitude of 'when I'm ready'. Shortly afterwards and before he was seen Mr Schneider coded and an hour later he died. Elizabeth was extremely upset and felt that she should have done more.

REFLECTIVE QUESTIONS

- Was there anything else Elizabeth should/could have done?
- What steps would you take to ensure safe patient care in a similar situation?
- What steps could be taken to improve interprofessional communication in your workplace?

CASE STUDY 18.2

The nurse manager of the orthopaedic ward was very pleased to recruit Sophie as a new graduate. Among Sophie's many strengths was the fact that she had been a student on the ward for a significant part of her final undergraduate year. The nurse manager expected that, since Sophie was very familiar with the hospital policies and procedures and the patient group and had been a very interested student, she would transition to her role as a registered nurse smoothly. Six weeks after commencing as a new graduate, the nurse manager identified an alarming pattern related to Sophie's performance. She has been receiving increasing reports that Sophie is frequently late for work, she leaves the ward for breaks without handing over her patients and she needs frequent reminders that patient care activities are to be completed on time.

REFLECTIVE QUESTIONS

- Identify the issues that are of concern to the nurse manager.
- What steps should be taken to ensure that Sophie is contributing fairly to the ward team?
- What support does Sophie need to improve her professional behaviour?

CASE STUDY 18.3

Jack is excited to be working as a registered nurse on the cardiac ward after graduating from university with a Bachelor of Nursing. Prior to graduation Jack worked as a volunteer in the quit-smoking campaign office. In preparation for the National Heart Foundation's Heart Week, Jack's nurse manager approaches him to see if he is interested in contributing to the planning and implementing of focused relevant health promotion activities for patients and families.

REFLECTIVE QUESTIONS

- What additional skills do your bring to your role as a new graduate that would advance patient care in your unit?
- How could you use your skills in your unit to improve patient outcomes, whether physical or psychological?
- How would you approach your nurse manager to offer your skills?

RECOMMENDED READING

Conway J, McMillan M. Connecting clinical and theoretical knowledge for practice. In: Daly JS, Jackson D, editors. Contexts of nursing. Sydney: Elsevier; 2010. p. 351–69.

Duchscher JB. A process of becoming: the stages of new nursing graduate professional role transition. Journal of Continuing Education in Nursing 2008;39:441–50.

Irurita V. Preserving integrity. In: Greenwood J, editor. Nursing theory in Australia: development and application. Sydney: Harper Education; 2000.

Maben J, Latter S, Macleod Clark J. The theory–practice gap: impact of professional–bureaucratic work conflict on newly-qualified nurses. Journal of Advanced Nursing 2006;55:465–77.

Schoessler M, Waldo M. The first 18 months in practice: a developmental transition model for the newly graduated nurse. Journal for Nurses in Staff Development 2006;22:47–52.

REFERENCES

1. Walker K. Dangerous liaisons: thinking, doing nursing. Collegian 1997;4: 4–14.

2. Walker K. On philosophy: nursing and the politics of truth. In: Daly JS, Jackson D, editors. Contexts of nursing. Sydney: Elsevier; 2006. p. 60–72.

3. Duchscher JB. A process of becoming: the stages of new nursing graduate professional role transition. Journal of Continuing Education in Nursing 2008;39: 441–50.

4. Dearmun AK. Supporting newly qualified staff nurses: the lecturer practitioner contribution. Journal of Nursing Mangament 2000;31:426–39.

5. Schoessler M, Waldo M. The first 18 months in practice: a developmental transition model for the newly graduated nurse. Journal for Nurses in Staff Development 2006;22:47–52.

6. Cheeks P, Dunn PS. A new-graduate program: empowering the novice nurse. Journal for Nurses in Staff Development 2010;26:223–7.

7. Nursing and Midwifery Board of Australia. National competencies standards for the registered nurse. Canberra: Nursing and Midwifery Board of Australia; 2010.

8. Hinds R, Harley J. Exploring the experiences of beginning registered nurses in the acute care setting. Contemporary Nurse 2001;10:110–116.

9. Fox R, Henderson A, Malko-Nyhan K. They survive despite the organizational culture, not because of it: a longitudinal study of new staff perceptions of what constitutes support during the transition to an acute tertiary facility. International Journal of Nursing Practice 2005;11:193–9.

10. Speedy S. Theory–practice debate: setting the scene. Australian Journal of Advanced Nursing 1989;6:12–20.

11. Daehlen M. Job satisfaction and job values among beginning nurses: a questionnaire survey. International Journal of Nursing Studies 2008;45:1789–99.

12. Victorian Department of Human Services, Nurse Policy Branch. Graduate nurse program guidelines. Melbourne: Nurse Policy Branch, Victorian Government Department of Human Services; 2003.

13. Kolb A. Experiential learning. New Jersey: Prentice Hall; 1984.

14. Johnstone M, Kanitsaki O, Currie T. The nature and implications of support in graduate nurse transition programs: an Australian study. Journal of Professional Nursing 2008;24:46–53.

15. Hayes J, Scott A. Mentoring partnerships as the wave of the future for new graduates. Nursing Education Perspectives 2007;28:27–9.

16. Maben J, Latter S, Macleod Clark J. The theory–practice gap: impact of professional–bureaucratic work conflict on newly-qualified nurses. Journal of Advanced Nursing 2006;55:465–77.

17. Rolfe G. The deconstructing angel: nursing, reflection and evidence-based practice. Nursing Inquiry 2005;12:78–86.

18. Rolfe G. The theory–practice gap in nursing: from research-based practice to practitioner-based research. Journal of Advanced Nursing 1998;28:672–9.

19. Schon D. The reflective practitioner. London: Temple Smith; 1983.

20. Rolfe G. Closing the theory practice gap. Oxford: Butterworth Heinemann; 1996.

21. Forneris S, Peden-McAlpine C. Evaluation of a reflective learning intervention to improve critical thinking in novice nurses. Journal of Advanced Nursing 2007;57:410–21.

22. Carper B. Fundamental patterns of knowing in nursing. Advances in Nursing Sciences 1978;1:13–23.

23. Maslow A. Motivation and personality. 2nd ed. New York: Harper & Row; 1970.

24. Brooks N, editor. Kozier and Erb's fundamentals of nursing. Australia: Pearson; 2010. p. 282.

25. Craven R, Hirnie C. Fundamentals of nursing: human health and function. 5th ed Philadelphia: Lippincott; 2006.

26. Siviter B. The newly qualified nurse's handbook. London: Baillière Tindall, Elsevier; 2004.

27. Waterworth S. Temporal reference frameworks and nurses' work organization. Time and Society 2003;12:41–54.

28. Benner P, Tanner C, Chesla C. Expertise in nursing practice: caring, clinical judgment and ethics? 2nd ed. New York: Springer; 2009.

29. Taylor C. Assessing patients' needs: does the same information guide expert and novice nurses? International Nursing Review 2002;49:11–19.

30. Hoffman K., Aitken L, Duffield C. A comparison of novice and expert nurses' cue collection during clinical decision-making: verbal protocol analysis. International Journal of Nursing Studies 2009;46:1335–44.

31. Phillips N, Duke M. The questioning skills of clinical teachers and preceptors: a comparative study. Journal of Advanced Nursing 2000;33:523–9.

32. Wolf Z. Nurses' work: the sacred and the profane. Philadelphia: University of Philadelphia Press; 1988.

CHAPTER 19

Reflective practice for the graduate

Kim Usher, Kim Foster and Lee Stewart

LEARNING OBJECTIVES

When you have completed this chapter you will be able to:

- understand the benefits of reflection and identify its importance to nursing practice, research and leadership
- appreciate the link between reflection, self-monitoring and improved client outcomes
- understand how reflection is linked to an effective and fulfilling career
- recognise the usefulness of using a reflective framework to assist in the development of your reflective processes
- apply the key elements of reflection to your practice.

Keywords: reflection, nursing practice, self-monitoring, leadership, research

---

INTRODUCTION

Nursing has embraced the idea of reflective practice to varying degrees and applied it across the areas of nursing practice, education, research and leadership with the intent of achieving best outcomes for clients. Reflection has been described as a process of going back over something after it has occurred with the aim of making sense of the situation so that necessary changes can be identified.[1,2] In other words, the purpose of reflection is that it leads to action that is better informed. This occurs via a process of learning through experience in a way that aids in the development of new insights about self and practice.[3] Reflection is also closely linked to critical thinking. Whilst not identical, it is paramount that reflection has a critical intent as being a critical thinker involves questioning the world and challenging assumptions that are taken for granted. In this chapter we have chosen to use the word 'reflection' but our intent is to convey the link between critical thinking and reflection at all times.

Reflection has also been linked to self-awareness or self-development. Johns[4] terms this as being 'mindful' of self. In this way he believes a practitioner can use reflection with the aim of confronting and resolving the contradiction between one's vision and actual practice. Through the development of this notion of contradiction, Johns[5] would say, we come to understand why things are the way they are, which allows us to develop new insights that assist us to respond more effectively in the future. The outcome is thus a process of continuous monitoring that leads to improvement of practice.[6] We assume you are interested in knowing and realising desirable and effective practice, but as Johns[7] reminds us, we sometimes work in conditions where such a realisation may be difficult or even impossible. In such cases, reflection takes on an even more important role in the goal of professional development. We hope this chapter will help you, as a new graduate, to recognise the importance of the ability to self-monitor and self-regulate and come to understand the benefit and reward reflective practice can bring to your role in the years ahead.

This chapter assumes you already have a basic understanding of reflective practice and have utilised many of the processes suggested as ways of enhancing reflection, such as keeping a journal and exploring critical incidents, during your undergraduate years.[6] Hence, we will not be offering a comprehensive theoretical overview of reflection here but will instead focus on what we believe to be of most importance to the graduate nurse from a practical perspective: the impact of reflection on practice, leadership and management, and research. We have focused on these areas because we believe reflection can help the new graduate to assimilate to the new practice environment and effectively manage the challenges of daily practice. It will also be important for you as you move on in your career and start to take on management and leadership roles, and likewise as you begin to become involved in research within the clinical arena. The first section of the chapter addresses reflection and how it can benefit your practice; the second section applies the usefulness of reflection to the areas of management and leadership; and the last section connects reflection to the research process.

If you feel your understanding of the theoretical underpinnings of reflective practice is not sufficient to appreciate this chapter fully, please read an introduction to the material, such as the chapter by Usher and Holmes.[6] In that chapter, the framework developed by Rolfe et al.[8] was used as an example of a framework to guide reflection. We have also referred to that framework throughout this chapter and have included it as Figure 19.1 for your reference. While we do not propose that frameworks are necessary for reflection to occur, many novice practitioners find them a useful starting point. There are a number of other frameworks or models of reflection that may be more suitable to your use, including those of Burrows[9] and Smith and Russell.[10] You will find helpful texts in the recommended reading at the end of this chapter.

Descriptive level of reflection	Theory- and knowledge-building level of reflection	Action-oriented (reflexive) level of reflection
What . . . ⟶	So what . . . ⟶	Now what . . .
. . . is the problem/difficulty/reason for being stuck/reason for feeling bad/reason we don't get on?	. . . does this tell me/teach me/imply/ mean about me/my patient/others/our relationship/my patient's care/the model of care I am using/my attitudes/my patient's attitudes?	. . . do I need to do in order to make things better/stop being stuck/improve my patient's care/resolve the situation/feel better/get on better?
. . . was my role in the situation?		. . . broader issues need to be considered if this action is to be successful?
. . . was I trying to achieve?	. . . was going through my mind as I acted?	. . . might be the consequences of this action?
. . . actions did I take?		
. . . was the response of others?	. . . did I base my actions on?	
. . . were the consequences	. . . other knowledge can I bring to the situation?	
• for the patient?	• experiential?	
• for myself?	• personal?	
• for others?	• scientific?	
. . . feelings did it evoke	. . . could/should I have done to make it better?	
• in the patient?		
• in myself?		
• in others?	. . . is my new understanding of the situation?	
. . . was good/bad about the experience?		
	. . . broader issues arise from the situation?	

Fig. 19.1 Framework for reflection. Source: Rolfe G, Freshwater D, Jasper M. Critical reflection for nursing and the helping professions: a user's guide. New York: Palgrave; 2001. p. 35.

NURSING PRACTICE IN THE FIRST YEAR AND BEYOND

This section addresses the usefulness of reflective practice for the graduate nurse during the transition year and beyond. Criticisms of reflection, as Usher and Holmes[6] remind us, include the notion that the reflective process is often viewed as simply an academic exercise. Graduate nurses often have memories of keeping a reflective journal as a tedious classroom assignment, but that 'it does not happen in the real world'. We are certain you have spent some time during your undergraduate or preregistration course completing classroom exercises and assessments of a reflective practice nature and you may have found these activities more or less helpful. However, we remain committed to the ideal of registered nurses who continue to think critically and to reflect upon their practice so they become the best practitioners possible. We hope that registered nurses will not only see the usefulness of reflection in their early years but consider it an important skill for the future where they will continue to reflect and mentor others, and that they retire from the profession with the knowledge of that contribution to nursing practice and to the care of their communities.

Consider your own situation now as a new graduate. Imagine that you have incorporated Rolfe et al.'s[8] framework into your practice so that it is almost second nature to what you do – it is part of your practice. An event occurs at work and you ask yourself: What is the problem here? What is my role in this situation – how have I contributed to what happened? So what does this teach me? Now what do I need to do to make things better next time? Using this framework to unpick everyday experiences allows us to describe events to ourselves more clearly, to build more knowledge from that description and to take action ourselves to improve situations. This is where we can truly become empowered as nurses: where we have the opportunity to use a reflective approach to unravel a complex situation, see it for what it is, identify ways to ensure it does not happen again, or identify strategies to improve the outcomes in the future. The alternative is to leave things as they are and go on as if nothing has happened. This usually means we go away, justify our actions in an uncritical or unreflective way and then find it difficult to move on. Taylor[1] reminds us that the practice arena may not always turn out to be what it first seemed and, as a result, nurses may struggle to hold on to the ideals of why they wanted to be a nurse in the first place, leading to people leaving. She states that reflection offers stability in this situation, something to which health professionals can turn to help make sense of the world and re-evaluate their practice. In other words, the reflective approach helps us habitually to self-correct, and assist others to do the same so that the whole notion of continuous improvement becomes part of who we are as nurses. Reflection on nursing practice then becomes 'a way of being, an active way of engaging practice towards realising desirable practice in whatever way it is known and understood'.[7]

This sort of knowledge – learning from practice, or practice wisdom[11] – began to an extent during your first clinical placement, and can become a habit (or not!) during your first year of practice and beyond. It is important that you realise the benefits, both personal and professional, of being a reflective practitioner from the outset of your career. We cannot persuade you to do this with what we might consider to be the power of the good logical argument. You are the one who will make that decision for yourself – we can simply provide you with guidance to arrive at that decision.

A key component of reflection is to remember what happened. Burton (cited in Usher and Holmes)[12] calls this 'a type of cognitive "postmortem" or an act of looking back at practice'. This is what is also termed reflection on action, which occurs after the event has taken place. This type of reflection can be extremely powerful and will greatly contribute to your effectiveness as a practitioner. Reflecting in action is also possible and this implies pausing within a particular situation with the intent of trying to make sense of or reframe a situation to enable a better outcome.[13,14] We know this is about persistently cycling through the testing of theories and hypotheses while you are actually engaged in practice.[15] Sound difficult? Of course it can be, and the challenge is to attempt this more advanced form of reflection so it becomes habitual, rather than being just another difficult task you have to turn your mind to in the midst of a busy working day. The issue here is that habitual unconscious action is largely replaced by habitual reflection by the self-aware nurse who, with customary self-monitoring, delivers the sort of nursing care leading to improved client outcomes.

You may be familiar with the term 'clinical supervision', for which there are varying definitions and models in practice. Whilst we recognise the lack of agreement as to the term, one way of understanding clinical supervision is that it is a formal, structured and systematic process of engaging in learning and reflection on action which occurs within the context of a supportive professional relationship between a supervisor and supervisee. You may be more familiar with the term 'preceptor' rather than 'clinical supervisor' and the processes for assisting the new graduate by either preceptor or clinical supervisor are generally readily comparable. The process seeks to enhance practice through supporting and developing the nurse's job identity, competence, knowledge, ethics and skills.[16] Clinical supervision is therefore one of a number of ways in which nurses can engage in reflective practice.[17] It is important to note, though, that the term 'supervisor' does not refer to the nurse's direct line manager or nursing supervisor (although it is possible the clinical supervisor role may be performed by this person), but rather, to the role of an experienced and competent health professional (often a nurse) with whom the supervisee works either individually or in a group.

Whilst it is most often associated with mental health nursing, clinical supervision has also been reported as an important facet of practice in midwifery, and for nurses working in settings such as hospices and palliative care, the community and medical/surgical areas. Clinical supervision can also offer a particularly helpful form of professional support for nurses working in isolated and/or rural and remote settings.[5,18,19] In this process, nurses meet with their supervisor on a regular basis to discuss various aspects of their practice (a form of dialogical reflection), which includes nurses' self-assessment of their performance in order to develop and sustain further competence in their work through transforming their knowledge.[5,17] While this may appear to be a rather daunting process, when managed in a constructive and supportive way, many nurses find that having an opportunity to reflect on their practice with a clinical supervisor brings significant benefits. Indeed, you might be aware that clinical supervision is viewed increasingly as an integral form of professional support for nurses that can assist in recruitment and retention and that some health services provide it for staff as a part of their employment package.

So, like many other nurses, reflecting on action and using clinical supervision in your practice may help to deepen your self-awareness and self-understanding, balance work and the rest of your life, reduce uncomfortable feelings of distress related to your work and explore problematic issues related to your practice.[19] The benefits extend to your clients through the enhanced nursing knowledge, skills and strategies you bring from engaging in this process.

Clinical supervision is not limited to clinical practice, however, and can also be a valuable aspect of nursing management and leadership, where it has been found to assist in the development of communication, coping and leadership skills.[20]

THE NURSING LEADER AND MANAGER

Remember, reflection is essentially concerned with thinking about what you do so you can learn to do it better. This is not something we tend to do naturally. Instead, as Johns[21] reminds us: 'as we go about our everyday business we take the world largely for granted and respond habitually'. We have already discussed the importance of reflection to the novice practitioner. This section explores how reflective practice may benefit you now in your work as a graduate nurse in your future career as you possibly take on management and leadership roles.

Taylor[1] has suggested that reflection can be emancipatory. Emancipation means freedom from your own and from other people's expectations and roles in order to adopt other ways of being.[1] This type of reflection is linked to empowerment, which is the process of giving and accepting power[1] and helps the practitioner take actions that are based on insights.[5] The aim of reflection can therefore be to 'free practitioners from the taken-for-granted assumptions and oppressive forces which limit them and their practice'.[22] This is particularly important when thinking about nursing leaders and managers as they have an important role in change.[1] Think about how nursing leaders and managers shape the organisation and how they go about improving patient or client care. Also consider how they influence you as a graduate nurse. Finally, think about the sort of nursing leader and manager you are going to be. Johns proposes that 'the Buddhist perspective would view reflection as a way to nurture and realise wise and compassionate practice within a strong ethic of doing good in the world'.[23] Sounds like something to aspire to, does it not? Likewise, reflection for nursing leaders and managers could assist them to realise why they do not always 'do good in the world' and would help them to explore how they could do more good.

Reflection requires that nursing leaders and managers take a critical approach to their practice. Essentially:

> critical theorising ... looks at the way life is and asks how it might be different and better for the majority of people, not just for the privileged few who hold and use power.[24]

Emancipatory and empowering reflection is important for nurses in leadership and management positions in healthcare. Think for a moment about your own life and how you live it, going about your everyday business with family, friends and work colleagues, perhaps not reflecting a great deal on the things that happen and why they happen – you just live. You do the sort of things that most other people do in your environment – you eat, sleep, talk with people, have disagreements, make up, fall in love, fall out of love, attend classes, study, work, party, go shopping, watch TV, go to the movies. Think of this as your 'everyday life'. That is, 'we just do stuff', and that 'stuff' of everyday life is nevertheless strongly influenced by elements such as the culture within which we live, family background, school education systems, and so on.

Now think about what happens, for example, in a hospital (or a school, or a university). Have you ever attended a formal meeting in one of these settings? If so, you will have noticed that 'everyday life' looks a bit different. There are rules for behaviour that seem to apply, and most people follow these rules. The rules will be about things such as what is said, what is permitted to be said, who speaks, whose voice is heard, who is not permitted to speak, maybe whose voice is not heard. From a critical perspective we would say that people in such a meeting are engaged in 'discourse', this being 'an unusual form of communication in which the participants subject themselves to the force of the better argument, with the view to coming to an agreement about the validity or invalidity of problematic claims'.[25] This sounds wonderful, that people might be able to get together and talk carefully, openly and freely about problems, and arrive together at good solutions to those problems. Remember those rules, however − does everyone get to speak in the same way? Obviously not, and that is the problem. Discourses like this become institutionalised,[26] that is, we make rules for what is allowed to be said, and these rules tend to govern the sort of decisions (sometimes very bad ones) that are allowed to be made to solve problems. We ask ourselves questions in these meetings about what is going on, questions such as, 'why aren't there enough beds for patients in our public hospitals?', but the answers to those questions are not always arrived at from free and open discussion; instead they are governed by the institutionalised rules that are in play. This is where it becomes interesting. Unless healthcare leaders and managers, in our case nursing leaders and managers, reflect upon how power is used or misused in this way, this tendency to control people and processes, so much of the creative thinking that happens in everyday life is lost. This is what reflection is all about − it is about nursing leaders and managers reflecting upon these social circumstances, and moving forward with this understanding. It is about encouraging those disparate voices at the level of discourse, for example, in formal meetings, rather than leaving people whispering in corridors.

Obviously, in healthcare organisations or universities, the nursing leaders and managers do not 'hold all the power'. They do have their share though. How do they use or misuse this power? Power can be power with others or power over others. The goal for the effective nursing leader and manager would be that of power with rather than over − the notion of empowerment of everyone − themselves, nurses, students, clients or patients, other members of the healthcare team. 'When leaders share power with others, they're demonstrating profound trust in and respect for others' abilities.'[27] In order to understand this good use of power, nursing leaders and managers need knowledge about how they themselves behave, that is, how they use or misuse their power.

Effective leadership and management always seem to start with self-knowledge,[28,29] and self-knowledge comes from reflection upon our thinking and behaviours. Knowing ourselves does not come from wandering rather sleepily through life, behaving in habitual ways that are often culturally determined and socially constructed. We need to be awake to the effects of these social and cultural factors, so we can change our responses when we need to. Kouzes and Posner[30] describe 'exploring your inner territory' as a key to effective leadership. Think about the nursing leader and manager who has clarified her values, figured out where she wants her organisation to go, what she wants for her clients or patients, what she wants for the nursing team. Compare this person with the nursing leader and manager who has never done this, never 'explored her inner territory', but rather, simply reacts to what happens on a daily, weekly, monthly, yearly basis. Can you begin to see the difference between the reflective and the non-reflective life? Ask yourself which of these lives you want. It is crucial at this stage to note that reflection itself is not simply another imposition by others on your precious time:

it is not an artificial technique that is imposed by regulatory authorities or universities; rather, it is the refinement of a natural process that is part of being human, and which needs to be nurtured and encouraged.[31]

Think about emancipatory reflection for a moment now in relation to your own nursing practice. How do nursing leaders and managers (and others) either empower you or disempower you in relation to your practice? It has been claimed that 'emancipatory reflection leads to "transformative action" which seeks to free nurses and midwives from taken-for-granted assumptions and oppressive forces which limit them and their practice'.[32] It may be that through the role of the nursing leader and/or manager you will use reflection as means to attain a higher level of self-awareness in order to be a more effective leader/manager.

So how can this help you now in your role as a new graduate? Perhaps it is first of all worth considering the idea that it is important for new graduates to accept that others will be their leaders. It is not always easy to follow others but at times we need to be able to accept leadership and learn from those with more experience, particularly when we begin our career. Imagine a graduate nurse who experiences a crisis at work, perhaps makes a mistake or becomes stressed due to workloads. This experience, this crisis, with the guidance of a reflective, wise and supportive nursing leader and manager, could be a means of developing higher levels of skill and better coping mechanisms for use in the future. The nursing leader and manager who utilises a framework such as that developed by Rolfe et al.[8] and guides you, through asking questions such as: What is the reason for this mistake that was made? What was my role in this? So what was going through my mind when I did this thing? What is my new understanding of this situation? Now what do I need to do in order to make it better the next time? is nurturing an environment where you can learn, and where the organisation also learns.[5] In essence, where members of the healthcare facility have ongoing experiences like this with their leaders and managers, then this becomes part of the culture of the organisation.

Reflective nursing leaders and managers are transformational in the way that they practise,[5] and transformational leadership cultures are reflective cultures. Getting better at what we do comes from reflecting upon what we do and making necessary adjustments to our thinking and behaviours for future situations. Emancipatory reflection is about, as Taylor[33] explains, daring, imagining, planning and acting 'in ways that are capable of transforming your world'. You may be thinking that becoming a leader or manager is far in your future. However, nurses in their graduate year are being socialised by those with whom they work. The culture of a ward, department or community health service is largely shaped by the leadership on offer in that particular environment, and it is the people in that environment who will be shaping the graduate's practice. That leadership, culture and nursing practice has an impact upon the type of care that clients are receiving. An environment of reflective practitioners is one resulting in better client outcomes, whether this be through the graduate nurse administering medications safely, or the nurse manager embedding reflection on action into the culture of the environment.

We have been focusing on the importance of reflection to your practice as a manager and leader. Research and the need to base our practice on valid evidence are also important to the role of the nurse in practice, management and leadership, so let us now move to consider the link between reflective practice and research.

RESEARCH

As a graduate nurse working in a practice profession, it is important you maintain your professional development throughout your career in order to remain up to date with advances in healthcare and nursing practice. Part of this development will include involvement with research. Most commonly, this will be through use of evidence from empirical or scientific research that informs your practice – evidence-based practice. You may also conduct research as part of your nursing role; through undertaking postgraduate study; and/or through an interest in exploring a particular clinical issue that arises in your practice. While you may not have considered that you would be conducting research as part of your work, it is increasingly common for registered nurses to be involved in research through practice development projects and collaborative research with experienced researchers. In this section, we explore how reflective practice may be useful in both conducting and using research for practice, for, as Taylor[34] suggests, the processes and thinking required in reflective practice are those required in any kind of practice, including research

A reflective approach privileges subjective experience and interrelated ways of knowing, and can be seen to blur the distinctions between knowing and doing, art and science, theory and practice.[34] In addition, if reflection can be considered a paradigm or framework for collecting, evaluating, understanding and applying knowledge, then it can also be seen as the standard for generating and judging knowledge for reflective practice. From this perspective, reflective practice and evidence-based practice may be viewed as complementary philosophies from which to examine nursing practice.[35] Reflective methods can therefore not only guide nursing practice, education and leadership; they can also provide evidence for supporting developments and changes in practice. Reflective processes may be used as the framework for a research project; they can be incorporated with other research approaches; and/or they can be the focus of research itself.[36] As a framework for research, the processes of reflective practice can be used to develop a research project. The framework of reflection proposed by Rolfe et al.,[8] for instance, could be applied to a clinical problem and used to facilitate the development of a clinical research project.

Reflective practice has also been incorporated with other research approaches such as qualitative, quantitative or mixed methods studies, and used to inform nursing practice.[36] While we will not be exploring the types of research in detail here, a brief review of the major types of research approaches may be useful. In qualitative research, the focus is on lived subjective (personal) experience and people's use of language to share their experiences. Qualitative researchers therefore focus on participants' experiences of events, situations and relationships and seek to interpret or uncover meanings they may have made of them. This is in contrast to quantitative research, which investigates objective (observable) data and seeks to quantify it through use of statistical methods. In mixed methods research, both qualitative and quantitative research methods are used in combination, or sequentially, to enrich the exploration of a specific issue.

Action research and reflection are a particularly effective combination. Reflection forms part of the action research method which involves cyclical stages of planning, acting, observing and reflecting.[37] The combination of reflective practice and action research can be a valuable tool for developing knowledge in nursing and reducing the theory–practice gap.[38] An illustration of this combination can be seen in a study by Taylor,[38] who used these methods to facilitate reflective practice processes in 12 registered nurses. In the study, the nurses worked collaboratively with the researcher to explore dysfunctional nurse–nurse relationships such as workplace bullying and violence. In a series of action cycles, they critically reflected on practice issues and their stories of these and looked for particular themes and issues. The thematic concern of dysfunctional nurse–nurse relationships was explored through a plan of action containing skills and strategies implemented to address this issue. As might be expected, the nurses encountered difficulties in addressing workplace relationships and in implementing the action plan, but also found significant benefits through engaging in this process, such as more effective personal communication, the use of leadership skills and recognising the complexities that can exist in workplace relationships.

In another example of how reflective practice may be included in research, Kim[39] developed a method of critical reflective inquiry that can be used to develop nursing knowledge and practice. This research method incorporates notions from reflective practice, action science and critical philosophy and involves three phases – descriptive, reflective and critical/emancipatory. In the descriptive phase, nurses provide narratives of their practice which describe their thoughts and feelings, actions and circumstances of the particular situation/s. In the reflective phase, these narratives are analysed in the context of the nurse's personal beliefs, assumptions and knowledge. In this phase, models of 'good' practice and knowledge may be developed from reflective analysis and exploration of the nurse's practice. In the critical/emancipatory phase, the focus is on the correction and change of less desirable or ineffective practice, and/or moving on to new innovations that may have emerged from practice. Kim[39] suggested this process can be used as a research method; can be adopted in practice and nursing education as a way of improving practice; and/or can be the basis for shared learning where clinicians hold regular case conferences to explore issues.

Reflective practice has itself been the focus of research.[40–42] Using a mixed methods design, Paget,[41] for instance, evaluated whether education on reflective practice resulted in changes to the clinical practice of 200 pre- and postregistration nurses. The study found that most of the nurses considered reflective practice very useful and could identify long-term changes to their day-to-day clinical practice as a result of engaging in it. These included changes to practice regimes, a greater level of analysis of clinical experiences, enhanced communication skills and the ability to apply research findings to specific aspects of their practice.

Reflection and reflexivity in research

As we have seen, reflective processes can frame the research process and/or be a valuable part of the research process, as well as being integral to the development of nursing practices. In research, particularly qualitative research, reflection is an important aspect of reflexivity. Although there are various definitions of reflexivity, it can be understood as being based in the notion of researcher self-awareness and self-reflection on their role in the research they are conducting. A reflexive orientation includes being conscious of the role the researcher plays in constructing meaning in the research.[43] Reflexivity requires that, for the duration of the study, researchers critically examine their actions through each stage of the research process. This includes issues such as the participants' responses to the researchers, how researchers are collecting their data or field text, what they are seeing and hearing and how they are making their interpretations of the data. It may lead to alterations to aspects of the design and/or implementation of the research. The resulting reflections are then written up as part of the research report in order to make reader evaluation of the research possible through the process of transparent and auditable documentation.[44] You may notice that this process bears a number of similarities to the reflective methods for practice discussed earlier in the chapter. Similarly to reflective processes used to reflect upon practice, reflexivity in research is a creative as well as analytical method which may include the keeping of written and/or audiotaped research diaries, journals or field notes whilst conducting research, and/or the writing of reflective narratives and poetry.

Research methods in nursing that have been particularly associated with reflective practice and reflexivity include narrative inquiry and autoethnography. As you will have seen throughout this section, narratives are often used in reflective processes as people can be seen to share the meanings they have made from their experiences through the stories they tell of them. While narratives can be found in many qualitative research studies, this is often in the form of data rather than as a research method. Narrative inquiry, however, is a specific research methodology which seeks to understand personal experiences by focusing on the stories that structure and recall those experiences and using narrative analytic methods to interpret them.

Narrative research can be considered particularly pertinent to nursing, as nursing is an oral culture and stories may resonate as research that is meaningful and relevant to nurses. The stories derived from research into nurses' practices can shed light not only on what nurses do in practice, but also why they have practised in a particular way.[45] Reflexive narratives of nursing practice, for example, are a form of self-inquiry which can assist in transforming practice through exploring and reflecting upon particular patients and situations. Jarrett[46] explains how her reflexive exploration of two narratives of patients she cared for assisted her to make changes to her nursing of people with a disability:

> Both experiences help[ed] me to focus on an important aspect of my role and development of skills: easing the path for people with complex disabilities to come in, through and out of hospital. Predominantly this was triggered by recognising that people with complex needs fear being admitted to hospital … Coming into hospital, a large disruption for most people can become an even bigger deal if you have complex needs. Often the impact is as big for the carer who may take the lead in trying to negotiate care rather than doing it.

Another form of narrative research which relies on reflexivity is autoethnography, also referred to as personal narratives or narratives of the self. Autoethnography is a form of critical inquiry about personal or professional issues where researchers focus on their own experience for narrative data collection and analysis.[47] The researcher's personal experience is important primarily in terms of how it sheds light on the issue that is being studied. Autoethnography can range from starting research from one's own experience, to studies where the researcher's experience is explored alongside those of the participants, through to stories where the researcher's experiences of conducting the research become the actual focus of investigation.[48] Although it has been used by a number of professional disciplines, autoethnography is considered an emergent method in nursing research, with relatively few studies conducted by nurses.[49] Foster, however, included her own story and experience for analysis along-side those of her participants when she explored what it was like to grow up with a parent with serious mental illness. She reflects on her experience and the benefit of using autoethnography as a research method:

> having a parent with a mental illness sometimes places me in tension with my identity as a psychiatric mental health nurse. Identity is clearly not fixed. Thus, wounds and difficulties received in childhood can be transmuted into opportunities for insight and growth. As I have prepared for the field text [data] collection and analysis phase of this research inquiry, I have come to see that experiences are diverse, and meaning is shaped by many things, including the experience, reflection on that experience, and conversing about it with those who might share points of similarity and those who do not.[50]

CONCLUSION

In summary, we have suggested that, as a practice-based profession, nursing requires reflection on practice so as to enhance and develop nurses' knowledge, skills and practice. Reflection, as described in this chapter, not only helps us to identify and question poor practices, but also allows us to identify strategies for improvement. In this way we can provide the most effective care for our patients. The chapter also outlined how reflective practice can help you to develop a higher level of self-awareness. The development of this awareness helps us become more aware of the needs of others and more aware of the impact of our behaviour on those around us. Yet reflective practice is useful not only for practice and leadership, but as a method for research into nursing issues and practice, and/or to be used in combination with other research methods. As a graduate nurse, you can therefore use reflective practice to undertake a research project on an issue of clinical significance for you; to reflect on your experiences in practice and leadership; and to reflect upon and implement findings from research which enhance your nursing of the patients in your care.

CASE STUDY 19.1

Hemlata's second rotation during her graduate year is to an operating theatre in a large tertiary hospital. When acting as 'scout' in the orthopaedic theatre, she accidentally leans on and unsterilises the instrument tray. The orthopaedic surgeon shouts at her; the instrument nurse asks him to calm down and immediately sets about organising a replacement instrument tray with Hemlata's assistance. Afterwards, she sits down privately with Hemlata and gently takes her through a reflection of the situation.

REFLECTIVE QUESTIONS

What is Hemlata learning about the different approaches to leadership in this situation? What impact might this have on her own attitudes to communicating with less experienced staff?

CASE STUDY 19.2

Sue is working in a mental health unit. A client is removed from the activity area and put into a secure room alone because of abusive behaviour. Sue is very upset by the removal of the client and the approach the nurses used when placing him in isolation.

REFLECTIVE QUESTION

How can Johns'[5] notion of contradiction between vision and actual practice help Sue to resolve her feelings?

CASE STUDY 19.3

Jo has just started working on a busy medical unit. In the unit, a small group of nurses have been developing an action research project on nurses' and patients' perspectives of handover practices. Jo has been invited by the clinical nurse consultant, the project leader, to join the team. Jo is interested in the issue of handover and is keen to learn about research but feels anxious about being involved because she doesn't think she has a good understanding of the research process. As part of the initial phase of the project the team meets to plan and discuss the phases of the project and the respective roles they will take. Jo notices that, although there are some very senior nurses in the team, all team members join in the discussion and everyone's opinion is valued.

REFLECTIVE QUESTIONS

- How might Jo use reflection and reflective practices as part of her involvement in this action research project?
- Through her involvement in the project and in working with the team, what might Jo learn about her own practice, the practice of other nurses and her ability to reflect critically on these?

REFLECTIVE QUESTIONS

1. Think of a particular situation with a patient or family which you found challenging and/or where you felt troubled or concerned by their behaviour and/or your responses to it. How might engaging in clinical supervision have been helpful in addressing this situation/issue and in developing your knowledge and skills for the future?
2. When you attend your next work unit meeting, take careful note of the 'rules' for behaviour that seem to apply. Notice who gets listened to respectfully by the person who is the leader and manager of your work unit, whose opinion the leader takes seriously and acts upon. Notice any team members who give an opinion, but whose opinion does not seem to be taken seriously by the nursing leader and manager. If you feel comfortable in doing so, ask the nursing leader and manager later in private about what causes that person to listen to some people, and not to others. Reflect later upon the 'rules' in your work unit, and ask yourself how you can function in transformational ways to improve your unit's culture.
3. Think again about the connection between reflection and research. How do you think reflection could be useful in a clinical research project? Think in particular about how reflection and reflexivity might help you to identify things about you that you bring to the research endeavour and the decisions that are made throughout the project.

RECOMMENDED READING

Clouder L, Sellars J. Reflective practice and clinical supervision: an interprofessional perspective. Journal of Advanced Nursing 2004;46:262–9.

Johns C. Becoming a reflective practitioner. 2nd ed. Oxford: Blackwell; 2004.

Kinsella EA. Professional knowledge and the epistemology of reflective practice. Nursing Philosophy 2009;11:3–14.

Rolfe G, Freshwater D, Jasper M. Critical reflection for nursing and the helping professions: a user's guide. New York: Palgrave; 2001.

Usher K, Holmes C. Reflective practice: what, why and how. In: Daly J, Speedy S, Jackson D, editors. Contexts of nursing. 3rd ed. Sydney: Churchill Livingstone; 2009. p. 110–27.

REFERENCES

1. Taylor BJ. Reflective practice: a guide for healthcare professionals. 3rd ed. Maidenhead: Open University Press; 2010.

2. Royds K. Using reflective practice to learn from good and bad experiences. Learning Disability Practice 2010;13:20–3.

3. Boud D, Keogh R, Walker D. Reflection: turning experience into learning. London: Kogan Page; 1985.

4. Johns C. Becoming a reflective practitioner. 2nd ed. Oxford: Blackwell; 2004. p. 3.

5. Johns C. Becoming a reflective practitioner. 2nd ed. Oxford: Blackwell; 2004.

6. Usher K, Holmes C. Reflective practice: what, why and how. In: Daly J, Speedy S, Jackson D, editors. Contexts of nursing. 3rd ed. Sydney: Churchill Livingstone; 2009. p. 110–27.

7. Johns C. Becoming a reflective practitioner. 2nd ed. Oxford: Blackwell; 2004. p. xiii.

8. Rolfe G, Freshwater D, Jasper M. Critical reflection for nursing and the helping professions: a user's guide. New York: Palgrave; 2001.

9. Burrows DE. The nurse teacher's role in the promotion of reflective practice. Nurse Education Today 1995;15:346–50.

10. Smith A, Russell J. Using critical incidents in nurse education. Nurse Education Today 1991;11:284–91.

11. White J. Becoming a competent, confident professional practitioner. In: Chang E, Daly J, editors. Transitions in nursing: preparing for professional practice. Sydney: MacLennan Petty; 2001. p. 15–28.

12. Usher K, Holmes C. Reflective practice: what, why and how. In: Daly J, Speedy S, Jackson D, editors. Contexts of nursing. 3rd ed. Sydney: Churchill Livingstone; 2009. p. 113.

13. Freshwater D, Rolfe G. Critical reflexivity: a politically and ethically engaged research method for nursing. Journal of Research in Nursing 2001;6:526–37.

14. Schon DA. The reflective practitioner. New York: Basic Books, 1983.

15. Rolfe G. Closing the theory–practice gap: a model of nursing praxis. Journal of Clinical Nursing 1993;2:173–7.

16. Berggren I, da Silva A, Severinsson E. Core ethical issues of clinical nursing supervision. Nursing and Health Sciences 2005;7:21–8.

17. Clouder L, Sellars J. Reflective practice and clinical supervision: an interprofessional perspective. Journal of Advanced Nursing 2004;46:262–9.

18. Coleman D, Lynch U. Professional isolation and the role of clinical supervision in rural and remote communities. Journal of Community Nursing 2006;20: 35–7.

19. Turner K, Laut S, Kempster J, et al. Group clinical supervision: supporting neurology clinical nurse specialists in practice. Journal of Community Nursing 2005;19:4–8.

20. Hyrkas K, Appelqvist-Schmidlechner K, Kivimaki K. First-line managers' views of the long-term effects of clinical supervision: how does clinical supervision support and develop leadership in health care? Journal of Nursing Management 2005;13:209–20.

21. Johns C. Expanding the gates of perception. In: Johns C, Freshwater D, editors. Transforming nursing through reflective practice. 2nd ed. Oxford: Blackwell; 2005. p. 1.

22. Taylor BJ. Reflective practice: a guide for healthcare professionals. 3rd ed. Maidenhead: Open University Press; 2010.

23. Johns C. Expanding the gates of perception. In: Johns C, Freshwater D, editors. Transforming nursing through reflective practice. 2nd ed. Oxford: Blackwell; 2005. p. 7.

24. Taylor BJ. Reflective practice: a guide for healthcare professionals. 3rd ed. Maidenhead: Open University Press; 2010.

25. Crotty M. The foundations of social research. Crows Nest, NSW: Allen Unwin; 1998. p. 144.

26. Crotty M. The foundations of social research. Crows Nest, NSW: Allen Unwin; 1998.

27. Kouzes JM, Posner BZ. The leadership challenge. 3rd ed. San Francisco: John Wiley; 2002. p. 287.

28. Covey SR. Principle-centered leadership. New York: Simon Schuster; 1990.

29. Goleman D, Boyatzis R, McKee A. The new leaders: transforming the art of leadership into the science of results. London: Little Brown; 2002.

30. Kouzes JM, Posner BZ. The leadership challenge. 3rd ed. San Francisco: John Wiley; 2002.

31. Usher K, Holmes C. Reflective practice: what, why and how. In: Daly J, Speedy S, Jackson D, editors. Contexts of nursing. 3rd ed. Sydney: Churchill Livingstone; 2009. p. 103, 1015.

32. Beam RJ, O'Brien RA, Neal M. Reflective practice enhances public health nurse implementation of nurse–family partnership. Public Health Nursing 2010;27: 131–9.

33. Taylor BJ. Reflective practice: a guide for healthcare professionals. 3rd ed. Maidenhead: Open University Press; 2010.

34. Taylor BJ. Reflective practice: a guide for healthcare professionals. 3rd ed. Maidenhead: Open University Press; 2010.

35. Bannigan K, Moores A. A model of professional thinking: integrating reflective practice and evidence based practice. Canadian Journal of Occupational Therapy 2009;76:342–50.

36. Rolfe G. Evidence, memory and truth: towards a deconstructive validation of reflective practice. In: Johns C, Freshwater D, editors. Transforming nursing through reflective practice. 2nd ed. Oxford: Blackwell; 2005. p. 13–26.

37. Sigma Theta Tau International. The scholarship of reflective practice position paper. 2005. Online. Available: http://www.nursingsociety.org/about/resource_reflective.doc; 26 December 2006.

38. Taylor B. Identifying and transforming dysfunctional nurse–nurse relationships through reflective practice and action research. International Journal of Nursing Practice 2001;7:406–11.

39. Kim HS. Critical reflective inquiry for knowledge development in nursing practice. Journal of Advanced Nursing 1999;29:1205–12.

40. Gustafsson C, Fagerberg I. Reflection, the way to professional development? Journal of Clinical Nursing 2004;3:271–80.

41. Paget T. Reflective practice and clinical outcomes: practitioners' views on how reflective practice has influenced their clinical practice. Journal of Clinical Nursing 2001;10:204–14.

42. Peden-McAlpine C, Tomlinson PS, Forneris SG, et al. Evaluation of a reflective practice intervention to enhance family care. Journal of Advanced Nursing 2005;49:494–501.

43. Foster K, McAllister M, O'Brien L. Extending the boundaries: autoethnography as an emergent method in mental health nursing research. International Journal of Mental Health Nursing 2006;15:44–53.

44. Finlay L. 'Outing' the researcher: the provenance, process, and practice of reflexivity. Qualitative Health Research 2002;12:531–45.

45. Kucera K, Higgins I, McMillan M. Advanced nursing practice: a futures model derived from narrative analysis of nurses' stories. Australian Journal of Advanced Nursing 2010;27:43–53.

46. Jarrett L, Johns C. Constructing the reflexive narrative. In: Johns C, Freshwater D, editors. Transforming nursing through reflective practice. 2nd ed. Oxford: Blackwell; 2005. p. 147.

47. McIlveen P. Autoethnography as a method for reflexive research and practice in vocational psychology. Australian Journal of Career Development 2008;17: 13–20.

48. Ellis C. The ethnographic I: a methodological novel about autoethnography. Walnut Creek: Altamira Press; 2004.

49. Foster K, McAllister M, O'Brien L. Extending the boundaries: autoethnography as an emergent method in mental health nursing research. International Journal of Mental Health Nursing 2006;15:44–53.

50. Foster K, McAllister M, O'Brien L. Coming to autoethnography: a mental health nurse's experience. International Journal of Qualitative Methods 2005;4, Article 1. Online. Available: http://www.ualberta.ca/~ijqm/backissues/4_4/html/foster.pdf 20 Jan 2006.

CHAPTER 20

Mentoring for new graduates

Stephen Neville and Denise Wilson

LEARNING OBJECTIVES

At the end of this chapter you should:

- know the difference between mentorship, preceptorship and clinical supervision
- understand the importance of mentoring in nursing
- be able to articulate the skills and attributes necessary for a successful mentor relationship to develop
- identify appropriate mentoring strategies and processes
- feel prepared to participate in a mentoring relationship.

Keywords: mentorship, new graduate, postregistration development, preceptor, clinical supervisor/supervision

INTRODUCTION AND BACKGROUND

The role of student nurse is one of being nurtured and supervised, contrasting with the role of registered nurse, which demands a role reversal to become the nurturer, supervisor and mentor of others. Embarking on this journey to become a fully fledged functioning registered nurse involves opportunities and challenges – some are exciting, others are daunting. Often making the transition from student to registered nurse occurs within practice environments that are busy and complex, with minimal support readily available. Mentoring as a new graduate can be overwhelming, especially when the demands of the practice environment encroach, a crisis of confidence ensues and an all-consuming desire to continue being nurtured surfaces.

The role and responsibilities of being a registered nurse include mentoring other nurses and health professionals, such as health and nursing assistants – it is a role that cannot be escaped. It is useful to have some knowledge about mentoring and developing strategies and processes to assist in undertaking this role, although time and experience will enrich knowledge and skills around mentoring. Nevertheless, new registered nurses who are mentoring more junior staff cannot realistically be expected to know everything. In this chapter, we stress the importance of mentoring in nursing and explain the differences between mentoring, preceptoring and clinical supervision. Various approaches to mentoring are described, and the skills and attributes necessary for successful mentoring are outlined, so that as a new registered nurse you will feel better prepared to participate in a mentoring relationship. We begin by exploring the reality of making the transition from student to registered nurse.

THE TRANSITION TO PRACTICE

The transition from student nurse to registered nurse is a time of great anticipation and excitement but also one that is rather scary as the notion of autonomous practice becomes a reality. It is also a time of being faced with self-doubt and questions about our readiness: Do I have the necessary abilities and capabilities to be a registered nurse? What will others expect of me? Will I be able to do what is expected of me? How will I be able to juggle a full patient load? How will I manage emergencies? Will I get the help that I need when I need it? Will people treat me kindly? Will other nurses recognise my need for help? How will I mentor and support others while I am learning? It is usual to question your ability, readiness and fitness to practise and to do what is expected without the protection associated with student status. This conflicting concoction of feelings and emotions is quite normal as at last the doing, thinking and being a nurse become reality.

The process of becoming a professional registered nurse is influenced by a number of contextual factors in the workplace that include the expectations of self and others, the perception of status by others, being accepted, and being assisted and advocated for by others. Unfortunately the practice reality is not always as it should be. Socialisation into the profession may not be a smooth path, and the experience is often described as 'transition shock', as the reality of being a student differs markedly.[1] During the transition to practice, the experience is discernible by any or all of the following:

- the effort of being a professional functioning registered nurse
- a practice environment that is busy, complex and unpredictable, making it difficult to reflect and learn from experiences as the new registered nurse aims to get from the beginning to the end of the shift
- unrealistic workloads to manage with little support
- working with less than helpful colleagues who at times may seem obstructive – this is often described as lateral or horizontal violence[2]
- the dissonance that occurs with trying to apply theoretical knowledge and skills to practice reality
- an inability to use acquired knowledge and evidence because of the barriers created by any of the above points

- not having beginning status recognised, as evident by the unrealistic expectation that new registered nurses 'hit the floor running' and function to the level of experienced registered nurses
- the expectation to mentor another registered nurse, enrolled nurse or healthcare assistant without the necessary knowledge, experience or mentorship.

Research into lateral or horizontal violence in nursing has identified that this phenomenon is manifest in the form of bullying behaviours, being undermined, intimidating behaviours, whether verbal or non-verbal, and withholding information.[2] All of these factors are a source of stress and anxiety experienced by many new registered nurses that may result in not achieving one's own practice expectations, especially when factors outside your control contribute to an inability to make appropriate choices and sound decisions. Although conflict is inevitable when working with people, their behaviours and frailties, if ongoing it can have a detrimental effect on health and wellbeing.[3] Moral distress is an example of the stresses that may occur, especially when a conflict with personal values is experienced in some situations that can lead to a plethora of negative feelings and behaviours if not managed. This is an example of a situation where a mentor can assist to explore sources of moral distress or conflict and develop strategies to help move forward,[4] particularly when required to mentor others.

The self-confidence and self-worth of beginning registered nurses are potentially fragile, and are at risk in response to some practice situations. Understanding your self-concept is important for job satisfaction and managing the stresses experienced from being a new registered nurse.[5] Cowin and Hengstberger-Sims[6] claim the following dimensions assist in understanding one's self-concept: nurse general self-concept, care, staff relations, communication, knowledge and leadership. Such self-reflection can be difficult when adapting to a new environment, learning a new role and functioning in a practice setting, especially when at times it is difficult to ascertain what is right and wrong. Participating in the mentoring process has the potential to support newly registered nurses through difficult situations. In addition, mentoring can assist with the identification of individual developmental needs as a newly graduated nurse, and is especially important when you are required to mentor others in clinical practice.

With the reality of becoming a registered nurse, the illusion of safety and security experienced as a student nurse increasingly fades. An expectation of being a registered nurse includes the requirement to mentor and supervise health assistants, enrolled nurses and other registered nurses. Despite having registered nurse status, mentoring involves yet another new journey as a 'beginning' registered nurse. Mentoring requires confidence that comes with experience and developing professional practice, yet the practice environment does not always afford this luxury. Understanding the acquirement of practice experience and wisdom can be helpful.

It is important to remember that, as a new registered nurse, the preparation you have undergone as a student nurse leads you to the status of beginning registered nurse, not an experienced one, despite the expectations of others within the workplace. This is an important reality to remember when the expectations from yourself, your colleagues and/or patients and their families are beyond what seems to be fair and reasonable. Recognising your beginning status and not being afraid to ask are not always luxuries afforded to beginning practitioners. This is when having an experienced respected registered nurse with wisdom and expertise to assist you in the mentoring role is helpful. Positive outcomes of mentoring for the mentor include: the development of collegial relationships, networking, sharing of ideas, reflection, personal fulfilment and growth; and for the mentee: support, understanding, encouragement, analysis and friendship.[7] The transition to registered nurse status can be a daunting prospect, especially when required to mentor. However, the value of mentoring others cannot be underestimated, especially the contribution it can make to improving client outcomes.[8]

EXERCISE 20.1

Think about being a mentor and fold a piece of paper into quarters. In each quarter write the following headings:

- Expectations I have of myself
- Expectations others may have of me (such as other registered nurses, patients, patients' family, doctors, other health professionals)
- My readiness to be a mentor and the supports I have in place
- My fears about being a mentor.

Identify the strengths that you have to support your development as a mentor, and the areas for development. Undertaking this exercise may help you develop some of the skills and attributes necessary to participate in a mentoring role successfully. This exercise will help you to identify your future learning needs regarding being a mentor.

MENTORING: WHAT IT IS AND ISN'T

Even though mentoring has been around for a considerable length of time it remains an elusive term that has been identified as difficult to define. For example, in nursing there appears to be some confusion regarding the difference between mentorship, preceptorship and clinical supervision. While there are some similarities between the three concepts, the differences are important and should therefore be teased out to ensure they are better understood.

A preceptor is someone who is well versed in the skills and attitudes needed to be clinically successful, as well as being esteemed as an expert practitioner.[9] A preceptor is frequently involved in teaching a preceptee new or different clinical skills, usually within a structure focused on meeting specific learning objectives within a specified period of time. The preceptor–preceptee model is frequently utilised to foster student learning in undergraduate nursing programs, enrolled nurses and other healthcare personnel (healthcare assistants) new to working in a particular healthcare organisation, as well as new graduates as they transition from student to registered nurse.

Not only does the preceptor–preceptee relationship offer a supportive role for those facing the challenges associated with providing a healthcare service, it also protects the general public from relatively inexperienced new practitioners. Therefore formal evaluation of the preceptored person's performance is frequently a component associated with the preceptor role to ensure that preceptees have the appropriate knowledge and skills to be safe to practise. Therefore preceptorship is both pragmatic and functional and can best be described as providing transitional support.[10]

Traditionally, the concept of clinical supervision has been associated with professional groups such as counselling, psychotherapy, mental health nurses and social work, and has only been valued and promoted within nursing in Australia and New Zealand in recent times.[9] Clinical supervision has been defined as regular, protected time for facilitated, indepth reflection on clinical practice.[11–13] The aims of clinical supervision include enabling the supervisee to achieve, sustain and continue to develop high-quality practice. Clinical supervision may include aspects of both mentoring and preceptorship at differing times, but is largely based around the specific encounters that take place between the nurse and the client or the nurse and co-workers. It is the encounter or interaction that is the focus of the supervisory session.

Butterworth et al.,[14] who are key writers on clinical supervision and mentoring, differentiate clinical supervision from mentoring by identifying mentoring as 'an experienced professional nurturing and guiding the novitiate', and clinical supervision as 'an exchange between practising professionals to enable the development of professional skills' (p 12). At the same time a mentor relationship differs from preceptorship in that there is no formal evaluation process involved in the mentor–mentee relationship. Because of the similarities between preceptorship, clinical supervision and mentoring it appears that a definitive definition of mentoring is challenging to find.

The concept of mentoring can be traced back centuries to ancient Greek times. The traditional term 'mentor' has its origins in the ancient Greek classic, Homer's *Odyssey*. In this story, Odysseus, who is about to fight in the Trojan war, asks Mentor, his best friend, to tutor and care for his son Telemachus. As a result, Mentor becomes Telemachus' trusted counsellor, advisor and friend, teaching him about life and the world as he transitions into adulthood. In keeping with Greek mythology, mentoring relationships continued to be utilised in academic institutions such as universities. Here postgraduate students were attached to a more senior and wise person, whose role was to support and guide their academic development.

Both of the above examples identify that a mentor is an older, trusted and wiser person who protects and encourages a younger person in a relationship that occurs over a period of time. In contemporary nursing practice mentoring can be defined as an enduring relationship 'in which a more experienced person acts as an advisor for someone less experienced to assist his or her personal growth and development' (p 18).[15] Others suggest that both the mentor and mentee share in the personal, as well as professional, growth and development that occur as a consequence of this relationship and subsequent interactions.[16]

How mentoring benefits nursing practice

Mentorship has many benefits that not only positively influence nursing practice but also have an impact on today's healthcare market. McCloughen and O'Brien[17] identify mentoring as necessary to assist with role transition and providing support to any registered nurse, whether newly registered or experienced, as well as those health personnel who are new to a particular clinical area. It has also been suggested that healthcare organisations should implement mentoring programs as a means of enhancing nursing satisfaction and the retention of staff, which ultimately will have a positive impact on patient health outcomes.[18] Successful mentorship can improve corporate knowledge within an organisation and make employees feel valued, as well as forming the foundations for the development of future nurse leaders.[9,15]

Characteristics of mentors/mentees

Although not essential, a mentor is usually someone who has professional and/or academic standing within his or her field who may or may not be a nurse. As nursing evolves and recognises its full potential, more nurses are now willing to become mentors and more nurses seeking mentorship choose nurses to fulfil this important role. However, the mentor–mentee relationship is both dynamic and dyadic. Not only do mentees seek the support and guidance from a mentor but equally mentors actively seek nurses to mentor. Barker[10] claims that often mentors seek potential protégés to mentor, those who may progress the nursing profession forward, change practice and ultimately improve health outcomes.

EXERCISE 20.2

Do you consider yourself:
- intelligent?
- motivated?
- articulate with good communication and interpersonal skills?
- not afraid to work hard or take risks?
- to be open to new ways of doing things and seeing the world?
- trustworthy and full of integrity?
- to have good professional presentation skills?
- willing to invest in your career?
- to be curious by nature?
- to have vision both for yourself and for nursing?
  (Adapted from Grossman and Valiga[19])
  If you answer yes to all of the above then you have the qualities necessary to enter a mentoring relationship either as a mentor or a mentee.

Mentoring approaches

Mentor relationships revolve around supporting, coaching, listening, challenging and encouraging the mentee, whether the relationship between the mentee and mentor is formal or informal.[20] Having an understanding of the mentoring approaches that can be used to model and develop relationships is useful. Mentoring can vary from country to country, and there are a number of approaches that can range from the more traditional concept of mentoring that is considered informal, to the structured and formalised approach. A structured or formalised approach, however, is often limited as it tends to be based on an organisation's interest in improving quality, practice outcomes for clients or the retention of staff, rather than on the nurse's or health worker's personal developmental needs.

Informal mentoring is a reciprocal process that occurs naturally, where two people are attracted and develop a relationship based on mutual respect, trust, patience and positive role modelling by the mentor, and have the commitment to nurturing and mutual sharing.[9,21] Informal mentoring has been described as an 'alliance between two people, which creates a space for dialogue, resulting in their reflection, action and learning'.[9] At times, the mentoring relationship is not recognised as such due to its unstructured nature, and the development of friendships over time. Many nurses and health workers have been informally mentored by someone who is an expert whom they have professionally admired and respected as a representation of how they would like to practise. They themselves have generally been mentored by someone they have admired, who has nurtured, supported, challenged and encouraged them in their practice development. However, it should be noted that, without some structure and infrastructure for the mentoring relationship, the process of mentoring may be 'serendipitous and ineffective' (p 111).[22]

Formal approaches to mentoring, however, differ in intention, the context in which the mentoring relationship occurs, the duration of the relationship and the outcomes expected of the mentoring process.[9] Formal mentoring programs are either a requirement or available depending upon the organisation's culture and aim. They are distinguishable by their structured nature and the purposeful assigning of mentee to mentor,[9] and may or may not differentiate between areas of practice. Also evident in formal approaches to mentoring is the selection of volunteers deemed appropriate to undertake training and the role of mentoring, and evaluation of the effectiveness of the program in some way.[7] Specific groups of healthcare workers are frequently targeted for mentoring of some type.[15] New graduate programs for newly registered nurses may be an example of a formalised mentoring program, where mentoring is a component of the program. Such approaches toward mentoring are criticised as they are not considered 'true mentoring' in the traditional sense, as when, for example, Mentor became a mentor to Telemachus, as discussed earlier in this chapter.[9]

There are a number of models for mentoring.[15] The following is an overview of a selection of mentoring models.

ONE-TO-ONE MENTORING

- Traditional – characterised by a mentor–mentee relationship that is usually based on the expert mentoring of the novice.
- Pair mentoring – there is a horizontal relationship between the mentee and the mentor where the mentoring relationship is predicated on sharing expertise. This type of relationship values the often current knowledge and skills that the mentee brings to the practice setting, but may not be valued by others.
- Mentoring forward – in this model there is a vertical relationship where the mentee is mentored, and a horizontal relationship where the mentee passes on the knowledge and skills learnt from the mentoring relationship to another mentee. In this model, the mentee is also learning to become a mentor.

CLUSTER MENTORING

- Team mentoring – there are generally a number of mentors who are experts for a mentee, and they usually function in a vertical relationship. An example of this would be the learning of independent practice, such as community nursing, where the registered nurse needs to acquire diverse knowledge and skills that may span across specialty areas and disciplines.

- Inclusion mentoring – in contrast to team mentoring, inclusion mentoring involves one expert mentor for several mentees, and the mentoring activities are shared. Notably with this model, relationships may not be key.
- Group mentoring – this type of mentoring involves a group of like-minded people getting together to discuss their work situations. This type of approach may be helpful for new registered nurses who can share like experiences and problem-solve how to manage future situations. However, the disadvantage of this approach for new registered nurses is that sometimes you 'don't know what you don't know'; you are still learning the networks and how to access sources of expertise and resources.

DISTANCE MENTORING

- This approach occurs when meeting face to face is difficult. Mentoring occurs via telephone, email or, more recently, using videocams on personal computers. This approach requires clear goals and sound communication skills as it has been reported to be difficult to maintain using telephone or email.[15]

Considerations for mentoring

Prior to embarking on an organisational mentoring program you should consider the following aspects[15]:

1. Choice – what choices do you have within the mentoring context offered? Are you able to choose your mentee? Do you have the freedom to meet when desired?
2. Relationships – is the mentoring relationship based on collegiality, discipline-specific, aimed at improving professional networks and relationships, and gaining knowledge about the various structures within which you have worked?
3. Structure – what does the mentoring experience promote and facilitate? For example, will it enhance your networks, or ethical practice? Does it function to develop professional practice, or psychosocial aspects of practice, or both?
4. Resources – does the organisational culture value and promote mentoring?

No matter what type or model of mentoring you engage in, the nature of the relationship you have with your mentee and the quality of communication are crucial to its success. Successful mentoring is a reciprocal process that relies on the mentee being self-motivated and using initiative to engage in the process actively, and is important to remember when working with a mentee. The old saying that 'you get out what you put in' holds true for most mentoring relationships. If you are opting for an informal mentoring process, or have the choice of mentee in a formal mentoring program, selecting a mentee that you respect and can relate to is vital for its success. Mentees will also be looking for a role model, someone they respect and who possesses knowledge of nursing and health practice, possibly in your specialty area of practice, who is sensitive of their needs.

In the situation where an employing organisation arranges a mentoring relationship, and a mentee is assigned, you need to ask yourself: 'Am I the best person for this role?' There is no doubt that participating in a mentoring relationship will personally influence both parties in relation to achieving career aspirations as a registered nurse, as well as positively influencing practice and professional development. Having an overview of approaches to mentoring will enable you to explore how to begin a mentoring relationship.

Operationalising the mentoring process

As a new graduate, you may find yourself in the position of intentionally or unintentionally being a mentor to other nurses and/or healthcare assistants. It is therefore essential that you prepare yourself to undertake this role. You may have formally or informally participated in mentoring programs either as a mentor or a mentee, or as both. However, the realities of contemporary clinical practice may mean that you bring to the mentor–mentee relationship little experience of either of these processes. Exercise 20.2 identified that you have the qualities to mentor another person. It is important to realise that your work as a mentor sits alongside your role as a registered nurse, a role that is responsible for the provision of a safe and appropriate healthcare experience to consumers of that service.

EXERCISE 20.3

Make a list of the knowledge, skills and attributes you think you need to be a good mentor. Then compare your list with the one in Table 20.1. You could use this list to assess the effectiveness of your mentor during your final placement, and to assess your capacity to become a mentor.

How does a nurse become a mentor? The first step in the process is to be willing to undertake this role. Once you have decided to commit yourself to being a mentor you then need to look out for someone who might benefit from your knowledge and skills no matter how vast or limited. You might choose a person who is new to the area where you work, or as identified earlier, you may be formally assigned someone to mentor by your employing organisation.

As previously discussed, a definitive definition of mentoring is hard to provide. However, the essential characteristics[9] associated with being a good mentor have been identified (Table 20.1).

Getting started

Agreeing on and formalising a mentoring agreement is the first place to start in the mentoring process. When establishing a mentoring relationship or agreement with a mentee it is important to discuss and explore how the individuals involved anticipate the relationship will work. Formalising the mentor–mentee relationship through the utilisation of an official agreement protects both parties by potentially preventing situations from occurring where either person may feel his or her expectations are not being met. Find out if your employing organisation has an existing mentoring

Table 20.1 Essential characteristics for mentoring

Characteristic	Description
Envisioner	Gives the mentee a picture of what nursing can be like
Energiser	Is dynamic, positive and enthusiastic
Investor	Invests time and energy in the mentee
Supporter	Supports the mentee through the highs and lows of providing a healthcare service
Prodder	Pushes the mentee to achieve/provide the highest standards of professional development and care
Challenger	Opens the mentee's eyes to other possibilities and encourages critical thinking
Connections maker	Opens doors and introduces mentees to people of influence
Career counsellor	Supports and encourages the mentee to develop and work towards future career aspirations and goals

agreement template that you could utilise. If not, the areas to be considered when establishing a mentoring relationship and agreement should include, but are by no means limited to, the following:

- Name and preferred contact details of both the mentor and mentee, including preferred postal address, cell phone number and email address.
- The frequency, venue and length of each meeting, as well as how the meetings will take place. For example, will they be face to face, via email, chat room, videocam or phone?
- A mechanism for contacting each other outside the scheduled meetings in case any issue arises that demands immediate attention.
- Determine the focus of the mentoring relationship. For example, will it focus on clinical practice or career development, or a combination of the two? A well-defined timeframe should accompany all mentoring activities.
- It is imperative to include a statement relating to the confidentiality of any communication between the mentor and mentee.
- A review date should be included. The review should encompass both the relationship as well as the process.
- As this is a formal mentoring agreement, both mentor and mentee should sign and date the document.

EXERCISE 20.4

Critique the above list of suggested items that could be included in a mentoring agreement. Do you agree with the points above? Are there any more you would like to add?

BUILDING AND DEVELOPING THE MENTORING RELATIONSHIP

All mentors need to be able to use effective verbal and non-verbal therapeutic communication skills to ensure that they are effective in their role. All new graduates understand and utilise therapeutic communication skills, which formed the foundation of their nursing degree program, as being integral to any interactions between them as registered nurses and consumers of their health service. These verbal and non-verbal therapeutic communication skills can also be utilised throughout all mentoring interactions (see Ch 11).

Integral to the mentoring relationship is mastering the skills necessary to build, develop and maintain a positive mentor–mentee relationship, fundamentally based on trust.[10] Although all nurses are familiar with developing these types of relationships with consumers of health services as well as their colleagues, it may be challenging in a mentor–mentee relationship. It is important that the mentor is honest with the mentee and acknowledges any feelings of nervousness about working closely with that person, in addition to any thoughts or feelings of needing to know more than the mentee, as part of the relationship. Acknowledging these thoughts and feelings will only assist with the development of trust and ensuring the success of the process for both parties.

Due to the globalisation of the nursing workforce, nurses are a multicultural entity. Not only do mentors need to communicate ensuring verbal clarity, and attending to non-verbal cues, including physical actions, it is imperative to ensure that any interactions and interpretations between both parties are cognisant of cultural variations. Borges and Clement-Smith[21] assert that developing a communication style that takes into account variations in culture and ethnicity ensures there is no room for misinterpretation. All mentors should therefore communicate clearly, while carefully observing the impact the information given has on the mentee.

A particularly useful and powerful strategy for beginning the mentor–mentee relationship is encouraging the mentee to set goals. Yoder-Wise[23] identifies that the setting of long-term goals may be difficult to formulate when nurses are early on in their career. However, the setting of short- and medium-term goals will greatly assist the mentor to get to know the mentee, and additionally helps with providing structure and direction to the process.

What to do when the mentoring relationship strikes trouble

As previously discussed, the setting of goals along with timelines is important for ensuring the success of the mentor–mentee relationship. Research studies have identified that lack of commitment and time, poor preparation of both mentor and mentee, and organisational constraints were all significant issues that contributed to the breakdown in the mentor–mentee relationship.[24,25] Due to these issues the relationship between the two parties can drift apart with contact becoming less frequent to the point where the mentoring process ceases to exist. This situation can be both hurtful and discouraging for all concerned, with both individuals left wondering what they did wrong.

Earlier in the chapter it was suggested that, as part of the contractual arrangement between mentor and mentee, a review process is undertaken to ensure each participant's needs are being met. In situations where there has been a breakdown in the mentor and mentee relationship, an external third party may be needed to act as a mediator to resolve any issues – ideally such a provision should be negotiated during the contractual process. However, illuminating any potential and actual problems with the mentoring relationship should be highlighted and addressed early. An integral part of any mentoring session should include opportunities for both parties to check in with each other and acknowledge the strengths and issues that relate to the mentor–mentee relationship. Although this may be difficult to do, all nurses, as part of their education, have been taught the skills of managing conflict within professional relationships. It is important to acknowledge the possibilities of either party wanting to discontinue the relationship and understanding from the outset that this is a possibility, and could be part of the process. Discussing the termination of the relationship should occur well in advance, preferably at the very beginning of the process. A useful time for this to happen would be when the guidelines and contract are discussed and agreed on.

Another issue that may have a negative impact on the mentoring relationship relates to confidentiality and how ethical dilemmas are to be managed. The literature recommends that guidelines should be incorporated into the contract to help manage and address instances where the mentee discloses unsafe and/or unprofessional practice.[14] Familiarity with relevant legislation or regulation (such as the Health Practitioners' Competency Assurance Act in New Zealand, or the Health Practitioner Regulation National Law (Victoria) Act 2009 in Australia) is crucial as it outlines the legal obligations with regard to unsafe or incompetent practice. Inherent in, and underpinning, the mentoring relationship is the professional development of the mentee. Others take this further by asserting that professional nurturing and development of nurses promote ethical competence.[11]

Challenges for the mentor therefore include deciding what issues disclosed in confidence are breaches of the law and/or the code of conduct associated with being a health worker and those where no harm has occurred but significant professional development has taken place. Ideally, when beginning a mentor relationship, limits to confidentiality should be made clear. For instance, when patients' safety is compromised by unsafe practice, such as working outside the registered nurse scope of practice, or incidents of incompetence such as making errors in drug calculations, there is a legal obligation to report such incidents so remedial action can be instituted as soon as possible.

EXERCISE 20.5

Take time to conceptualise and then identify how you would manage moral and ethical dilemmas[26,27] that may arise as part of the mentoring process.

Support for mentors

Just as mentees need support and guidance from mentors, the reverse is also true. Successfully undertaking the role of mentor does not occur within a vacuum; it requires considerable financial investment on the part of the employing organisation, as well as a personal investment on the behalf of both mentor and mentee. Any financial investment by the organisation may not materialise as compensation to the mentor directly but should at least include either clinical supervision or mentoring for the mentor, or both.

If there is no formal support structures offered, such as clinical supervision or mentoring for the mentor, self-mentoring could be considered.[28] Self-mentoring requires that nurses, as a starting point, be self-reliant, believe in themselves, be innately reflective and have the confidence to ask questions. Many of these skills are fostered and encouraged in undergraduate nursing programs. Although not ideal, self-mentoring could be used to 'plug a gap' until appropriate resources and/or people are available to support the mentor formally.

EXERCISE 20.6

Identify things important for your own personal, professional and clinical practice development as a nurse, and list these. For example, your list may include items that relate to being:

1. a newly registered nurse
2. in the position of mentoring another nurse or healthcare assistant.

From this list, write personal, professional and clinical practice development goals. For example: Undertake clinical supervision in relation to mentorship development, or Complete a beginning registered nurse professional portfolio by the end of my first year of practice.

These goals will form the basis of your future clinical supervision and/or mentoring needs.

CONCLUSION

The process of becoming a confident and professional registered nurse occurs within an often chaotic practice environment. It is a process of moving from practising in an 'adequate' manner to becoming more confident and competent, to feeling able to contribute to the advancement of nursing. The requirement to be a mentor to others occurs during this process. Often new registered nurses may feel inadequate to assume and undertake this important role. However, having knowledge about mentoring and its various approaches can provide the basis for developing the skills and attributes to be a positive mentor.

The mentor–mentee relationship is dynamic and dyadic, and is based on the characteristics required of all registered nurses – that is, trust, effective verbal and non-verbal communication and the ability to share information and support development. A positive mentoring relationship contributes to improvements in practice, and ultimately health outcomes. Mentoring others can be a source of personal and professional satisfaction, derived from seeing others grow professionally in their practice. Informal mentoring approaches bring the added bonus of the development of long-term friendships that can be an ongoing source of support.

CASE STUDY 20.1

Rosie is excited to be a new registered nurse and has been assigned a mentor, Lilly, by the nurse manager in the area. Lilly is an experienced registered nurse and is enthusiastic about nursing and patient care. While Lilly has been excellent at introducing Rosie to various people of relative importance and modelling networking behaviour, Rosie is really committed to improving the standard of her nursing practice and being exposed to challenging questions to make her think critically about various aspects of her practice. She suddenly realises she should have talked to the nurse manager about her needs earlier when she had the opportunity.

REFLECTIVE QUESTIONS

- What strategies could Rosie use to ensure that her mentoring needs are met by Lilly?
- Why should Rosie have determined the characteristics needed in a mentor and her mentoring needs before getting into a situation where a mentor is assigned for her?
- Who could Rosie have talked to about her mentoring needs?

CASE STUDY 20.2

Craig is a newly registered nurse who is working in an assessment, treatment and rehabilitation ward in a large metropolitan hospital. He is being mentored by a very experienced registered nurse and is very happy with the mentoring he has received. Two enrolled nurses have just been employed to work on the ward and Craig has been asked to mentor one of these people.

REFLECTIVE QUESTIONS

- How should Craig prepare for his new role as mentor?
- How should he now use his time with his mentor?

CASE STUDY 20.3

Cassie is new to her clinical area, which is a busy surgical ward in a medium-sized acute hospital in a small city where most people know each other. Cassie has been assigned a mentor who was reluctant to take on the role. They have been meeting irregularly and, when they have met, the mentor constantly complains about how busy she is and consequently rushes the arranged sessions. Cassie feels unsupported and dissatisfied, and would like to be mentored by a different registered nurse.

REFLECTIVE QUESTION

- What steps should Cassie take to address her feelings of being unsupported and dissatisfied, taking into consideration that she is a newly registered nurse who is new to the clinical area and part of a small well-connected community, and is at risk of being isolated if she speaks out?

RECOMMENDED READING

Beecroft P, Santner S, Lacy M, et al. New graduates' perceptions of mentoring: six-year programme evaluation. Journal of Advanced Nursing 2006;55:736–47.

Cross W, Moore A, Ockerby S. Clinical supervision of general nurses in a busy medical ward of a teaching hospital. Contemporary Nurse 2010;35:245–53.

Latham CL, Hogan M, Ringl K. Nurses supporting nurses: creating a mentoring program for staff nurses to improve the workforce environment. Nursing Administration Quarterly 2008;32:27–39.

McCloughen A, O'Brien L, Jackson D. Positioning mentorship within Australian nursing contexts: a literature review. Contemporary Nurse 2006;23:120–34.

O'Keefe T, Forrester DA. A successful online mentoring program for nurses. Administration Quarterly 2009;33:245–50.

REFERENCES

1. Boychuk-Duchscher J. Transition shock: the initial stage of role adaptation for newly graduated registered nurses. Journal of Advanced Nursing 2009;65: 1103–13.

2. Stanley K, Martin M, Michel Y, et al. Examining lateral violence in the nursing workforce. Issues in Mental Health Nursing 2007;28:1247–65.

3. Almost J. Conflict within nursing work environments: concept analysis. Journal of Advanced Nursing 2005;53:444–53.

4. Nathaniel A. Moral reckoning in nursing. Western Journal of Nursing Research 2006;28:419–38.

5. Arthur D, Yong-Loo L. The professional self-concept of nurses: a review of the literature from 1992–2006. Australian Journal of Advanced Nursing 2007;24: 60–4.

6. Cowin L, Hengstberger-Sims C. New graduate nurse self-concept and retention: a longitudinal study. International Journal of Nursing Studies 2006;43: 59–70.

7. Ehrich L, Hansford B, Tennet L. Formal mentoring programs in education and other professions: a review of the literature. Educational Administration Quarterly 2004;40:518–40.

8. Funderburk A. Mentoring: the retention factor in the acute care setting. Journal of Nursing Staff Development 2008;24:1–5.

9. McCloughen A, O'Brien L, Jackson D. Positioning mentorship within Australian nursing contexts: a literature review. Contemporary Nurse 2006;23:120–34.

10. Barker E. Mentoring – a complex relationship. Journal of the American Academy of Nurse Practitioners 2006;18:56–61.

11. Berggren I, da Silva A, Severinsson E. Core ethical issues of clinical nursing supervision. Nursing and Health Sciences 2005;7:21–8.

12. Cross W, Moore A, Ockerby S. Clinical supervision of general nurses in a busy medical ward of a teaching hospital. Contemporary Nurse 2010;35:245–53.

13. Lakeman R, Glasgow C. Introducing peer-group clinical supervision: an action research project. International Journal of Mental Health Nursing 2009;18: 204–10.

14. Butterworth T, Faugier J, Burnard P. Clinical supervision and mentorship in nursing. 2nd ed. Chelthenham: Stanley Thornes; 1998.

15. Heartfield M, Gibson T. Mentoring for nurses in general practice: national issues and challenges. Collegian 2005;12:17–21.

16. Dorsey L, Barker C. Mentoring undergraduate nursing students. Nurse Educator 2004;29:260–5.
17. McCloughen A, O'Brien L. Development of a mentorship programme for new graduate nurses in mental health. International Journal of Mental Health Nursing 2005;14:276–84.
18. Block L, Claffey C, Korow M, et al. The value of mentorship within nursing organizations. Nursing Forum 2005;40:134–40.
19. Grossman S, Valiga T. The new leadership challenge. Creating the future of nursing. Philadelphia: F A Davis; 2008.
20. Donner G, Wheeler M. Taking control of your nursing career. A handbook for health professionals. Canada: Mosby; 2009.
21. Borges J, Clement-Smith B. So you think you're ready to mentor? Strategies for mentoring a diverse nursing workforce. Nurse Leader 2004;2:45–8.
22. Kerfoot K, Cox M. The synergy model: the ultimate mentoring model. Critical Care Nursing Clinics of North America 2005;17:109–19.
23. Yoder-Wise P. Leading and managing in nursing. 5th ed. Missouri: Mosby; 2010.
24. Beecroft P, Santner S, Lacy M, et al. New graduate nurses' perceptions of mentoring: six-year programme evaluation. Journal of Advanced Nursing 2006;55:736–47.
25. Gilmour J, Kopeikin A, Douche J. Student nurses as peer-mentors: collegiality in practice. Nurse Education in Practice 2007;7:36–43.
26. Johnstone M-J. Bioethics: a nursing perspective. 5th ed. Sydney: Churchill Livingstone/Elsevier; 2009.
27. Fry ST, Johnstone M-J. Ethics in nursing practice: a guide to ethical decision making. Chichester, UK: Wiley-Blackwell; 2008.
28. Cherry B, Jacob S. Contemporary nursing. Issues, trends and management. 5th ed. Philadelphia: Mosby; 2011.

CHAPTER 21

Professional career development: development of the CAPABLE nursing professional

Jane Conway and Margaret McMillan

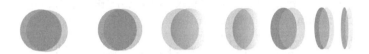

LEARNING OBJECTIVES

When you have completed this chapter you will be able to:

- differentiate between professional career development and career progression
- identify factors that result in changing career development opportunities for nurses
- apply the CAPABLE framework to thinking about your professional career development
- identify interrelationships among professional career development, reflective practice and lifelong learning
- identify a range of strategies for career development.

Keywords: career, capability, lifelong learning, career pathway, role transition

---

INTRODUCTION

This chapter explores the concept of professional career development in nursing. It identifies the need to view professional career development as uniquely personal yet aligned to the directions of the nursing profession and responsive to community and organisational expectations. The chapter introduces the CAPABLE framework in order to assist those in transition to examine, reflect upon and validate their professional careers. The framework has been derived from key concepts related to career development in nursing and other literature.

DEFINING PROFESSIONAL CAREER DEVELOPMENT

A career can be defined as the lifelong process of aligning individual interests and the opportunities (or limitations) present in the external work-related environment, in order to meet both individual and environmental needs.[1] Career planning is the process through which individuals evaluate the opportunities that exist, determine their career goals and take advantage of employment experience, education and other developmental opportunities that will help them reach these goals.[2] Career progression involves developing through a frequently hierarchical career pathway where each new position is viewed as having greater responsibility, authority and remuneration. Historically, measures of success in a career have often valued extrinsic factors such as status, remuneration and opportunity for further promotion.[3] Career progression can be one outcome of career development. However, career development is a process which is far more broad-reaching than achieving career progression. Career development is directed to meeting subjective as well as objective determinants of success and satisfaction. It is the process of managing life, learning and work over the lifespan and involves life planning, career exploration, career building and skill building.[4]

The view of a career as a contract between employer and employee, which is based on long-term mutual commitment and establishment of a profound relationship within which there are well-defined opportunities for hierarchical promotion, is increasingly superseded by a view of a career as a series of shorter-term interactions between employers and employees based on exchange of services and benefits. Reasons for this include increased mobility in the workforce, increasing flexibility in patterns of work, flattened organisational structures and differing expectations among generations of workers.[5] There has been significant change in both the availability and retention of workers in all industries,[6] including nursing and other health professions.[7]

In addition to this global change there has been a marked change within nursing from the model of the 1950s, in which nurses' practices were directed largely within a medically dominated paradigm, to contemporary times which have seen significant changes in the roles nurses can fulfil as a result of policy reform.[8] Nursing is also increasingly governed by nurses. Nursing remains informed by other disciplines but is transmitted and co-created through a range of strategies framed by a consciousness of the uniqueness of the knowledge, skills and attitudes that constitute the practice of nursing. Over the last few decades, nursing has emerged as a profession with curricula that emphasise nursing as a discipline distinguished from others.[9]

New nursing career paths and roles have emerged and evolved.[10] These new career paths and roles place emphasis on professional achievements which are inclusive of, but not limited to, educational achievements. Moreover, the dominant concept of professional career development as progression up a career ladder with hierarchical promotion, which pervades male-dominated conceptions of career development, has to coexist with more contemporary thinking which identifies professional career development, particularly for women, as fluid, zig-zag, up and down, and at times static. There is increasing emphasis placed on acknowledging the desire for work–life balance and wellbeing as part of career planning, as well as recognition that workplaces and employees are altering patterns of work to include casual, part-time and contracted work arrangements.[11] Those engaged in research related to the careers of nurses have also begun to turn their attention to the career trajectories of men in what continues to be a female-dominated profession.[12]

Professional career development for new and experienced nurses is directly linked to the maintenance of high-quality care delivery. Quality care and sustainable career development are integral to health workforce development, and must be supported and sustained through educational systems and processes, career structures and pathways that are aligned to organisational need yet are sufficiently flexible and responsive to accommodate individual goals, aspirations and circumstances. There is a need to examine the extent to which both career development and progression foster fitness for purpose within an environment of changed, and continuously changing, expectations of nurses and nursing.[13]

The outcomes of professional career development for nursing include enhanced capacity, competence, confidence and cohesion within the health workforce.[14] There is acknowledgment that career opportunities are shaped at least as much by personal aspirations, expectations and confidence as they are by factors such as economics, employment opportunities and societal views about the interdependence among employers and employees.[15] A confident, competent nursing workforce that has the capacity to provide comprehensive, person-centred care and is part of a cohesive, interprofessional healthcare team is dependent upon the professional career development opportunities undertaken by nurses. In writing this chapter, we have concluded that the chapter should focus on presenting a framework for professional development that can be used to guide transition and promote excellence in current and future roles and positions.

While we do not intend to focus specifically on career progression per se, it is necessary to acknowledge that over the past five decades career pathways in nursing have changed in response to the changing role of nurses and other health professions within healthcare.

We concur with others that career development is an iterative rather than a linear process that requires nurses to take responsibility for themselves and their careers. It is important to acknowledge that every nurse's career will consist of periods of 'exploration, establishment, maintenance, and disengagement'[16] and each of these necessitates some type of transition. The response to transition should be both directed towards and emerge from personal, professional and organisational strategy. According to Mintzberg,[17] strategy is a combination of:

1. a direction – a guide or course of action into the future
2. a pattern – consistency of behaviour over time
3. positioning – examination of relative and competitive advantage
4. perspective – ways of doing things.

In this chapter, we propose the CAPABLE framework as a mechanism to configure a professional career development strategy in a way that involves examination of the dynamic interplay among personal, professional and organisational factors. In doing so, we commit to professional career development as strategic rather than positional, and nest the CAPABLE framework within a humanistic rather than mechanistic view of career development.

THE CAPABLE FRAMEWORK: A MECHANISM FOR PROFESSIONAL CAREER DEVELOPMENT

The curriculum vitae (CV) is the formal record of career development used when applying for positions. We propose that the concept of curriculum can be readily used to frame professional career development, as professional career development is both the process and culmination of a range of learning experiences.

Many readers of this chapter will be familiar with the notion of a curriculum as the overarching structure of formal courses in nursing. A curriculum determines the content, the outcomes which should be achieved and the processes by which these should be achieved. Learning experiences are fundamental to building knowledge, developing skills and fostering professional behaviours. A curriculum is the blueprint against which learning experiences occur. Sound curriculum frameworks integrate learning experiences and the outcomes of those experiences. They are responsive to both the needs and the expectations of learners and other stakeholders such as employers, communities, professional bodies and regulatory authorities. Furthermore, in practice-oriented professions such as nursing, a curriculum provides the nexus between the expectations of the workplace and the outcomes of the learning experience. The challenge for many nurses is to use what Moore[18] has termed the 'curriculum of experience' to create personalised learning that enhances professional career development.

The CAPABLE framework provides a mechanism for nurses to individualise a 'curriculum of work experience' in order to identify and respond to their professional career development needs. CAPABLE is an acronym for interrelated aspects of professional career development. The aspects involve an ability to explore and align:

Context
Appraisal
Personal and professional conditions
Authenticity
Beneficence
Lifelong learning
Evidence.

It has been observed that traditional approaches to career management that were based in formalised career structures embedded in industrial and regulatory frameworks will not be sustained in the future as both workplaces and workers become boundaryless.[19] This will require nurses to have strategies to respond to increased diversity and flexibility, not only in career structures but also in their professional career development. There is widespread and longstanding recognition that both the individual and the organisation have joint responsibility in career development; however, there is increasing emphasis on individual ownership, control and direction of one's professional career. CAPABLE is an iterative and integrated framework that acknowledges that personal and professional contexts are the crucial moderators of professional career development and that each of these is dynamic. In the remainder of this chapter, we discuss each of the aspects of the framework and elaborate on the application of each of these to the curriculum of work experience.

Exploring context

In a seminal work Kanter[20] described a career as an event that is connected, in a dynamic relationship, with economic, social or political issues within a society and plays a role in outcomes for that and other societies. Thus, professional career development within nursing both directs and emerges from practice and has a need to be responsive to a range of stakeholder interests. Just as effective clinicians are aware that context is the crucial moderator in nursing practice and have developed mechanisms for managing situations contextually rather than seeking to manage all situations in the same way, those who have effective careers transfer this concept to recognition of how context has an impact on professional career development and make wise and informed decisions.

The context in which professional career development occurs can be viewed from personal and macro and micro workplace levels. In the CAPABLE framework, we discuss the impact of personal context as part of aligning personal and professional conditions. Initially, we encourage exploration of the workplace context as a first step in framing professional career development, as many people may have outmoded or unrealistic expectations of the workplace or limited understanding of how the context of the workplace shapes opportunities for professional career development.

At a macro level, access to professional development for nurses is shaped by a number of factors in the broader healthcare and social policy context.

CASE STUDY 21.1

Three student nurses were given an assignment which required each student to interview a nurse about his or her career.

STUDENT A

The person I interviewed was a nurse with over 40 years' experience. When she was at school, she was not sure about her future and the job she wanted. Here is part of her story.

Someone who studied science, maths and languages and stayed on to complete high school in my day was not usually encouraged to take nursing as a career option. After I left school I had a range of experiences. I worked in a factory with educated migrant workers, a delicatessen in an affluent suburb – becoming familiar with gourmet foods, demeaning clientele and a demanding boss – and had a stint in a bank. I became an assistant in nursing, caring for terminally ill cancer patients. Despite never having considered nursing as a career, I was exposed to articulate, resourceful women [registered nurses] who seemed to like what they did, to be truly engaged with the people for whom they were caring and who displayed a willingness to invest in me as a 'novice' in a fairly confronting environment. They made a difference!

Once I had decided to become a registered nurse, success in nursing studies was of utmost importance to me and has provided me with many opportunities for exciting work with the health sector. Once I had completed a Bachelor of Arts and Masters degrees I realised I had a sound set of skills.

As the first person in my immediate family to complete a degree, I identify strongly with those for whom attending university is something that is both an aspiration and motivation. Nurses and nursing have to overcome an initial sense of being an impostor in academic environments.

I entered nursing and stayed in that profession because it enabled me to really deploy my skills in problem solving, in dealing with novel situations; it provided me with a reason to pursue further studies that were relevant to my work and meaningful to me; enabled me to seek answers to the larger questions about people and societal challenges over 40 years. I was exposed to a range of cultures and situations, always learning more about myself and others. I made myself highly employable through further study. Numerous colleagues have invested in me over the years and I have learnt a great deal from a number of key people, some of whom have been my own students. As you move through your career you should reflect on the learning you have experienced as an investment, by others, in you and my challenge to you is to pass that investment on by continuing to learn and share your learning with others.

The only person who can truly direct your professional future is you. What really matters is that we cherish the people who are co-travellers on any life journey that we choose to take.

STUDENT B

The person I interviewed was a registered nurse who had 12 years of postgraduate experience. He has been working as a clinician in the same area of practice since graduating. I asked him whether he had ever considered a career change. He told me that he had been approached by others to consider working in management or education but he did not want to do that. He said his passion was for clinical work and that the things he really enjoyed were being able to work as part of an interdisciplinary team and to develop and refine his clinical knowledge and help others develop theirs. He said he felt it was very important to him that I did not make assumptions about people who had been in the same job role for a long period of time. He thought some people might see this as reflecting a lack of ambition or commitment to nursing but, for him, the essence of nursing work is being able to provide excellent care and maintain practice standards as a role model in clinical practice. He said that, to him, knowing what he wanted to achieve and getting work–life balance were important and that he had seem some people end up dissatisfied in either their work or personal life when they made unwise choices.

He said that he had undertaken another degree in a field other than nursing because he wanted some different intellectual stimulation and to mix with people who were from a range of backgrounds. I asked him if he felt it was important that nurses had lots of experience to be able to provide care with confidence. He thought about this and said that, while experience was important, it was how you thought about what you did in practice and your willingness to maintain and develop your knowledge and skills that were important. He told me he spent at least 5 hours each month in independent professional reading. This was very important to him because he enjoyed learning but also because he discussed what he had learnt with others in the workplace. He told me that his proudest moments in recent times were when the wardsmen voted him the nurse in his workplace that they would most like to have provide care to them or their families and when he had been able to support an undergraduate student gain confidence in the work unit.

STUDENT C

The person I interviewed was a recently graduated nurse. She came to nursing because she was not sure what she wanted to do when she left school and thought it would provide her with a starting point and she could transfer to another degree if she wanted to. After the first 6 months of study, she came to realise that nursing was far more interesting than she had initially thought. She liked the exposure she had to a range of practice areas as an undergraduate student and used this to identify what she liked and did not like. Since graduating 12 months ago, she has decided she will aim toward a nurse practitioner position. She told me she is in the process of finding a workplace mentor and has a 5-year career plan drafted.

REFLECTIVE QUESTIONS

- Are there similarities between any or all of these people's stories and your own or that of other nurses? What is similar and what is different?

- When you read these nurses' experiences, what aspects reflect the utility of the CAPABLE framework as an approach to career development?
- When you read these people's experiences, how do they cause you to think about:
  - the contextual and personal factors that shape your professional career development?
  - the opportunities you have for career consolidation?
  - new career opportunities developing in nursing?
  - best positioning yourself to gain access to these?
  - the extent to which the role you work in or aspire to demands knowledge, skills, attitudes and circumstances consistent with your present ones?
  - things you might need to change or learn in order to fulfil the role?
  - ways you can demonstrate your accomplishments?
  - seeking and responding to feedback you have received about your performance?
  - the enablers and barriers to professional career development?
  - strategies to make the most effective use of the enablers and reduce the barriers?

EXERCISE 21.1

Interview a nurse in the workplace and ask: 'What opportunities for career development exist in nursing now that may not have been previously available? How do you think career opportunities for nurses will change over the next decade?'

Nurses are regarded as a trustworthy group of professionals. Perceptions of inherent 'good' prevail, but must be re-examined in light of the needs of clientele in the contemporary environment. According to a report, *Modernising Nursing Careers: Setting the Direction*,[21] the nursing workforce in the UK should.

- organise care around the needs of patients
- ensure patients have a good experience of nursing, as reputations of organisations and patient choice will rest on the quality of nursing
- work in a range of settings, crossing hospital and community care, and use telemedicine
- have the skills and competencies to care for older people and people with long-term conditions, who may have both physical and mental health needs
- be able to use preventive and health promotion interventions
- work for diverse employers, and take opportunities for self-employment where appropriate
- have sufficient numbers of nurses with advanced-level skills to meet demand
- work as leaders and members of multidisciplinary teams inside and outside hospital, and across healthcare and social care teams
- work with new forms of practitioners, for example assistant practitioners and anaesthesia practitioners
- deliver high productivity and best value for money.

Similar demands of nursing workforces are being made in other countries, including Australia and New Zealand.

Initiatives related to professional career development in nursing are intrinsically linked to the broader societal context, and nurses have to be cognisant of factors that have an impact on policy and expectations. Nursing is a dynamic and goal-oriented activity which results from individual and group needs and the problems associated with health breakdown or a need to maintain health. It takes place within and across different societies. The organisation and delivery of nursing services, and therefore the nature of professional career development in nursing, are profoundly influenced by the community expectations of the profession. The context of nursing is as extensive as the population or communities served.

Organisational theorists have developed PEST, a schema for examining the political, economic, sociocultural and technological factors that have an impact on a given activity. Figure 21.1 indicates some of the macro-level factors that have an impact on the profession of nursing and hence professional career imperatives, aspirations and development.

At the more micro or local level, the 'curriculum of work experience' is shaped by many factors, including the kind of learning that people engage in during organised

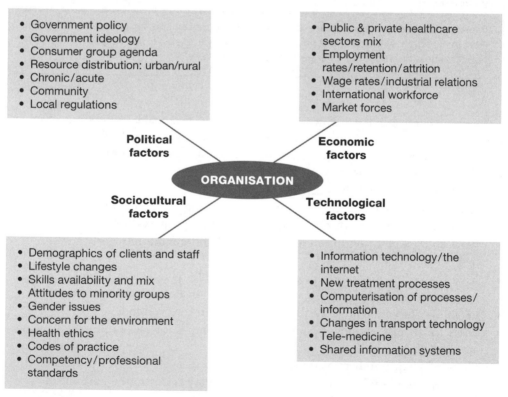

Fig 21.1 Contextual impacts on professional change – application of the political, economic, sociocultural and technological (PEST) analysis. Source: Conway J, McMillan M. Connecting clinical and theoretical knowledge for practice. In: Daly J, Speedy S, Jackson D, editors. Contexts of nursing. Sydney: Churchill Livingstone; 2005. p. 317–31.

or productive activities.[18] Many nurses seek formal career development opportunities, including support to attend professional development courses within their place of employment, and undertake programs leading to qualifications through university and other providers.[22] This should be actively encouraged and supported by management. However, access to these formal learning opportunities can be limited by a number of constraints, including clinical, organisational and personal factors wherever nurses work.[23] There is a particular need to consider a range of factors in the clinical context, including the patient, when seeking support for professional development opportunities out of the workplace.

Selecting the most appropriate approach to professional career development requires an ability to scan the environment and determine where opportunities for consolidation of existing knowledge, skills and behaviours or creation of new career directions arise. There are a range of other professional career development opportunities in the workplace that nurses should capitalise upon, including peer supervision, mentorship, secondment, reflective practice and self-directed learning. While the ability to be conscious of the environment in which professional career development occurs is important, professional career development requires individuals to possess a range of other skills and abilities. These align with the remainder of the elements within the CAPABLE framework.

Appraisal of conduct

The ability to examine our own performance critically and be accountable for our actions is essential to professional career development. Career transition is often marked by a process of exploration of achievements and aspirations and requires the ability to conduct a realistic self-appraisal. Appraisal is a process by which people can:

- confirm outcomes of previous experience
- identify areas of strength
- identify areas for development
- remotivate and energise
- help predict and identify personal potential
- acknowledge performance against existing standards.

Appraisal is an ongoing process that can be informed by, but is not limited to, the formalised performance development meetings that should occur between nurses and their managers. Appraisal consists of assessing accomplishments and performance to make an informed judgment about strengths and limitations in order to identify areas for improvement. It is a mechanism through which nurses can self-manage their professional career development.

It is rare that one assessment strategy provides sufficient or valid evidence for the range of knowledge, skills and behaviour that underpins professional practice. Assessment can be individual or team-based; it can focus on the products of learning or the process of learning; it can be conducted by yourself, a peer, a supervisor or another expert. Of critical importance in selecting the assessment strategies you will use to inform your appraisal is an awareness of the purpose of the appraisal and the criteria against which you wish to make your judgment. These criteria should include those that are both general to the profession of nursing and specific to your local situation.

Generic criteria against which to appraise your professional career development include codes of conduct and ethics, legislative frameworks, professional competency standards and evidence-based/best-practice standards. More specific criteria against which to make a judgment can be found in specific position descriptions and expectations of particular roles. It is important that you ground your professional career development in the criteria for a given role or position that you seek further development in or aspire towards. If you are considering applying for a new position, it is essential that you address each of these criteria specifically in your application; too often, applications from nurses include a cover letter and a CV but no indication that the nurse has been able to link the CV to the specified criteria.

Conducting an appraisal can be a process that involves both openness and vulnerability. Feedback is considered an essential part of the appraisal process. You should seek feedback that is constructive and balanced. It should include comments both about things you have done well and about areas and suggested strategies for improvement where necessary.

Nurses should be proactive in seeking and offering feedback that is supportive and constructive. All too often, feedback is perceived as reactive and punitive. Sadly this often has much to do with the way feedback is delivered or received rather than the feedback itself. The principles of giving feedback are that it is fair, timely, specific, accurate and supportive.

Genuine feedback is not the same as validation or unconditional positive regard; it can sometimes be painful to hear, but you should enter into receiving feedback with a mindset that the feedback is intended to assist you to develop professionally. Those who receive feedback should respond in ways that demonstrate not only a valuing of the feedback itself but also respect and valuing of the person providing the feedback and an ability to control any defensiveness to the feedback through being approachable, suspending judgment and maintaining objectivity.

The individual who is appraising strengths, limitations and aspirations through reflective practice, as well as in response to feedback from others, may need validation and support. Such support should be collegial and external to the assessment and feedback process in order to avoid blurring of boundaries.

Appraisal is not only about personal performance and ability; it is also about your capacity given personal and professional conditions. These need to be aligned in order to have realistic expectations of yourself and others and maximise opportunities at various times of your professional career.

EXERCISE 21.2

You are being interviewed for a position. How would you respond to an interviewer who posed the following questions?

- What would you identify as two areas of strength and one area for improvement in your professional practice?
- If I asked your peers the same question, how would they respond?
- Imagine you are being asked to give feedback to a fellow nurse who is considering applying for another position. What would you include in that feedback?

Aligning personal and professional conditions

The interdependence of both personal and professional conditions on career development cannot be underestimated.[24] Indeed, over 20 years ago Hall[25] noted that a career constitutes a 'bundle' of socialisation experiences as a person moves into, undertakes and moves within and from work roles.

Individual life and work priorities influence choices about professional career development. These priorities may be determined by factors such as the criteria for career satisfaction, financial necessity, and social and familial responsibility. Work–life balance is imperative in creating and maintaining personal and career effectiveness. We encourage those who are challenged to align personal and professional conditions to engage in a simple risk–benefit analysis when making decisions about career development and progression.

In our experience, people in transition may have an expectation that a series of concessions can or ought to be made on the basis of personal conditions. While it is not unreasonable to seek to test the extent to which professional conditions can accommodate personal circumstances through processes such as flexible work practice, there are situations in which these cannot be accommodated and to do so for an individual may compromise principles of patient safety, optimal use of resources and fairness to others.

It is widely recognised in the literature related to career development that the timing and sequencing of career transitions are influenced by a person's ability and means to match decisions, commitments and context. However, the importance of individual agency and the interplay of an individual's resilience and attitude to risk-taking cannot be overlooked when examining life and career transitions.[26] Individual agency is based on the interaction of individual and relational needs and an ability to capitalise on opportunities for career mobility.

Historically nurses have viewed career development as synonymous with progression through a hierarchy, as the shape of organisational structures has a direct and significant impact on career opportunities. This has placed what we consider to be an unrealistic emphasis on vertical mobility as the measure of professional success. However, the focus on vertical mobility as the criterion for success and the key contributor to employee attachment and satisfaction represents a tradition that can no longer be supported as organisational and career structures in contemporary healthcare become increasingly less hierarchical. This is consistent with trends in other industries and organisations where research has identified that employees are redefining career success as multidimensional, shaped by the individual and linked to broader factors such as happiness and personal values.[27–29]

Lateral mobility has been noted as an alternative to vertical mobility. In nursing this is exemplified by the expansion of the roles and functions within the scope of nurses' clinical practice which has seen a renewed valuing of clinical practice roles as career development opportunities, rather than the longstanding view that management or education roles constitute career progression in nursing. These increased lateral mobility opportunities substitute for reduced opportunities for upward mobility and are a mechanism for career growth and success. While they can provide an antidote to experiencing a career plateau, more importantly they maintain nursing expertise in direct client care roles.

As we see it, those engaging in professional career development make one of three choices at various stages of their career depending upon personal and professional conditions: (1) remain and consolidate in an existing role; (2) realign and commit to a different role; and (3) remove and commence a new role. Irrespective of which of these choices is made, the motivation for the decision and the methods used to acquire professional career development must be authentic.

EXERCISE 21.3

List factors in your personal life that may have an impact on the realisation of your professional aspirations.

Determining authenticity

The workplace enables professional career development to remain authentic and congruent with client, personal and workplace needs. Experiences within the workplace establish the curriculum of work. In doing so they define the goal-directed activity of nursing which underpins the direction for professional career development. Authentic development opportunities are active, meaningful and constructive both for nurses and for those with whom they work as clients and peers.

It is not enough to take a minimalist approach to do what needs to be done to keep a job. Authenticity is grounded in contemporary practice and based in sound evidence of what the clientele, the organisation and the health service need with respect to optimal outcomes with minimal risk. Hence seeking or taking any opportunity for career development needs to be authentic on several levels – organisational, process and personal.

Organisational authenticity can be determined through examining the PEST framework (Fig 21.1) and your particular context of practice, including the strategic plan for the area in which you work.

On matters of process, there is a need to relate policy on human resource management to practice. This applies to application for positions or promotion within the workforce or workplace. The manner in which a CV is developed and the claims presented need to be valid so that objective referees can attest to their authenticity.

Personal authenticity suggests an open mindset to the development of yourself and others – not a hidden curriculum. Personal authenticity can be determined through exploring your personal commitment and motivation, your willingness to invest in your professional career and your ability to be realistic about your accomplishments, goals, expectations and intent. Personal authenticity is an inherently ethical endeavour and should assist in being not only non-maleficent, but in enacting beneficence as you develop your career.

EXERCISE 21.4

Think about your career aspirations. Examine what motivates you and what you need to do to meet these. Explore how realistic you are about your accomplishments, goals, expectations and intent.

Enacting beneficence

The intent of beneficence is to achieve 'good'. In terms of professional career development, this means having an ability to identify one's own and others' strengths, avail yourself and others of opportunity and operate within, and accept, processes.

The ultimate goal of professional career development in nursing is to achieve increased capacity in the profession to respond to complexities in client needs and enhance the profession's ability to address these needs. Professional career development activity should contribute to the maintenance of quality and the reforms necessary to optimise healthcare delivery. Nurses are expected to practise in ways that are safe, competent, culturally appropriate, supported by a sound knowledge base and that enhance the generation and dissemination of new knowledge and learning.

Frequently, position descriptions and interview processes require demonstration of application of knowledge about ethical practice and personal and professional standards. Individuals, employers, supervisors, education bodies and regulatory authorities have a collective responsibility to ensure that the knowledge and skills base from which a nurse operates are not only extensive enough for the roles and functions of a given position, but also up to date, within the law and directed towards client benefit. This provides a series of safeguards, enhances risk management and contributes to quality improvement through promoting application of the principles of ethics, which include doing good, not doing harm, justice and autonomy.

As fully developed professionals, nurses should demonstrate that they include ethical behaviour as part of their repertoire for practice. Just as it is an expectation that care should be in the patient or community's best interest, professional career development should also be in the best interest of the patient/community and profession. Those who seek professional career development should ensure that the processes through which they seek and gain development are ethical. Most workplaces have a range of rules, policies and guidelines shaped by various acts and other legislative frameworks that govern procedures for professional career development. The principles of confidentiality, privacy and equity are enshrined in many of these.

Although both the employer and the individual are responsible for ethical behaviour, nurses, as professionals, should operate ethically in all facets of their working lives. In our experience many nurses are not fully aware of the governance processes surrounding professional career development and seek opportunity or advancement outside the usual parameters of merit, equal opportunity, objective review and competitive appointment. Nurses should be conscious of the potential for there to be a contradiction between their professional commitment to ethical practice in client care and some of the processes through which they seek and provide professional career development and progression.

Professional development experiences underpin a range of functions in the healthcare environment and are critical to enhanced patient care as well as to developing the confidence and competence necessary for a career in nursing. Engaging in lifelong learning is part of the ethical nurse's repertoire, as lifelong learning is oriented to maximising individual potential in order to optimise practice and performance and reduce and avoid risk.

EXERCISE 21.5

Imagine you are involved in a selection process. What criteria would you use to determine the ethical behaviours of others in both clinical practice and their professional lives?

Engaging in lifelong learning

The Nursing and Midwifery Board of Australia has identified the need for continuing professional development (CPD) within its standards. In doing so, it has determined the minimum requirements for demonstration of CPD for registration.[30] The Board uses the Australian Nursing and Midwifery Council's definition of CPD to define CPD as:

> the means by which members of the profession maintain, improve and broaden their knowledge, expertise and competence, and develop the personal and professional qualities required throughout their professional lives. The CPD cycle involves reviewing practice, identifying learning needs, planning and participating in relevant learning activities, and reflecting on the value of those activities.[31]

When transitioning from formal, institutionalised education such as experienced in universities and other training environments, many people fail to transfer the structure previously provided by the curriculum within that educational experience to their personal professional development in the workplace.[32] Moreover, they fail to recognise that experience, when framed appropriately, results in learning, internalisation and professional development.

A plan for lifelong learning is the formalised and systematic procedure that is the outcome of the rational and analytical processes within context analysis and the conduct of appraisal. The lifelong learning plan for career progression is an integrated set of decisions focused on moving from the critical thinking and problem solving that underpin effective clinical performance to strategic thinking and problem framing.

Development activities, including formal learning opportunities, membership of professional associations and collegial networks, experience that is deconstructed through reflective practice, and developmental relationships are required for professional career development. While there are numerous terms for and approaches to developmental relationships such as mentoring, coaching, critical companionship and clinical supervision, we concur with the views of Rock and Garavan[33] on the four key elements that dictate the:

> conceptual and operational aspects of developmental relationships. These focus on self-insight, self-efficacy and self-determination; learner motivation and capability; social capital theory; and learning and feedback culture.

Irrespective of the term used to describe a developmental relationship, the key outcome of such a developmental relationship is that nurses are, both personally and professionally, constantly transformed and emancipated from their previous ways of thinking and acting.[34–36]

Considerable intellectual, human and financial investment is made in clinical teaching and professional development in nursing. Effective professional career development requires the ability to develop and demonstrate psychomotor skills, clinical reasoning and decision making, and attitudinal attributes such as accountability, respect for others and professionalism. Nurses, as lifelong learners, require information fluency, mindset and commitment to nursing. They are required to be knowledgeable rather than simply knowledgable. That is, they should be procedurally competent, information-fluent personnel who are able to coordinate client throughput and care processes; make meaningful contributions to systems review; manage consumer expectations, competing value systems and tensions in resource allocation; and be active and influential participants in healthcare teams.

In order to achieve this, nurses should be able to articulate and conceptualise the nature of their discipline in order to develop both themselves and the profession. As knowledgeable, lifelong learners, nurses should seek, and provide to others, professional career development opportunities which:

- incorporate learning opportunities that maximise exploration of the elements of evidence-based practice in nursing
- include discipline-specific application of knowledge to practice
- integrate knowledge from other sources to inform the practice of nursing
- have a spiral effect through continual conceptualisation and reconceptualisation of nursing practice in context
- centralise the concept of inquiry into and about practice
- align 'thinking about nursing' with 'knowing how to nurse'
- result in thoughtful, skilled and efficient nursing actions
- promote the notion of 'ongoing inquiry'.

Nurses who have effective careers have the ability to question and justify practice, and emphasise the ability to think about nursing as well as the ability to perform nursing actions to manage nursing situations best. They have developed thoughtful, highly skilled and efficient actions, can integrate knowledge from other disciplines with nursing-specific knowledge and continue with lifelong learning as part of their professional career development. In addition, they are proficient at collecting evidence of their professional career development and presenting this for scrutiny and evaluation.

EXERCISE 21.6

List two activities you are engaged in that provide evidence of your commitment to lifelong learning.

Gathering evidence

The workplace should be seen as a knowledge-building site – a place in which people heighten awareness, skills and experience in order to gain insight, take action, review and reflect and demonstrate tangible outcomes.

In order to demonstrate outcomes that support claims of professional career development, evidence must be collected and presented. The evidence must be of sufficient quality and related to its intended purpose. We recommend all nurses maintain a portfolio of evidence about their practice and development. This can be used both to guide personal reflection and analysis of professional career development needs, and to present evidence to others at performance review or when applying for a position.

EXERCISE 21.7

Locate a description for a position to which you aspire. Identify two criteria and collect evidence to support the extent to which you satisfy these.

A portfolio offers a legitimate basis on which to judge personal competence. It can be a powerful reflective mechanism through which to identify additional education or expansion goals while incorporating critical thinking, reflection and theory–practice integration.[37]

The presentation and organisation of a professional portfolio are critical to its impact and utility. A portfolio is more than a collection of statements of attendance at professional development sessions, or a log of activity. It is a well-structured communication of critical reflection on practice and development that requires continuous investment. Effective portfolio development requires that the 'rules of evidence' are met. That is, the evidence within the portfolio must be current, relevant, accurate, objective and of sufficient scope to support meaningful decision making. It should also be well organised and presented professionally.

The way in which a portfolio is structured and presented can reflect a person's thinking about (or lack of thinking about) his or her work and career as a nurse. It should demonstrate an ability to analyse and relate to context, appraise personal professional performance, make judicious decisions regarding personal and professional conditions, commit to authenticity and beneficence and engage in lifelong learning. It is, after all, the evidence of a CAPABLE professional.

EXERCISE 21.8

Examine your professional career aspirations and apply the CAPABLE framework by asking yourself the key questions related to each element of the framework, as presented below.

Aspects for exploration and alignment	Have I/will I?
Context	fully explored contemporary economic, social and political issues that have an impact on opportunities for optimal role enactment as a nurse?
Appraisal	critically examined my own performance and accepted accountability for my own actions?
Personal and professional conditions	explored the extent to which individual life and work aspirations and priorities align and are sustainable?
Authenticity	represented myself accurately and realistically and behaved in a manner consistent with codes of conduct and within organisational processes?
Beneficence	ensured my motivations and expectations are ethical and client-focused?
Lifelong learning	actively sought and engaged in career development opportunities?
Evidence	collected sufficient evidence to support claims I make about my current capabilities and career experience?

CONCLUSION

It is acknowledged that there is no single path or simple recipe for professional career development and that the next decade will see the emergence of new career paths and structures for nurses.

Any approach to career development needs to include an overall understanding of the expectations of the future health workforce and identify a set of personal and professional principles and goals to be progressed on a consistent basis. The CAPABLE framework provides an integrated approach to minimise dissonance among career aspirations, educational achievement, personal goals and contemporary workplace needs.

RECOMMENDED READING

Conway J, McMillan M. Connecting clinical and theoretical knowledge for practice. In: Daly J, Speedy S, Jackson D, editors. Contexts of nursing. Sydney: Churchill Livingstone; 2005. p. 317–31.

Dyess SM, Sherman RO. The first year of practice: new graduate nurses' transition and learning needs. Journal of Continuing Education in Nursing 2009;40: 403–10.

Price B. Professional development opportunities in changing times. Nursing Standard 2007;21:29–33.

Shirey MR. Building an extraordinary career in nursing: promise, momentum, and harvest. Journal of Continuing Education in Nursing 2009;40:394–402.

Turner SO. The nursing career guide. Sudbury, Massachusetts: Jones and Bartlett; 2007.

REFERENCES

1. Tams S, Arthur M. New directions for boundaryless careers: agency and interdependence in a changing world. Journal of Organizational Behavior 2010;31; 629–46.
2. Somnez B, Yildirim A. What are the career planning and development practices for nurses in hospitals? Journal of Clinical Nursing 2010;18:3461–71.
3. Bradley L, Brown K, Dower J. Career progression in the public sector: gender differences in career success. International Journal of Employment Studies 2009; 17:102–34.
4. Lindgren A. Career development month: let's review career development. Online. Available: http://www.cica.org.au November 2010.
5. Davis A, Blass E. The future workplace: views from the floor. Futures 2007;39: 38–52.
6. Sheehan C, Holland P, DeCieri H. Current developments in HRM in Australian organisations. Asia Pacific Journal of Human Resources 2006;44:132–52.
7. International Council of Nurses. Country overview report 2006. International Council of Nurses Workforce Forum; 2006. Online. Available: http://www.icn.ch/forum2006overview.pdf 28 Jun 2007.
8. Keleher H, Parker R, Abdulwadud O, et al. Review of primary and community care nursing. Melbourne: Monash University; 2007.

9. Gould D, Berridge E, Kelly D. The national health service knowledge and skills framework and its implications for continuing professional development in nursing. Nurse Education Today 2007;27:26–34.

10. National Health Workforce Taskforce. Health Workforce in Australia and Factors for Current Shortages, 2009. Online. Available: http://www.ahwo.gov.au/publications.asp.

11. Patton W, McIlveen P. Practice and research in career counseling and development – 2008. Career Development Quarterly 2009;118–57.

12. Jiunn-Homg L, Hsing-Yi Y, Sheng-Hwang, C. Factors affecting the career development of male nurses: a structural equation model. Journal of Advanced Nursing 2010;66:900–10.

13. Jasper M. Editorial. Life at work – modernizing nursing careers. Journal of Nursing Management 2007;15:1–3.

14. Conway J, McMillan M, Becker J. Implementing workforce development in health care: a conceptual framework to guide and evaluate health service reform. Human Resource Development International 2006;9:129–39.

15. Roberts CA, Ward-Smith P. Choosing a career in nursing: development of a career search instrument. International Journal of Nursing Education Scholarship 2010;7:1.

16. Chang PL, Chou YC, Cheng FC. Designing career development programs through understanding of nurses' career needs. Journal of Nurses in Staff Development 2006;22:246–53.

17. Mintzberg H. The rise and fall of strategic planning. New York: Free Press; 1994.

18. Moore D. Analyzing learning at work: an interdisciplinary framework. Learning Inquiry 2007;1:175–88.

19. Walsh K, Gordon JR. Creating an individual work identity. Human Resource Management Review 2008;18:46–61.

20. Kanter E. Careers and the wealth of nations: a macro-perspective on the structure and implications of career forms. In: Arthur M, Hall D, Lawrence B, editors. Handbook of career theory. Cambridge: Cambridge University Press; 1989. p. 506–22.

21. Scottish Executive. Modernising nursing careers: setting the direction. Edinburgh, Scotland: Scottish Executive; 2006.

22. Joyce P, Cowman S. Continuing professional development: investment or expectation? Journal of Nursing Management 2007;15:626–33.

23. Price B. Professional development opportunities in changing times. Nursing Standard 2007;21:29–33.

24. Smith-Ruig T. Exploring career plateau as a multi-faceted phenomenon: understanding the types of career plateaux experienced by accounting professionals. British Journal of Management 2009;20:610–22.

25. Hall D. Careers and socialization. Journal of Management 1987;13:301–21.

26. Schoon I. Risk and resilience: adaptations in changing time. Cambridge: Cambridge University Press; 2006.

27. Dries N, Pepermans R, Carlier, O. Career success: constructing a multidimensional model. Journal of Vocational Behavior 2008;73:254–67.

28. De Vos A, Soens N. Protean attitude and career success: the mediating role of self-management. Journal of Vocational Behavior 2008;73:449–56.

29. Blustein DL, Kenna AC, Gil N, et al. The psychology of working: a new framework for counseling practice and public policy. Career Development Quarterly 2008;56:294–308.

30. Nursing and Midwifery Board of Australia. Continuing professional development registration standard, 2010. Online. Available at: http://www.nursingmidwiferyboard.gov.au/Registration-Standards.aspx.

31. ANMC (Australian Nursing and Midwifery Council). Continuing Competence Framework for Nursing and Midwives 2009. Online. Available at: http://www.anmc.org.au.

32. Hofler L. Nursing education and transition to the work environment: a synthesis of national reports. Journal of Nursing Education 2008;47:5–12.

33. Rock A, Garavan T. Reconceptualizing development relationships. Human Resource Development Review 2006;5:330–54.

34. Freire P. The pedagogy of oppression. Harmondsworth: Penguin; 1972.

35. Mezirow J. A critical theory of self directed learning. New Directions for Continuing Education 1985;25:17–30.

36. Faulk DR, Parker FM, Morris AH. Reforming perspectives: MSN graduates' knowledge, attitudes and awareness of self-transformation. International Journal of Nursing Education Scholarship 2010;7:Art 24.

37. Buckley S, Coleman J, Davison I, et al. The educational effects of portfolios on undergraduate student learning: a best evidence medical education (BEME) systematic review. Medical Teacher 2009;31:282–98.

CHAPTER 22

Continuing competence for practice

Rachael Vernon, Elaine Papps and Denise Dignam

LEARNING OBJECTIVES

When you have completed this chapter you will be able to:

- differentiate between continuing competence and professional development
- examine your professional accountability for continuing competence
- recognise that there are some international differences in the responsibilities of regulatory authorities and professional bodies in relation to continuing competence
- identify the types of evidence around continuing competence requirements
- critically consider the types of evidence you might use to demonstrate your continuing competence.

Keywords: competence, continuing competence, continuing competence frameworks, continuing professional development, regulation

INTRODUCTION

As you are considering starting your first year of practice you may well think that once you have demonstrated competence sufficient to become registered you can now take a well-earned rest from scrutiny over your practice. However, it is now no longer possible just to return the self-declaration form and pay the money to continue to have a current nursing registration to practise. It is a worldwide trend for all registered health practitioners to continue to demonstrate competence to satisfy the relevant registration authority that you remain safe to practise.

This chapter focuses on the notions of competence and continuing competence in relation to contemporary nursing practice. It provides an international perspective and utilises current and other important literature to discuss the difference between continuing competence and professional development, the types of evidence that might be required to satisfy the registration authority of competence to practise and the practical ways you might gather and keep continuing competence evidence as you are transitioning from a student to a registered nurse.

We hope that after reading this chapter you will be able to start the process of information gathering to support your practice as a continuing competent and safe practitioner.

REGULATION

Competence and continuing competence for nurses are closely associated with regulation. It is helpful to understand the context of this, so we have provided a brief overview to assist you. Nurses, like other health practitioners, are regulated by legislation. In general, the purpose of regulation is to protect the public who are cared for or treated by a registered health practitioner. An important document, published in 1992 by the International Council of Nurses, and cited by Bryant (2005), identified that regulation is concerned with the governance of occupations.[1] For nurses this means that the public is protected from individuals who may call themselves nurses, but in fact are not nurses. The title of 'nurse' can only be used if a person is registered with the organisation with responsibility for regulating nurses. Bryant[1] notes that one way of protecting the public through regulation is to ensure that the health professionals who are regulated are competent to practise. This responsibility is generally the role of regulatory authorities.

Most regulatory authorities for nurses take the form of a board or council. In Australia, the various state and territory boards had responsibility for revalidating registration for nurse and midwives until 2010. The Australian Nursing and Midwifery Council (ANMC) set the national standards. The UK has a Nursing and Midwifery Council, and the USA has a National College of State Boards of Nursing. However, Canada has a different system, and we refer to this later in the chapter.

Initially, these regulatory authorities were concerned with the initial registration of nurses, and the accreditation of courses that prepare nurses to practise. Through the maintenance of a register of nurses, there was confirmation that a nurse was continuing to practise. However, in most developed countries, nurses are now required to maintain continuing competence, which means that regulatory authorities now have continuing competence-reporting mechanisms in place. In the next section we explore the notion of competence before moving on to discuss continuing competence requirements for nurses.

What is competence?

Competence has become part of the language of nursing, but what this means for nurses and nursing is not necessarily agreed on in terms of one single international definition. The regulatory authorities for nursing in several different countries have developed similar, but different, definitions.

The ANMC defines competence as:

the combination of skills, knowledge, attitudes, values and abilities that underpin effective and/or superior performance in a profession/occupational area and context of practice.[2]

The Nursing Council of New Zealand's (NCNZ's) definition is that competence is 'the combination of skills, knowledge, attitudes, values and abilities that underpin effective performance as a nurse'.[3]

The National Council of State Boards of Nursing in the USA defines competence as: 'the application of knowledge and the interpersonal decision-making required for the practice role, within the context of public health'.[4] Similarly, the Canadian Nurses Association defines competence as:

the ability of a registered nurse to integrate and apply the knowledge, skills, judgement and personal attributes required to practise safely and ethically in a designated role and setting.[5]

EXERCISE 22.1

- What are the common features of each of these definitions?
- What are the differences?
- If you were to explain to a consumer of nursing care what competence means, how would you describe competence?

Competency standards have been developed internationally as a basis for assessing competence for entry to the register as well as a way of differentiating and standardising the variations in scopes and levels of practice within the nursing profession.[6,7] However, in some countries the demonstration of competence in order to fulfil that part of the registration requirement is not only through meeting competence requirements of a particular nursing education program. Entry to the register of registered nurses in New Zealand is through successful completion of a Nursing Council-approved undergraduate degree in nursing program. The competencies for the registered nurse scope of practice must be met to complete this program. This is followed by a pass grade in the Nursing Council state examinations. Interestingly, with the enactment of the Health Practitioners Competence Assurance Act 2003 (HPCA Act NZ), the requirement for a 'state examination' (currently comprising two multiple-choice examinations) is no longer enshrined in the legislation, and is now at the discretion of the regulatory authority. This issue alone has promoted much discussion amongst nursing academics and professional groups as the question must be asked: 'how does a pass grade in two multiple-choice examinations ensure a safe and competent practitioner?' Surely a more credible measure of competence is graduates' ability to complete successfully all specified requirements of a Nursing Council-approved and audited nursing program. This, by virtue of its ongoing approval, requires the awarding educational institution to ensure that the graduate meets the competencies for entry to the register of nurses.

Although examinations for entry to the register are used in the USA, they were discontinued in Australia several years ago. There has, however, been recent debate about their reinstatement in Australia.[8]

EXERCISE 22.2

Look at the competencies for registered nurses on a website relevant to you:
- Australia – Nursing and Midwifery Board of Australia (www.nursingmidwiferyboard.gov.au)
- New Zealand – NCNZ (www.nursingcouncil.org.nz)
- Canada – Canadian Nurses Association (www.cna-nurses.ca).

Continuing competence

Eight international reviews relating to competence and continuing competence in nursing have been completed since 2000.[1,2,4,5,7,9–11] These reviews tell us, among other things, that whilst standards for entry-level competence are clearly articulated and relatively well understood, the way that nurses interpret continuing or continued competence is not well understood.

The regulatory authorities in most developed countries clearly expect that nurses will be competent to practise nursing on registration, and will maintain that competence in respect of their chosen area or scope of practice as their careers develop and when they renew their registration.[7] However, the literature identifies that there is confusion between the meaning of competence, performance and continuing competence.[12,13] As a result, in addition to definitions of competence, regulatory authorities have developed definitions of continuing competence.

In 2009, the ANMC defined continuing competence as:

> the ability of nurses and midwives to demonstrate that they have maintained their competence to practise in relation to their context of practice, and the relevant ANMC competency standards under which they gain and retain their licence to practise.[14]

In New Zealand there is not an actual definition of continuing competence as such. Instead, the NCNZ has defined what nursing practice is in order to determine whether a nurse requires an annual practising certificate (APC) and whether the required standard of practice has been maintained. This definition of practising states that a nurse:

> is using nursing knowledge in a direct relationship with clients or working in nursing management, nursing administration, nursing education, nursing research, nursing professional advice or nursing policy development roles, which impact on public safety.[15]

There is also confusion over the difference between competence at entry level of practice and continuing competence.[7,11,16–18] Many nurses consider that continuing competence should reflect the basic level of practice competence similar to that demonstrated when first registered. Others consider that continuing competence should reflect the context and setting of the practitioner and thus is more than just basic beginning competence.[18–20] However, there is general agreement in the literature that frameworks, standards for, and assessment of, continuing competence should relate to the individual's particular scope of practice and area of practice.[2]

Continuing competence frameworks

The main purpose of a continuing competence framework (CCF) is that of quality assurance – a mechanism to ensure that health professionals are competent in their practice and thereby protect the public.[2,5,21] For health consumers and employers, CCFs and their associated standards and monitoring activities offer a level of assurance that practitioners are competent as well as providing a mechanism for identifying those who are not. CCFs are considered to be tools that have an important function in regulating and guiding the profession.[1,2,5] Frameworks involve the setting of standards for competence assessment and ensuring there is consistency in the monitoring and ongoing assessment of competence.

It is important to be aware that CCFs are about continuing competence requirements for the ongoing right to practise as a nurse. This is not the same as competency standards for specialist and advanced nursing practice roles. Countries such as Australia, New Zealand and Canada have developed CCFs. These are outlined below, so you can determine the similarities and differences.

CONTINUING COMPETENCE FRAMEWORK IN AUSTRALIA

The ANMC framework has previously set the standards for competence and professional development. This framework included four main elements, which have been used as a model in some states, such as Western Australia, where a CCF was introduced. The four components are: (1) a professional portfolio; (2) recency of practice; (3) assessment of practice; and (4) continuing professional development (CPD). The Western Australian scheme involved 5% of nurses and invited them to respond within 6 weeks to an electronic audit tool indicating the four ANMC components. Registrants are required to complete three sections: the first on personal details, the second on CPD activities and the third reporting on their regency of practice and practice hours. Nurses who did not meet the standards were classified as: CPD deficit, exemption granted, incomplete response or no response. The audit resulted in a number of inquiries and a 37% response by the due date, which improved to 75% by 2 weeks past the due date. Late responses, incomplete responses and resistance to the process were evident.[22] It may be that this work indicates a number of issues that will need to be addressed in the profession, as an Australian national scheme is further developed – not least an understanding of how continuing competence is not the same as professional development.

As discussed earlier, continuing competence in Australia up until 2010 has been part of the mandate of the various state and territory regulatory authorities. With the introduction of the national regulatory framework effective from 1 July 2010, under the Health Practitioner Regulation National Law Act 2009, there is now one registration and accreditation scheme for health professionals. The Australian Health Practitioner Regulation Agency (AHPRA) is responsible for the registration and accreditation of 10 health professions across Australia, including nurses. The nursing profession is represented by the newly formed (August 2009) National Nursing and Midwifery Board of Australia. This national board sets policy and standards and enacts the work of the AHPRA, while the devolved work of individual notification and registration decisions is enacted by the state and territory boards. The concern of continuing competence for registered nurses is part of the national scheme, and under the new law all health practitioners must undertake CPD: this is detailed by each national board under the standards for each profession. A range of other standards exist, including topics such as English-language skills, criminal history, recency of practice and medication endorsement.

The Nursing and Midwifery Board of Australia published a document on its website, entitled 'Continuing professional development registration standard'.[23] There is also a frequently asked question section on the website about CPD. These standards apply to registered and enrolled nurses, registered nurses endorsed as nurse practitioners, registered midwives and registered midwives endorsed as midwife practitioners. They do not apply to students or non-practising registered nurses or midwives. The standards include specific reference to the context of nursing practice and include 20 hours of professional development. The document outlines how to verify and count the hours and indicates that an annual audit of a number of nurses will be undertaken by the board.

Prior to the new national registration and accreditation scheme the state and territory nursing regulatory authorities all had slightly different approaches to continuing competence. Perhaps most interesting is that the West Australia Board developed a continuing competence audit and in 2009 piloted the ANMC framework for competence. The requirements of the National Nursing and Midwifery Board of Australia are set out in a national framework, which requires that nurses revalidate their registration on an annual basis. They must also maintain a professional portfolio and make an annual formal self-declaration of competence. A minimum of 20 hours' CPD must have been undertaken annually, and nurses must have practised in theprevious 5 years or completed a return-to-practice program. Verification of hours spent in practice is required through a statutory declaration from the individual or evidence from an employer of practice hours. Two per cent of nurses are audited annually.

CONTINUING COMPETENCE FRAMEWORK IN CANADA

The professional nursing jurisdictions across Canada have continuing competence programs. While each jurisdiction may differ slightly there is agreement by way of a joint position statement that:

- continuing competence is the ongoing ability of a nurse to integrate and apply the knowledge, skills, judgement and personal attributes required to practise safely and ethically in a designated role and setting
- enhancing continuing competence through lifelong learning is essential to professional nursing practice because it contributes to the quality of patient outcomes and to the evidence base for nursing practice.[24]

The position statement references the Canadian Nurses Association position statements and provincial and territorial documents from the Alberta Association of Registered Nurses, College of Registered Nurses of Manitoba, College of Registered Nurses of Nova Scotia, Nurses Association of New Brunswick, Registered Nurses Association of British Columbia and Registered Nurses Association of the Northwest Territories and Nunavut. These professional bodies involved in the regulatory function of the profession all have guides for continuing competence requirements. The

Canadian Nurses Association[5] published an earlier document entitled *A National Framework for Continuing Competence Programmes for Registered Nurses* (2000). Those involved in the development of this document included the professional bodies listed above and also the Yukon Registered Nurses Association, Saskatchewan Registered Nurses Association, College of Nurses Ontario, Association of Prince Edward Island and the Association of Registered Nurses of Newfoundland and Labrador. The number of professional bodies involved in supporting continuing competence programs indicates the need to hold joint agreement on the essential elements that reflect continuing competence in Canada. The various bodies agree that provincial and territorial codes of ethics and standards of practice are the foundation for continuing competence programs.[5] The range of evidence required across the provinces and states includes: self-assessment, peer feedback, continuing education, professional portfolios, certification (of specialty credentials), written examinations, interviews, observed structures, clinical examination and hours of practice.[5]

CONTINUING COMPETENCE FRAMEWORK IN NEW ZEALAND

In New Zealand, the NCNZ is responsible for education and registration requirements for nurses, and there is a separate Midwifery Council as a result of the introduction of the HPCA Act NZ in 2003. While nurses have been regulated in New Zealand for over a century, beginning with the enactment of the Nurses Registration Act 1901, the enactment of the HPCA Act NZ in 2003 brought 15 health professional groups under one statute and repealed 11 separate statutes relating to 13 individual regulatory authorities. The purpose of the HPCA Act is the clearly stated:

> to protect the health and safety of members of the public by providing for mechanisms to ensure that health practitioners are competent and fit to practise their professions (HPCA Act NZ 2003 s1).

Following the enactment of the HPCA Act NZ 2003, in 2004 the NCNZ established and implemented a national CCF.[25] The primary purpose of this CCF is to provide mechanisms to ensure that nurses are competent and fit to practise in their profession, as stipulated in the HPCA Act NZ 2003. This new requirement meant there was a significant change to the process for nurses to renew their APC. Before this statute was enacted, the only requirement under the old legislation (the Nurses Act 1977) for nurses to renew their APC was that they paid the annual fee and signed a renewal form. There was no requirement for a nurse either to declare competence or provide evidence of being competent.[26] The NCNZ now has responsibility for the ongoing monitoring of the continuing competence of nurses, and can decline to issue an APC if the applicant has at any time failed to meet the required standard of competence, failed to comply with conditions, not completed an ordered competence program or not held an APC (or practised) for 3 years preceding application.[27] The 'required standard of competence' is defined under the HPCA Act 2003 NZ s5(1) as 'the standard of competence reasonably to be expected of a health practitioner practising within that health practitioner's scope of practice'.

When a nurse receives the annual APC renewal form, a declaration must be signed that the competencies for the registered nurse scope of practice (or competencies for enrolled nurses if that is the case) have been met. The current requirements for CCF involve evidence in three areas. Firstly, there has to be evidence of ongoing professional practice, which is stated as:

> Nursing practice is using nursing knowledge in a direct relationship with clients or working in nursing management, nursing administration, nursing education, nursing research, nursing professional advice or nursing policy development roles, which impact on public safety.[15]

Secondly, there has to be evidence of ongoing professional development. The requirement for this is a minimum of 60 hours in the last 3 years, relevant to work environment and practice as a nurse. The third requirement is providing evidence of meeting the NCNZ's competencies for the nurse's scope of practice. This involves a self-declaration that states the individual meets the competencies for his or her particular scope of practice – for example, registered nurse.[24]

Five per cent of nurses are audited annually. This is a random audit, and when nurses receive their annual APC renewal information, they are advised at that time if they will be audited. Nurses, however, can be exempt from audit if they participate in a professional development and recognition program (PDRP) which has been accredited by the NCNZ. These programs are administered by health employer groups, such as district health boards. Those nurses who choose to participate in a PDRP accredited by NCNZ have a portfolio which is assessed within their employing organisation. Nurses who choose not to participate or do not have access to a PDRP are subject to selection by the NCNZ in the random recertification audit of 5% of nurses who apply for renewal of their APC.

Evaluation of CCFs is emergent. In New Zealand, the NCNZ's CCF has recently been evaluated, primarily in order to:

- explore the validity of the stipulated hours of professional development and days/hours of practice over a 3-year period, as indicators of competence
- provide information on the efficacy of undertaking a random audit of 5% of the nursing workforce to meet recertification requirements
- document and track the different forms of written evidence that are currently acceptable to the Council to demonstrate competence
- identify issues related to peer assessment of competence.[28]

In Australia and New Zealand, then, there is a legal mandate for regulatory authorities to have processes in place to meet the requirements of the HPCA Act. However, this is not yet the case internationally.

Clearly different countries have similar requirements for continuing competence. What is important to understand, however, is that various organisations have different roles and responsibilities, that is, individual nurses, employers, regulatory authorities and professional bodies. While it is evident from the literature that individuals are responsible for their own competence, there is debate and a level of confusion about employers' responsibility in terms of identifying, facilitating and supporting continued competence.[2,5,21,29] But it is the nurse who is responsible and accountable for maintaining continuing competence. Employers have a role in ensuring that nurses have a current practising certificate, and are performance-managed and developed in their workplace. Regulatory authorities are responsible for quality assurance mechanisms that ensure nurses meet specific competencies. The next section outlines how continuing competence is assessed.

COMPETENCE ASSESSMENT

Assessing the competence of practising nurses is an important part of maintaining professional standards[13] and as such has a role in professional regulation.[7] However, there is no international consensus about the meaning of continuing competence, and how and what aspects should be assessed. As identified by National Education Framework Cancer Nursing (EdCaN),[9] the literature identifies a tension between academic qualifications and a professional's competence to practise.[19] Generally, there is agreement in the literature that competence assessment in nursing cannot be based only on demonstration of theoretical knowledge or technical skills, but should also involve some inference about a nurse's attitudes and professional practice.[9]

The most common indicator of competence in nursing practice is demonstration of practice. However, there is considerable debate about the assessment and adequacy of performance as a valid indicator.[11,13] The difficulty with performance is whether demonstrating a particular skill or activity, in one area or on a particular day, indicates competence in all situations on any given day,[19] and whether competence is directly observable in terms of performance of an activity.[20,30] The literature suggests that observed competent performance of tasks can only be inferred, as the measurement of underpinning competencies requires evaluation of aspects such as behaviours, attitudes and insights that are not readily amenable to quantification.[20] Similar issues have been identified in relation to assessment of the different levels of nursing practice.[16,31]

In any competence assessment process the challenge is to ensure objectivity.[19] Pearson et al.[18] note that measurement of competence is a form of regulation that may be limiting and failure to achieve competence in postregistration nursing can have a negative effect on the nurse, the assessor and the profession. Standardisation of nursing practice through the development of generic competencies that do not take account of the specific context, or the diversity of practice environments, is cautioned against.[30] Many assessment tools outlined in CCFs are based on self-assessment or direct observations by a peer, a mentor, a manager or an assessor, and include some level of subjectivity.[11] Interrater reliability means that two or more assessors reach the same result. Therefore the need for assessment approaches to encourage interrater reliability is very important.[30]

Numerous competence assessment tools are identified in the literature.[9,11,17,28,32–34] However, in general there is agreement that assessment of competence should include more than one competence indicator and assessment process.[2,5,9,18,28,35] Few research studies discuss competence assessment tools which provide approaches to ensure validity and reliability,[28,30,35] although there is consensus that standardised assessment tools can be used to measure technical skills. However, decision-making and behavioural skills require a level of judgment from the assessor, as they are subjective and difficult to quantify.[30,36] Pearson et al.[37] caution that, if the aspect of nursing practice is subjective, then it is more difficult to specify a generic assessment criterion with which to measure the activity.

CONTINUING COMPETENCE INDICATORS

Indicators of continuing competence are not easily defined and go beyond measurement of entry-level skills. Additionally, it is not possible to make a valid inference about continuing competence using a single indicator in isolation. These issues have been identified by several authors[2,5,9,11,21,28,29,38] who have also summarised the most commonly used indicators of continuing competence. These are outlined and discussed further below. It may be easier to understand the types of evidence used in assessing competence if you consider those that are self-reported such as self-assessment and those that can be peer-reviewed or audited or observed by others.

Self-assessment and self-declaration of competence

Nurses can make a self-assessment of their nursing practice, and show that they reflect on their practice. This self-assessment is against the relevant required standards or competencies for practice, and usually involves the individual signing a self-declaration of competence. Self-assessment has been criticised for its subjectivity,[28] as it relies on the ability of an individual assessor to make a critical assessment. Therefore in order to be valid, there needs to be a formal feedback mechanism to ensure there is a connection to any issues identified that are relevant to the context of practice for the nurse.

Recency of practice and hours of practice

The number of hours that a nurse has worked in clinical practice, and how recent that clinical experience is, infer that knowledge and skills are current and quantifiable in terms of assessment of a skill or task and verification of hours of practice. Usually the practitioner is asked to declare these hours and may or may not be asked to have verification, such as sign-off from a manager. Used independently, however, hours are not an adequate indicator of continued competence or safety to practise.[2,11,28,29]

Continuing professional development

One indicator of the continuing competence of a nurse is CPD, which ensures that the continuing competence of an individual is relevant to current nursing practice.[28,39] There are issues around CPD: for example, what exactly can be considered as CPD, and whether it is different from maintaining currency of skills such as intravenous and cardiopulmonary resuscitation.

Professional knowledge is not static in nursing and CPD is primarily concerned with the maintenance and updating of such knowledge. CPD is an indicator which appears in many CCFs.[5,9,11,14,25,28,40] CPD is considered to be a valid indicator and has the potential to improve currency of knowledge, skills, reflective activity and insight, but used independently it is not a reliable indicator of competence.

Portfolio

A portfolio is a tool used to record practice and develop an individual's reflective thinking. It is subjective in nature and can lack interrater reliability. When used on its own it is not a reliable measure of competence or safety to practise,[2,9] although technological improvements, such as the ePortfolio, suggest that numerous types of data can be stored electronically. The ePortfolio can be used for competence evidence, professional development, promotion or career plans, teaching tools and risk assessment.[41]

Learning plan

Some CCFs[13,24] require the inclusion of a learning plan as part of the professional development record. A learning plan is a written document that reflects two elements of your personal nursing practice: what you need to learn and how you can learn it.[42] The professional bodies often offer guides on how to prepare the learning plan and may have templates for nurses to follow. Typical aspects to a learning plan include individual development needs, what activities might address these and when that should happen.

Contributing to the profession

Participation in research, involvement in committees, policy development, quality assurance programs and publication infer involvement in current practice and professional networks, but do not presume competence or safety to practise.[9,11]

Peer review

Peer review is identified as a feasible way of assessing competence, although it is time-consuming for the individual and the reviewer, and can have issues of interrater reliability. It is cautioned that the peer reviewer must have a clear understanding of the criteria for assessment and the context of practice. There is ongoing debate in the literature as to the meaning of 'peer'. Should a peer reviewer have the same professional education, qualifications, scope of practice and be in a similar position, or be a colleague with equal or higher status from another work area/discipline[2,5,21,25,28,43]? Regardless of the selected option, the peer-review process must produce an auditable trail that demonstrates a valid assessment of competence that would meet requirements of public accountability.[2,5,25,28] This is now a more accepted element of competence assessment among medical practitioners. The feasibility of using peer review for assessing competence in nursing is questionable when considering the numbers of registered nurses.

Performance appraisal

Performance appraisal occurs in employment settings. It involves the evaluation of an employee by an employer/manager and is generally undertaken to identify the ongoing development of employees, to identify learning needs, as well as for promotion and salary increments. Validity and reliability of performance appraisal depend on the assessment mechanism, tools and criteria used. Used in conjunction with a formal peer review of the individual's performance, performance appraisal may be used to demonstrate continuing competence in practice.[2,5] As a measure of competence for continuing practice, however, performance appraisal may have very different criteria to those that could be used for promotion or development.

Document audit

The physical audit of clinical case notes and documentation is another type of evidence that is directly verifiable. As a source of evidence for competence, document audit requires valid and standardised criteria used consistently between practitioners as a standard measure. However, it is time-consuming and expensive given the large numbers of nurses. Document audit may be included as evidence to support competence; however, any documentation used as evidence for direct patient care must have all patient identification information removed to respect privacy and confidentiality.

Objective structured competence assessment or evaluation (OSCE)

There is debate in the literature as to the validity and reliability of simulated clinical skill assessments such as OSCEs in assessing continued competence.[5,11,21] In addition the expense of administering OSCEs is high, given the number of registered nurses.

Examination

This is a commonly used indicator in the USA and in New Zealand for entry to the register of nurses. Fitzgerald et al.,[11] however, report that there is no research to support that it is an effective indicator of continuing competence to practise.

Patient feedback

Patient feedback as a measure of continuing competence is considered subjective and unreliable. It is also more often associated with quality improvement data. However, it has been suggested that patient feedback might provide some customer-focused information that is currently missing from evidence used to demonstrate continuing competence. Certainly patient outcome data is one aspect of customer-focused evidence that might be considered as evidence of competence,[44] as it could identify the extent of an individual's impact on patent care.

In summary, evidence for continuing competence should always be valid, reliable and measurable. It should include a variety of indicators of evidence, and the section above has provided discussion of the strengths and weaknesses of various continuing competence indicators.

EXERCISE 22.3

What type of evidence do you think is the best combination to demonstrate continuing competence? Write a list of each type and draw up a column of pros and cons for each type of evidence.

CONCLUSION

This chapter has provided an overview of competence, continuing competence and CCFs in three countries – Australia, New Zealand and Canada. This overview, as well as other information about a range of continuing competence indicators, may assist you to understand the ongoing complexity of the evolving requirement for registered nurses to demonstrate continuing competence to practise nursing. If you have completed the learning activities, you should be able to identify how competence and continuing competence relate to you personally. Finally, the case studies outlined below may be useful in assisting you to think further about some of the scenarios that relate to meeting continuing competence requirements and appropriate ways to provide evidence of your continuing competence.

CASE STUDY 22.1

One of your colleagues comes to you for advice. She tells you that she knows a registered nurse who is a clinical nurse specialist, and that this nurse says she is not going to do any work on continuing competence requirements. She told your colleague that she has already met the competencies for her specialist role and there is no need for her to demonstrate that she meets any others to revalidate her registration.

REFLECTIVE QUESTION

- What advice will you give your colleague?

CASE STUDY 22.2

A study undertaken by the New Zealand Nurses Organisation in November 2008 provides information about what New Zealand nurses understand about the issues of CPD. The study found that nurses were overwhelmingly in favour of CPD in the workplace. Additionally, the study found that issues such as work–life balance, access to resources, time and travel were barriers to professional development.

REFLECTIVE QUESTIONS

- List the enablers and barriers in your area of practice.
- What strategies could you use to address any barriers you have identified?

CASE STUDY 22.3

You need to provide evidence of an aspect of your nursing practice that relates directly to patient feedback that they have been consulted about their plan of care. It seems that the only way you can do this is to ask some patients you have cared for to write a letter about this.

REFLECTIVE QUESTIONS

- What specific issues are there in relation to patient feedback as a way of demonstrating continuing competence?
- What other options might there be to provide evidence of your practice?
- Where would you go for assistance in this matter?

RECOMMENDED READING

Byrne M, Schroeter K, Carter S, et al. The professional portfolio: an evidence-based assessment method. Journal of Continuing Education 2009;40:545–52.

Chiarella M, Thoms D, Lau C, et al. An overview of the competency movement in nursing and midwifery. Collegian 2008;15:45–53.

Hughes E. Nurses' perceptions of continuing professional development. Nursing Standard 2005;19:41–9.

National Nursing Research Unit. Nursing competence: what are we assessing and how should it be measured? Policy plus evidence, issues and opinions in healthcare 2009;18:2.

Vernon R, Chiarella M, Papps E, Dignam D. Evaluation of the continuing competence framework. Wellington, New Zealand: Nursing Council of New Zealand; 2010.

REFERENCES

1. Bryant R. Regulation, roles and competency development. The global nursing review initiative. Geneva: International Council of Nurses; 2005.

2. Australian Nursing and Midwifery Council. Development of a national framework for the demonstration of continuing competence for nurses and midwives – literature review. Canberra, Australia: Australian Nursing and Midwifery Council; 2007.

3. Nursing Council of New Zealand Definition of Competence. Wellington: Nursing Council of New Zealand; 2009. Online. Available: http://www.nursingcouncil.org.nz/contcomp.html 8 November 2009.

4. National Council of State Boards of Nursing. Assuring competence: a regulatory responsibility. Chicago, USA: National Council of State Boards of Nursing; 2009.

5. Canadian Nurses Association. A national framework for continuing competence programmes for registered nurses. September 2009. Contract No. 1. Ottawa: Canadian Nurses Association; 2000.

6. Vernon R. Literature review – competence and the regulation of nurses [chapter contributing to PhD thesis]. Sydney: University of Sydney; 2010.

7. Chiarella M, Thoms D, Lau C, et al. An overview of the competency movement in nursing and midwifery. Collegian 2008;15:45–53.

8. Wellard S, Bethune E, Heggen K. Assessment of learning in contemporary nurse education: do we need standardised examination for nurse registration? Nurse Education Today. 2007;27:68–72.

9. EdCaN. Competency assessment in nursing: a summary of literature published since 2000. Report prepared on behalf of EDCaN (National Education Framework Cancer Nursing) by Alison Evans Consulting 2008.

10. Vernon R, Chiarella M, Papps E, Dignam D. Evaluation of the continuing competence framework. Wellington: Nursing Council of New Zealand; 2010.

11. FitzGerald M, Walsh K, McCutcheon H. An integrative systematic review of indicators of competence for practice and protocol for validation of indicators of competence. Report commissioned by the Queensland Nursing Council 2001. Adelaide, South Australia: Adelaide University in conjunction with the Joanna Briggs Institute.

12. Flanagan J, Baldwin S, Clarke D. Work-based learning as a means of developing and assessing nursing competence. Journal of Clinical Nursing 2000;9:360–8.

13. McMullan M. Students' perceptions on the use of portfolios in pre-registration nursing education: a questionnaire survey. International Journal of Nursing Studies 2006;43:333–43.

14. Australian Nursing and Midwifery Council. Continuing competence framework. February 2009. Online. Available: http://www.anmc.org.au/professional_ standards February 2009.
15. Nursing Council of New Zealand. Definition of practising. Online. Available: http://www.nursingcouncil.org.nz/index.cfm/1,32,html/Practising-Certificates September 2011.
16. Benner P. From novice to expert: excellence and power in clinical nursing practice. London: Addison-Wesley; 1984.
17. Hendry C, Lauder W, Roxburgh M. The dissemination and uptake of competency frameworks. Journal of Research in Nursing 2007;12:689–700.
18. Pearson A, FitzGerald M, Walsh K, et al. Continuing competence and the regulation of nursing practice. Journal of Nursing Management 2002;10: 357–64.
19. Gibson F, Soanes L. The development of clinical competencies for use on a paediatric oncology nursing course using a nominal group technique. Journal of Clinical Nursing 2000;9:459–69.
20. National Nursing Research Unit. Nursing competence: what are we assessing and how should it be measured? Policy plus evidence, issues and opinions in healthcare. Online. Available: www.kcl.ac.uk/schools/nursing/nnru/policy 2009.
21. Goodridge JM. Continuing competence programmes for registered nurses: ARNNL background paper. Canada: Association of Registered Nurses of Newfoundland and Labrador; 2007.
22. Gillett H, Horgan L, editors. Demonstrating competence …. The good, the bad and the ugly. Western Pacific and South East Asian Regulators (WPSEAR) meeting Singapore, October 2010. Singapore: Nurses and Midwives Board Western Australia; 2010.
23. The Nursing and Midwifery Board of Australia Registration Standard. Continuing professional development and registration standard. Online. Available: http:// www.nursingmidwiferyboard.gov.au/Search.aspx?q=continuing%20 professional%20development%20and%20registration%20standards 2011.
24. Canadian Nurses Association and Canadian Association of Schools of Nursing. Joint position statement. Promoting continuing competence for registered nurses. Ontario, Canada: Canadian Nurses Association, 2004.
25. Nursing Council of New Zealand. Continuing competence framework. Wellington, New Zealand: Nursing Council of New Zealand; 2004
26. Papps E. Knowledge, power, and nursing education in New Zealand: a critical analysis of the construction of the nursing identity. Unpublished PhD thesis. Dunedin: University of Otago; 1997.
27. Health Practitoners Competence Assurance Act, (2003, s12(4)).
28. Vernon R, Chiarella M, Papps E, Dignam D. Evaluation of the continuing competence framework. Wellington: Nursing Council of New Zealand; 2010.
29. Campbell B, MacKay G. Continuing competence: an Ontario nursing regulatory programme that supports nurses and employers. Nursing Administration Quarterly 2001;25:22–30.
30. McGrath P, Fox Young S, Moxham L, et al. Collaborative voices: ongoing reflections on nursing competencies. Contemporary Nurse 2006;22:46–58.

31. Calman L, Watson R, Norman I, et al. Assessing practice of student nurses: methods, preparation of assessment and student views. Journal of Advanced Nursing 2002;38:516–23.
32. Centre for Innovation in Professional Health Education and Research. Review of work-based assessment methods. Sydney: University of Sydney; 2007.
33. Watson R, Stimpson A, Topping A, et al. Clinical competence assessment in nursing: a systematic review of the literature. Journal of Advanced Nursing 2002;39:421–31.
34. McMullan M, Endacott R, Gray MA, et al. Portfolios and assessment of competence: a review of the literature. Journal of Advanced Nursing 2003;41:283–94.
35. Scott Tilley DD. Competency in nursing: a concept analysis. Journal of Continuing Education in Nursing. 2008;39:58–64.
36. Davis R, Turner E, Hicks D, et al. Developing competency framework for diabetes nursing. Journal of Clinical Nursing. 2008;17:168–74.
37. Pearson A, FitzGerald M, Walsh K. Nurses' views on competency indicators for Australian nursing. Collegian 2002;9:36–40.
38. Pearson A, Fitzgerald M. A survey of nurses' views on indicators for continuing competence in nursing. Australian Journal of Advanced Nursing 2001;19:20–6.
39. Meretoja R, Isoaho H, Leino-Kilpi H. Nurse Competence Scale: development and psychometric testing. Journal of Advanced Nursing. 2004;47:124–33.
40. Nursing and Midwifery Council. The prep handbook. London, United Kingdom: United Kingdom Nursing and Midwifery Council; 2008.
41. Andre K. E-Portfolios for the aspiring professional. Collegian 2010. in press;doi:10.1016/j.colegen.2009.10.006.
42. Foster S. Developing a continuing competence learning plan. Nursing BC 2007;39:13.
43. Gopee N. The role of peer assessment and peer review in nursing. British Journal of Nursing 2001;10:115–21.
44. Nelson S. Careful what you wish for: resolving uncertainty in the assessment and regulation for continuing competence. Melbourne: University of Melbourne; 2010.

STATUTES

Health Practitioners Competence Assurance (HPCA) Act 2003 (NZ)
Health Practitioner Regulation National Law Act 2009
Nurses Act 1977 (NZ)
Nurses Registration Act 1901 (NZ)

INDEX